Energy Balance and Cancer

Series Editor:
Nathan A. Berger,
Case Western Reserve University,
Cleveland, OH, USA

For further volumes:
http://www.springer.com/series/8282

I. George Fantus
Editor

Insulin Resistance and Cancer

Epidemiology, Cellular and Molecular Mechanisms and Clinical Implications

Springer

Editor
I. George Fantus
Departments of Medicine and Physiology
University of Toronto
Toronto, ON, Canada
and
Division of Cellular and Molecular Biology
Toronto General Research Institute
University Health Network and
Banting and Best Diabetes Centre
Toronto, ON, Canada
and
Centre for Modeling Human Disease
Samuel Lunenfeld Research Institute
Mount Sinai Hospital
Toronto, ON, Canada
gfantus@mtsinai.on.ca

ISBN 978-1-4419-9910-8 e-ISBN 978-1-4419-9911-5
DOI 10.1007/978-1-4419-9911-5
Springer New York Dordrecht Heidelberg London

Library of Congress Control Number: 2011933469

Printed on acid-free paper

Springer is part of Springer Science+Business Media (www.springer.com)

Preface

The recent and rapid "Westernization" of developing nations characterized by movement from rural to urban environments, growth of manufacturing industries and increased use of motorized transport, have resulted in better education and job opportunities, and increased average income that has clearly been welcomed as an improved quality of life. At the same time, these changes have been accompanied by a significant decrease in physical activity, a departure from traditional diets to consumption of "fast," prepared, high-fat and calorie-dense foods and, as a consequence, increased rates of obesity. The global obesity epidemic has been well-documented in the medical and lay press. It has also been established that obesity is the leading cause of insulin resistance and the accompanying "metabolic syndrome" associated with elevated levels of circulating insulin, and frequently, glucose intolerance, hypertension, and dyslipidemia. Indeed obesity and insulin resistance are the leading risk factors for the development of type 2 diabetes mellitus, also rapidly increasing worldwide.

A more recent discovery, now receiving increasing attention, is that obesity and these same metabolic perturbations are associated with an increased incidence of several forms of cancer. The precise causes or mechanistic links which explain this association are not completely clear. There may be one critical element, but there are data which suggest that multiple different factors contribute.

This book reviews the epidemiological associations between insulin resistance and cancer. This is followed by reviews of animal models which support this relationship and provide insight into potential mechanisms. Several chapters then provide detailed examination of the metabolic, cellular and molecular changes characterizing the insulin resistant state, such as hyperinsulinemia, abnormal metabolism and hormone signaling, and how these interact with various tumor characteristics. For example, some tumors present increased quantities of the fetal form of the insulin receptor, unique regulation of oxidative (Krebs' cycle) metabolism (Warburg effect), as well as mutations in various relevant signaling pathways. Finally, the clinical implications of these data are integrated with considerations of insulin "sensitization" and potential metabolic interventions to prevent and treat cancer. It should be noted that while a number of cancers are associated with obesity, the authors here have focused primarily on breast cancer as a key and significant model.

As this book is designed for a broad audience, early chapters provide reviews of metabolic homeostasis and the molecular details of insulin signaling to provide a framework and understanding for the nonexpert of the concepts and data presented in the later chapters.

On behalf of all the authors, I would like to thank the staff at Springer for their advice and support throughout the preparation of this issue and we sincerely hope you find it a valuable reference and enjoyable to read.

Toronto, ON I. George Fantus, M.D., F.R.C.P.(C)

Contents

1 **Insulin and the Physiology of Carbohydrate Metabolism** 1
Sandra Pereira and Adria Giacca

2 **Insulin/IGF-1 Signaling Nodes and their Role in Carcinogenesis** 53
Cullen M. Taniguchi and C. Ronald Kahn

3 **The Mechanisms and Impact of Obesity and Insulin Resistance on Breast Cancer Incidence** 77
Deborah J. Clegg

4 **Obesity and Cancer: Epidemiology** 101
Melinda L. Irwin

5 **Insulin, Insulin Resistance, and Cancer Associations** 111
Lorraine Lipscombe

6 **Animal Models of Hyperinsulinemia, Insulin Resistance, and Cancer** 141
Ruslan Novosyadlyy, Archana Vijayakumar, Yvonne Fierz, and Derek LeRoith

7 **Potential Mechanisms Linking Insulin to Cancer** 159
Yael Babichev, Sarah Khalid, and I. George Fantus

8 **Actions of Insulin As a Survival and Growth Factor: Akt, mTOR, and Regulation of Translation** 181
Luc Furic, Mark Livingstone, Ivan Topisirovic, and Nahum Sonenberg

9 **AMP-Activated Protein Kinase and Cancer Cell Metabolism** 193
Bin Zheng and Lewis C. Cantley

10 **The Role of the IGF Axis in Human Malignancy: Evidence from Epidemiological Studies and Tissue Analysis** 213
Julia V. Burnier, Shun Li, and Pnina Brodt

11 IGF-I and Insulin Receptor Families in Cancer 243
Antonino Belfiore, Ira D. Goldfine, and Roberta Malaguarnera

12 Insulin Resistance: Clinical Implications for Cancer Treatment and Prevention 269
Saroj Niraula and Pamela J. Goodwin

Index 293

Contributors

Yael Babichev Division of Cellular and Molecular Biology, Toronto General Research Institute, University Health Network and Banting and Best Diabetes Centre, Toronto, ON, Canada

Centre for Modeling Human Disease, Samuel Lunenfeld Research Institute, Mount Sinai Hospital, Toronto, ON, Canada

Antonino Belfiore Department of Clinical and Experimental Medicine, University of Catanzaro, Campus Universitario, loc. Germaneto, 88100 Catanzaro, Italy
belfiore@unicz.it

Pnina Brodt Department of Medicine, McGill University, Montreal, QC, Canada H3A 1A1

Department of Oncology, McGill University, Montreal, QC, Canada H3A 1A1

Department of Surgery, McGill University, Surgical Labs, Royal Victoria Hospital, Room H6.25 687 Pine Avenue, Montreal, QC, Canada H3A 1A1
pnina.brodt@muhc.mcgill.ca

Julia V. Burnier Department of Medicine, McGill University, Montreal, QC, Canada H3A 1A1

Lewis C. Cantley Division of Signal Transduction, Beth Israel Deaconess Medical Center, Center for Life Sciences, Room 417, 330 Brookline Avenue, Boston, MA 02115, USA

Department of Systems Biology, Harvard Medical School, Boston, MA 02115, USA
lewis_cantley@hms.harvard.edu

Deborah J. Clegg Department of Internal Medicine, University of Texas Southwestern Medical Center, 5323 Harry Hines Blvd., Dallas, TX 75390–8854, USA
deborah.clegg@utsouthwestern.edu

I. George Fantus Departments of Medicine and Physiology, University of Toronto, Toronto, ON, Canada

Division of Cellular and Molecular Biology, Toronto General Research Institute, University Health Network and Banting and Best Diabetes Centre, Toronto, ON, Canada

Centre for Modeling Human Disease, Samuel Lunenfeld Research Institute, Mount Sinai Hospital, Toronto, ON, Canada
gfantus@mtsinai.on.ca

Yvonne Fierz Division of Endocrinology, Diabetes and Bone Diseases, Department of Medicine, Mount Sinai School of Medicine, New York, NY 10029, USA

Luc Furic Department of Anatomy and developmental biology, Monash University, Wellington Road, Clayton, Victoria, Australia, 3800
luc.furic@monash.edu

Ira D. Goldfine Department of Medicine and Diabetes Center, University of California, San Francisco/Mt. Zion Medical Center, San Francisco, CA, USA

Adria Giacca Department of Physiology, University of Toronto, Toronto, ON, Canada
adria.giacca@utoronto.ca

Pamela J. Goodwin Samuel Lunenfeld Research Institute, Mount Sinai Hospital and Princess Margaret Hospital, University of Toronto, Toronto, ON, Canada
pgoodwin@mtsinai.on.ca

Melinda L. Irwin Department of Epidemiology and Public Health, Yale School of Public Health, 60 College Street, New Haven, CT 06520-8034, USA
elinda.irwin@yale.edu

Sarah Khalid Departments of Medicine and Physiology, University of Toronto, Toronto, ON, Canada

Division of Cellular and Molecular Biology, Toronto General Research Institute, University Health Network and Banting and Best Diabetes Centre, Toronto, ON, Canada

Derek LeRoith Division of Endocrinology, Diabetes and Bone Diseases, Department of Medicine, Mount Sinai School of Medicine, New York, NY 10029, USA
derek.leroith@mssm.edu

Shun Li Department of Medicine, McGill University, Montreal, QC, Canada H3A 1A1

Lorraine Lipscombe Department of Medicine, University of Toronto, Toronto, ON, Canada
lorraine.lipscombe@wchospital.ca

Mark Livingstone Department of Biochemistry and Goodman Cancer Centre, M cGill University, 1160 Avenue des Pins Ouest, Montréal, QC, Canada H3A 1A3

Roberta Malaguarnera Department of Clinical and Experimental Medicine, University of Catanzaro, Campus Universitario, loc. Germaneto, 88100 Catanzaro, Italy

Saroj Niraula Samuel Lunenfeld Research Institute, Mount Sinai Hospital and Princess Margaret Hospital, University of Toronto, Toronto, ON, Canada

Ruslan Novosyadlyy Division of Endocrinology, Diabetes and Bone Diseases, Department of Medicine, Mount Sinai School of Medicine, New York, NY 10029, USA

Sandra Pereira Department of Physiology, University of Toronto, Toronto, ON, Canada

C. Ronald Kahn Department of Medicine, Joslin Diabetes Center, Harvard Medical School, Boston, MA 02215, USA

Division of Signal Transduction, Department of Medicine, Beth Israel Deaconess Medical Center, Boston, MA, USA
c.ronald.kahn@joslin.harvard.edu

Nahum Sonenberg Department of Biochemistry and Goodman Cancer Centre, McGill University, 1160 Avenue des Pins Ouest, Montréal, QC, Canada H3A 1A3
Nahum.Sonenberg@mcgill.ca

Cullen M. Taniguchi Department of Medicine, Joslin Diabetes Center, Harvard Medical School, Boston, MA 02215, USA

Ivan Topisirovic Department of Biochemistry and Goodman Cancer Centre, McGill University, 1160 Avenue des Pins Ouest Montréal, QC, Canada H3A 1A3

Archana Vijayakumar Division of Endocrinology, Diabetes and Bone Diseases, Department of Medicine, Mount Sinai School of Medicine, New York, NY 10029, USA

Bin Zheng Division of Signal Transduction, Beth Israel Deaconess Medical Center, Center for Life Sciences, Room 417, 330 Brookline Avenue, Boston, MA 02115, USA

Department of Systems Biology, Harvard Medical School, Boston, MA 02115, USA

Chapter 1
Insulin and the Physiology of Carbohydrate Metabolism

Sandra Pereira and Adria Giacca

Introduction

The discovery of insulin nearly a century ago revolutionized the treatment of diabetes mellitus, particularly type 1 diabetes mellitus (T1DM), and initiated extensive research into the effects of insulin. At approximately the same time, it was shown that patients with cancer were characterized by glucose intolerance and impaired insulin sensitivity of glucose metabolism has been subsequently found in cancer [1, 2]. Insulin, a peptide hormone produced by the β cells in the pancreas, is anabolic, as it stimulates synthesis of glycogen, protein, and triglycerides and it suppresses glucose production by the body, while stimulating glucose uptake from the circulation [3]. Moreover, insulin action is tissue-specific, since it depends on the binding of insulin to its cell-surface receptor. The insulin receptor, which is composed of two transmembrane β chains and two extracellular α chains, has intrinsic tyrosine kinase activity [4, 5] and binding of insulin to its receptor initiates a signaling cascade characterized by phosphorylation events and genomic effects. The insulin receptor is expressed in various tissues, including the most widely studied insulin sensitive tissues, namely liver, skeletal muscle, adipose tissue, and selective regions of the brain. Insulin has mitogenic effects [6], but the ensuing discussion will highlight the metabolic actions of insulin. Furthermore, although insulin regulates the metabolism of all three macronutrients [7], which is interlinked, the focus will be on insulin's effect on carbohydrate metabolism.

A. Giacca (✉)
Department of Physiology, University of Toronto, Toronto, ON, Canada
e-mail: adria.giacca@utoronto.ca

I.G. Fantus (ed.), *Insulin Resistance and Cancer: Epidemiology, Cellular and Molecular Mechanisms and Clinical Implications*, Energy Balance and Cancer 1,
DOI 10.1007/978-1-4419-9911-5_1,

Assessment of Insulin Sensitivity of Glucose Metabolism

The Hyperinsulinemic Euglycemic Clamp

The gold standard for determination of insulin sensitivity in humans and animal models is the hyperinsulinemic euglycemic clamp. This protocol is typically performed in the fasting (postabsorptive) state, which usually occurs after an overnight fast in humans, and it involves elevating plasma insulin levels via a constant insulin infusion and maintaining postabsorptive plasma glucose concentrations by altering the rate of glucose infusion [8] (Fig. 1.1). The name of the protocol itself describes the steps and endpoints involved: "hyperinsulinemic" refers to increased insulin concentrations, "euglycemic" indicates normal glucose concentrations [9], and "clamp" is used figuratively to indicate maintaining the same glucose concentrations throughout the procedure [8, 10]. The term hyperinsulinemic isoglycemic clamp is analogous to hyperinsulinemic euglycemic clamp, except that the former is performed in subjects with elevated fasting glucose concentrations resulting from dysregulated glucose metabolism; therefore, the prefix *iso-* (simply meaning same glucose concentration as basal) is used instead of the prefix *eu-* (meaning good glucose concentration and same glucose concentration as basal) [11–14]. The clamp is based on the principle that insulin decreases circulating glucose by stimulating glucose uptake into tissues and suppressing glucose production in the body and glucose infusion is, therefore, necessary to neutralize the effect of insulin [8, 15]. Hence, glucose infusion is an index of whole body insulin sensitivity (Fig. 1.2). Indeed, glucose infusion corresponds to the classical DeFronzo's M index [8] when glucose

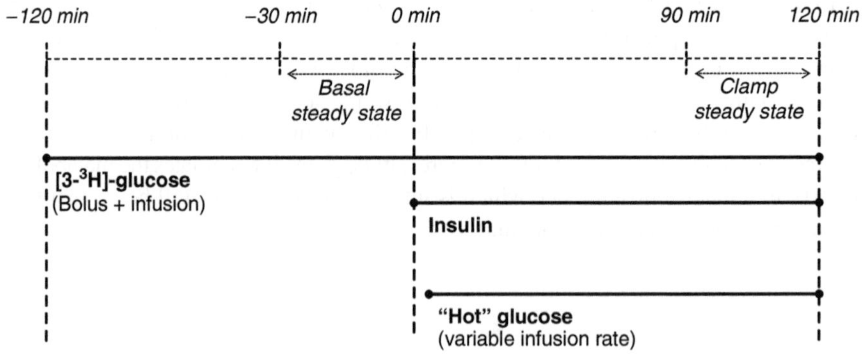

Fig. 1.1 A typical hyperinsulinemic euglycemic clamp protocol with concomitant [3-^{3}H]-glucose methodology [15]. The *solid lines* represent infusates, namely the tracer [3-^{3}H]-glucose, insulin, and "hot" glucose. A bolus followed by constant infusion is used for the tracer to reach steady state faster. The *dashed lines* represent time. "Hot" glucose also contains the tracer [3-^{3}H]-glucose to prevent a drop in plasma specific activity. Using this protocol, two physiological and isotopic steady states are achieved, one before (basal) and the other (clamp) after insulin infusion

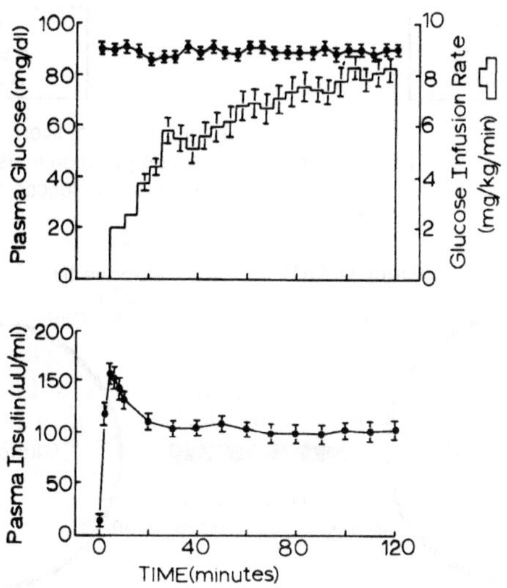

Fig. 1.2 Plasma insulin, plasma glucose, and glucose infusion rate (Ginf) during the hyperinsulinemic euglycemic clamp. Insulin infusion was started at 0 min. The goal of the hyperinsulinemic euglycemic clamp protocol is to maintain constant, basal glucose concentrations (euglycemia) in the presence of elevated plasma insulin concentrations (hyperinsulinemia). Adapted from DeFronzo et al. [8]

is perfectly clamped. When the hyperinsulinemic euglycemic clamp is combined with tracer glucose methodology, it allows endogenous glucose production (EGP), which is also known as endogenous rate of glucose appearance (endogenous Ra), to be distinguished from peripheral glucose utilization (Rd, rate of glucose disappearance), which indicates glucose uptake into tissues from the circulation [16–18]. EGP occurs mostly in the liver and the kidney is a minor contributor in overnight-fasted humans [19, 20] and both hepatic and renal EGP are suppressed by insulin in humans [20, 21]. EGP is the sum of two processes: gluconeogensis (GNG), whereby glucose is newly formed from precursors such as amino acid-derived pyruvate, amino acid-derived oxaloacetate, and lipolysis-derived glycerol, and glycogenolysis, which involves the breakdown of glycogen to its glucose subunits [22, 23]. Postabsorptive Rd is mostly insulin-independent and localized to tissues other than skeletal muscle, such as the central nervous system (CNS), in healthy humans [24]. In hyperinsulinemic euglycemic conditions, most Rd takes place in skeletal muscle [24]. Once insulin is elevated, the extent of EGP suppression and Rd elevation are indicative of hepatic and peripheral insulin sensitivity, respectively. Maximal suppression of EGP occurs at lower insulin concentrations than maximal increase in Rd, as the dose–response curves differ for these two variables [25]. Depending on the physiological state of the subject, supraphysiological levels of insulin will likely completely suppress EGP and this will make the study of hepatic insulin action inadequate.

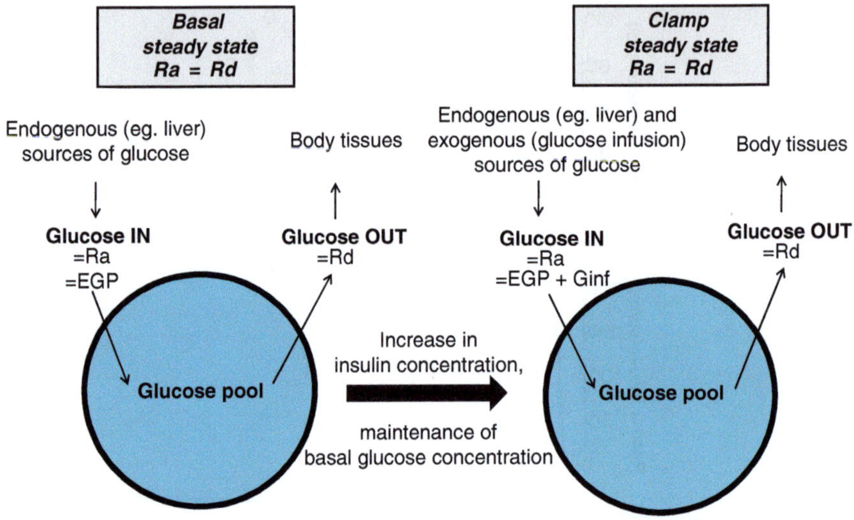

Fig. 1.3 The single pool model of glucose kinetics in the context of the hyperinsulinemic euglycemic clamp protocol. The single pool model is a simplification that is used to calculate glucose kinetics; the glucose pool refers to glucose in plasma and interstitial fluid [16, 26, 27]. At steady state, the rate of glucose appearance in the glucose pool (Ra) equals the rate of glucose disappearance (Rd) from the pool. *EGP* endogenous glucose production; *Ginf* glucose infusion rate

The most common evaluation of glucose kinetics is based on a single pool model, where the pool corresponds to glucose in plasma and interstitial fluid [16, 26, 27] (Fig. 1.3). The single pool model is a simplification and adjustments to the calculations have been made to take into account the fact that glucose is present in compartments with different rates of turnover [16]. Protocols involving the hyperinsulinemic euglycemic clamp establish two physiological and isotopic steady states: a basal steady state, immediately before insulin infusion starts and a clamp steady state, a period of time (typically at least 90 min in humans) after the start of insulin infusion [15, 16, 28–30]. At each steady state, total Ra (subsequently referred to simply as Ra in this chapter) is the rate at which glucose enters the glucose pool and it equals Rd, which is the rate at which glucose leaves the glucose pool [26]. At basal steady state, the only source of glucose is endogenous and, therefore, EGP equals Rd [16]. In the clamp steady state, Ra is made equal to Rd by the exogenous glucose infusion (Ginf), which adds to EGP [16]. Accordingly, Rd = EGP + Ginf and, therefore, EGP = Ra − Ginf.

Calculation of Rd and EGP relies upon the quantification of the glucose tracer plasma enrichment, if a stable isotope of glucose containing ^{2}H or ^{13}C is used, or the plasma glucose specific activity (SA), if a radioactive isotope of glucose containing ^{3}H or ^{14}C is utilized. The methodology underlying quantification of plasma glucose enrichment and plasma glucose SA includes mass spectrometry and scintillation counting, respectively [26]. SA refers to the number of disintegrations per minute (dpm) in the plasma sample, as a result of infusion of a radioactive glucose tracer, divided by the amount of glucose (tracee) in that sample [26]. There are various units for isotopic enrichment of a sample, but an example is tracer/tracee ratio (TTR) [26]. In simplest terms, postabsorptive Ra and Rd are essentially calculated by dividing the glucose tracer infusion rate by the enrichment or SA of the glucose tracer in plasma [26]. Accordingly, the EGP calculation is based on the principle of dilution: since newly produced glucose is not labeled, it dilutes the radioactivity in the pool of glucose and lowers plasma glucose SA, such that at a given tracer infusion rate, the greater the drop in plasma glucose SA, the greater the EGP. During the hyperinsulinemic clamp, Ginf would also have to be taken into account, as per the equations above.

To minimize error in the estimates of EGP, tracer (in addition to the constant tracer infusion rate) is also to be added to the glucose infusate used to maintain postabsorptive glucose levels during hyperinsulinemia; due to the presence of radioactivity in the glucose infusate, it is called "hot" Ginf [16]. Specifically, the addition of tracer to the glucose infusate avoids the decrease in the SA of glucose in plasma with "cold" Ginf (Ginf that does not contain radioactive tracer) and the related reflux of tracer from remote compartments, which affects plasma SA independent of Ra and underestimates Ra until equilibrium is reached [16].

Glucose tracers, either radioactive or stable isotopes, can be used to determine different endogenous Ra endpoints, depending on the atom labeled (carbon or hydrogen) and the location of the atom labeled [26]. Any tracer methodology relies upon a series of assumptions, such as lack of discrimination between the tracer and the tracee by the body's biochemical pathways and lack of tracer recycling, although the latter is not always the case [16, 26]. Carbon tracers give slightly lower estimates of endogenous Ra than ^{3}H (trititium) or ^{2}H (deuterium)-containing tracers as labeled carbon is retained in recycled glucose from 3 carbon precursors derived from labeled glucose [26]. The most widely used hydrogen-labeled tracers are 3-^{3}H-glucose, 2-^{3}H-glucose, or 6-^{3}H-glucose and 6,6-$^2H_2$-glucose. Tritium or deuterium are exchanged with unlabeled water protons during GNG and are, therefore, not affected by recycling. The exception, however, is hydrogen labeled glucose on position 6, which may not lose one of its labeled hydrogens in reactions between citric acid cycle intermediates and could be recycled as singly labeled glucose on position 6 [26]. Estimates of EGP have been found to be comparable between hydrogen- and carbon-labeled glucose tracers upon quantification of labeled carbon recycling [31]. Depending on the tracer utilized, endogenous Ra may not only reflect the rate of GNG and glycogenolysis, but also the rate of cycling of substrates, especially the glucose cycle [26]. The glucose cycle exists because the conversion of glucose to glucose 6-phosphate by glucokinase occurs at the same time as the reverse reaction, which is catalyzed by glucose 6-phosphatase [26]. For example, 2-^{3}H-glucose or 2-^{2}H-glucose loses its label in the futile cycling between glucose and glucose-6-phosphate and it also loses its label when glucose cycles to glycogen and back (glycogen cycling). When glycogen stores are low, as after an overnight fast, the rate of glucose cycling can be quantified by subtracting the estimate of endogenous Ra obtained using 6-^{3}H-glucose from the estimate of endogenous Ra obtained using

2-^{3}H-glucose (also referred to as total glucose output) [32]. Glucose cycling is an indicator of flux through glucokinase and insulin, during the hyperinsulinemic euglycemic clamp, elevates glucose cycling [32].

In the literature, parameters of glucose kinetics (usually Rd and Ginf) are often adjusted for circulating glucose or insulin concentrations during the clamp steady state or for the change in circulating insulin concentrations from baseline to the clamp steady states. The physiological rationale is that both the level of glycemia during the clamp and the insulin concentration (or its change) affect glucose metabolism and, hence, an adjustment should be made. The adjustment can be achieved by using the glucose or insulin concentrations as covariates during statistical analysis or simply by dividing the endpoint by the glucose or insulin concentrations. During the hyperinsulinemic euglycemic clamp, the increase in glucose disposal and suppression of EGP are proportional to, but have a non-linear relationship with, circulating insulin ranging from physiological to supraphysiological concentrations, and maximal responses are obtained [33]. When parameters of glucose kinetics are divided by insulin concentrations or changes in insulin concentrations in a study population, an underlying assumption must be that since the range of insulin concentrations (or changes in insulin concentrations) is small, the relationship between insulin concentrations and the endpoints is essentially linear within that range. When Ginf or Rd is divided by the plasma glucose concentration, the result is called the metabolic clearance rate [34]. Glucose kinetics are also usually adjusted for body composition, such as body weight or lean tissue, because body composition affects glucose metabolism [15, 35, 36].

Peripheral glucose utilization can be subdivided into oxidative and non-oxidative metabolism using indirect calorimetry [37]. Non-oxidative glucose disposal consists of non-oxidative glycolysis and glycogen synthesis [38]. In addition, determination of glucose uptake in specific insulin sensitive tissues in vivo is possible with the use of 2-[^{14}C]-deoxyglucose [39]. The protocol, which is routinely used in animal studies, assumes that 2-[^{14}C]-deoxyglucose cannot be metabolized beyond phosphorylation at the 6 position and it requires assessment of 2-[^{14}C]-deoxyglucose in plasma and 2-deoxyglucose-6-phosphate in tissues [39–42].

Assessment of Gluconeogenesis In Vivo

Insulin-mediated suppression of EGP occurs as a result of inhibition of glycogenolysis and GNG, although glycogenolysis is suppressed at lower insulin concentrations than GNG in healthy subjects [43]. Moreover, as fasting is extended, the proportion of EGP from GNG increases [44–46]. Currently, there is no gold standard for assessment of GNG in vivo [47, 48]. Methods of quantifying GNG in vivo can be broadly categorized into techniques using carbon-labeled precursors (radioactive ^{14}C and stable ^{13}C tracers) for the synthesis of glucose, mass isotopomer distribution analysis (MIDA) using carbon-labeled precursors, mass isotopomer methods using U-^{13}C-glucose, and the deuterated water ($^{2}H_2O$) method [22, 26]. ^{13}C nuclear magnetic resonance (NMR) spectroscopy has also been utilized to determine net glycogenolysis, based on hepatic glycogen content, and GNG is calculated indirectly, as the difference between EGP (calculated with another methodology, such as [6-^{3}H]glucose) and net glycogenolysis [22, 44, 49, 50]. The high cost of the apparatus does not make this technique a routinely viable option for the quantification of GNG [22, 44, 49, 50].

Calculation of GNG using ^{14}C- or ^{13}C-containing tracers involves the use of labeled gluconeogenic precursors, such as alanine, and it depends on the plasma glucose SA (or enrichment if stable isotopes are used) and SA (or enrichment) of precursor in plasma [26, 51]. An example of this technique is the constant infusion of labeled precursor that results in an isotopic steady state (labeled tracer and labeled glucose); at steady state, the proportion of GNG in EGP is the ratio of glucose SA (or glucose enrichment) to precursor SA (or precursor enrichment) [51]. The gluconeogenic pathway has various points of entry and the estimate of GNG using this technique depends on the labeled precursor utilized. The technique relies upon enrichment measurements of precursors in plasma, since the SA (or enrichment) of GNG precursors cannot be measured directly [52]. The result is an underestimation of GNG, mainly because of dilution of the gluconeogenic precursor pool enrichment by production of unlabeled intracellular precursor and because of dilution of tracer in the oxaloacetate pool due to mixing of precursor-derived oxaloacetate with oxaloacetate from the Krebs cycle [22, 26, 51].

MIDA overcomes this limitation by determining gluconeogenic precursor pool enrichment indirectly [22, 26, 53]. MIDA calculates GNG based on the different mass isotopomers of glucose, a polymer, formed from infused labeled molecules, such as [^{13}C]glycerol and [^{13}C]lactate [22, 52]. An example of how MIDA can be utilized to calculate GNG is as follows: the frequencies of glucose mass isotopomers, specifically the ratio of doubly labeled glucose enrichment to singly labeled glucose enrichment, are used to determine the enrichment of the precursor pool, consisting of the monomers triose phosphates and not the tracer molecule per se [22, 26, 52, 54], and the GNG calculation (as percent of EGP) is then based on the ratio of product enrichment to precursor enrichment [26]. MIDA using labeled precursors assumes that enrichment of gluconeogenic precursors (triose phosphates) is constant across the liver, but when [^{13}C]glycerol is infused at low rates, the enrichment of the triose phosphate pool is not uniform, which leads to underestimations of GNG [22, 26, 49, 54–56]. MIDA accuracy in the determination of GNG, however, may be improved if higher infusion rates of [^{13}C]glycerol or if carbon tracers other than [^{13}C]glycerol are used [22, 54, 57].

Quantification of mass isotopomers of glucose and lactacte in plasma, resulting from [U-^{13}C]glucose administration, has also been used to calculate GNG based on glucose carbon recycling [22, 26, 50, 58]. Tayek and Katz [58] initially used this technique to calculate GNG as the product of glucose production, percent of glucose carbon recycled, factor for dilution of labeled pyruvate (using plasma lactate, which is assumed to have the same enrichment as intracellular pyruvate [59]), and factor for dilution by the Krebs cycle. Other equations have been subsequently published [60, 61]. The relative superiority of the equations is questionable [59, 62, 63] and they have been found to underestimate GNG in some studies [58, 61, 64]; potential explanations include the fact that only pyruvate-derived glucose is taken into account [50, 61] and the fact that neither lactate nor glucose reach isotopic steady state [65].

Quantification of GNG associated with [U-^{13}C]glucose administration has also been achieved via equations that use mass isotopomer analysis of glucose, but do not utilize assessment of mass isotopomers of lactate, referred to as the reciprocal pool model, and GNG does not appear to be underestimated [26, 66].

The $^{2}H_2O$ method is considered as probably the most reliable technique for GNG quantification in vivo [22, 49, 50]. Deuterated water is typically ingested by humans and injected i.p. in rats, thereby enriching body water [50, 67, 68]. The underlying principle is that ^{2}H from $^{2}H_2O$ is incorporated into specific carbons of glucose along the gluconeogenic pathway, thereby allowing the calculation of the proportion of total GNG in EGP and by subtraction the proportion of glycogenolysis in EGP, as well as the separate contribution to total GNG of the gluconeogenic precursors glycerol and phosphoenolpyruvate (PEP) [36, 68]. The ^{2}H enrichment at C2 of glucose (H2) is indicative of total EGP, namely GNG and glycogenolysis [45, 50]. ^{2}H from $^{2}H_2O$ is incorporated at C2 of glucose 6-phosphate in the reaction catalyzed by phosphoglucose isomerase, whereby fructose 6-phosphate is converted to glucose 6-phosphate [23, 45, 50]. This reaction is completely reversible so that glucose 6-phosphate derived from glycogenolysis also becomes labeled at C2; labeling at C2 of glucose 6-phosphate results in labeling at C2 of glucose [23, 45, 50]. On the other hand, the calculation of GNG is based on ^{2}H enrichment at C5 of glucose (H5), which results from ^{2}H at C2 of glyceraldehyde 3-phosphate in the following ways: ^{2}H from $^{2}H_2O$ becomes attached to (1) C2 of 2-phosphoglycerate in the reaction where PEP is converted to 2-phosphoglycerate (2-phosphoglycerate is subsequently converted to glyceraldehyde 3-phosphate) and to (2) C2 of glyceraldehyde 3-phosphate in the conversion of dihydroxyacetone phosphate (dihydroxyacetone phosphate is the first common intermediate of glycerol-derived GNG and other sources of GNG) to glyceraldehyde 3-phosphate by triose phosphate isomerase [23, 45, 50]. ^{2}H enrichment at C6 of glucose (H6) results from C3 enrichment of PEP, which in turn results from interconversions between alanine and pyruvate as well as between oxaloacetate and fumarate, and hence, the fraction of GNG from PEP can be estimated as the ratio of H6 to H2 [36, 45, 50, 68–70]. Moreover, the difference between H5/H2 and H6/H2 represents the fraction of GNG from glycerol [36, 45, 50, 68–70].

The ^{2}H enrichment at C3 (H3) has also been used instead of H5 in the equation for the fraction of GNG in EGP [71]. When triose phosphate isomerase produces dihydroxyacetone phosphate from glyceraldehyde 3-phosphate, ^{2}H becomes incorporated into one of dihydroxyacetone phosphate's carbons, which corresponds to C3 of glucose [71]. The ratio H3/H2 includes the contribution of glycerol to GNG because triose phosphate isomerase catalyzes a reversible reaction, although the fraction of GNG in EGP can be underestimated using the H3/H2 ratio if this reaction is not completely reversible [71].

The ^{2}H enrichment at C2 of glucose reaches equilibrium with plasma $^{2}H_2O$ enrichment approximately within 5 h in fasting, healthy humans and once such steady state is achieved, plasma $^{2}H_2O$ enrichment, which is easier to determine, can be used instead of H2 in the above equations [48, 67]. The $^{2}H_2O$ method can determine GNG during the fasting state and the hyperinsulinemic euglycemic clamp, although in the latter case H2 must be used instead of $^{2}H_2O$ if H5 is not in isotopic equilibrium because plasma C5 and C2 enrichment diminish due to insulin-induced glucose disposal, but insulin does not affect plasma ^2H_2O enrichment [48].

In general, the limitations of the ^2H_2O method are considered minimal [22, 50]. Recently, however, there has been concern over the use of H3 or H5 in the calculation of the fraction of GNG in EGP, as ^2H enrichment at C5 of glucose could be increased by the transaldolase reaction and ^2H enrichment at C3 of glucose could be decreased by isotope discrimination during the triose phosphate isomerase reaction, whereby labeling of dihydroxyacetone phosphate would decrease the rate at which it is converted to glyceraldehyde 3-phosphate [47, 72]. The consequence of the former (increased H5) would be overestimation of GNG, while that of the latter (decreased H3) would be underestimation of GNG [47, 72].

More invasive techniques, utilizing liver tissue collection and blood vessel cannulation, have been applied to the calculation of GNG in animal models. First, one method involves the infusion of a labeled precursor, such as [U-^{14}C]lactate in vivo [73–77]. The fraction of GNG can be determined from the ratio of [^{14}C]UDP-glucose SA and 2×[^{14}C]PEP SA, a precursor-product relationship [73–77]. This method is advantageous because SA of PEP, a gluconeogenic precursor, is measured directly within liver tissue, which avoids the problem of dilution of precursor in oxaloacetate pool, but it is limited by the fact that glycerol-derived glucose is excluded from the GNG calculation [75, 77]. Second, the arteriovenous (a–v) difference technique, which involves catheter placement in portal and hepatic veins as well as a femoral artery, has been used to calculate maximum and minimum estimates of GNG in dogs [77, 78]. The basic principle of both estimates is that the concentration of gluconeogenic precursors are compared in blood vessels entering and exiting the liver to determine their hepatic uptake [77, 78]. The maximum GNG is obtained when it is assumed that all of the gluconeogenic precursors taken up by the liver are transformed into glucose [77]. In contrast, the minimum GNG is the product of maximum GNG and gluconeogenic efficiency, which is the ratio of [^{14}C]glucose production to [^{14}C]alanine uptake by the liver and is less than 100% as a result of dilution of the oxaloacetate pool SA [77, 78]. Although this approach also includes circulating glycerol as a gluconeogenic precursor, intrahepatic gluconeogenic precursors such as amino acids are not included in the GNG calculation [77]. The two techniques for GNG quantification in animals described above, namely the techniques utilizing [^{14}C]PEP or a–v difference, have been used together and the results show that the [^{14}C]PEP-derived value of GNG is closer to the maximum estimate of GNG [77, 78].

Indices of In Vivo Insulin Sensitivity not derived from hyperinsulinemic clamps

In large population studies, it is impractical to perform hyperinsulinemic euglycemic clamps for financial, logistic, and technical reasons. Instead, other indices of insulin sensitivity have been devised and utilized and their accuracy has been typically compared to whole body and peripheral insulin sensitivity obtained with the hyperinsulinemic euglycemic clamp (Reviewed in [79, 80]). The following is intended as a discussion of the principles and validity of the most widely used and novel indices of in vivo insulin sensitivity, but it is not an exhaustive list.

Fasting Insulin

Fasting insulin concentration is among the simplest measures of insulin sensitivity because in the presence of insulin resistance the normal β cell compensates by increasing insulin secretion to maintain glucose homeostasis. The correlation of fasting insulin with whole body insulin resistance (inverse of insulin sensitivity) tends to be stronger among healthy subjects in some studies ($r \approx 0.4$–0.7) and it is rather poor among in type 2 diabetes mellitus (T2DM) subjects ($r \approx 0.5$) because insulin secretion is insufficient to counteract hyperglycemia and, hence, plasma insulin is not only dictated by insulin sensitivity, but also by the extent of β function [79, 81, 82]. In rats, the correlation of fasting insulin with whole body insulin resistance has been found not to be significant [83]. Fasting insulin correlates poorly with whole body insulin resistance in mice ($r \approx 0.3$) [84].

Homeostasis Model Assessment and Quantitative Insulin Sensitivity Check Index

Homeostasis model assessment (HOMA) and quantitative insulin sensitivity check index (QUICKI) are mathematical manipulations of circulating glucose and insulin concentrations. The basic underlying principle of HOMA, which incorporates experimental data, is that during fasting, plasma insulin concentrations dictate plasma glucose concentrations and vice versa [79, 85–87]. Thus, if a change in insulin levels is not adequate to maintain normal glucose levels, the change in glucose levels should also be taken into account. HOMA uses fasting plasma insulin and glucose concentrations to calculate combined hepatic and peripheral insulin resistance (HOMA-IR), and β cell function (HOMA – %B) [85, 87]. The simplified equations commonly used [85] were initially published by Matthews et al. [87]:

$$\text{HOMA} - \text{IR} = (\text{FPI} \times \text{FPG}) / 22.5$$

$$\text{HOMA} - \%\text{B} = (20 \times \text{FPI}) / (\text{FPG} - 3.5)$$

FPI and FPG represent fasting plasma insulin (mU/L) and glucose (mmol/L) concentrations, respectively [85, 87]. The number 22.5 in the HOMA-IR equation is obtained by multiplying 5 mU/L of fasting insulin by 4.5 mmol/L of fasting glucose, which represent concentrations in healthy individuals [79, 87]. Substitution of these concentrations for FPI and FPG into the above equations result in HOMA-IR = 1 and HOMA−%B=100% for healthy individuals [85, 87]. Continuous infusion of glucose with model assessment (CIGMA), which applies the principles of HOMA in the context of a continuous 60 min i.v. glucose infusion, shows better precision than HOMA for insulin sensitivity [87, 88], as expected due to its evaluation in an insulin-stimulated state. Nevertheless, HOMA is a useful index of insulin sensitivity in studies with large sample sizes [85]. HOMA-IR correlates well ($r \approx 0.7$–0.9) with whole body and peripheral insulin resistance determined using the hyperinsulinemic euglycemic clamp technique in populations with different levels of insulin sensitivity [87, 89]. Tripathy et al. [90], however, did not find a significant correlation between HOMA-IR and whole body insulin resistance among subjects with impaired fasting glucose.

Various derivations of HOMA exist. The inverse of HOMA-IR (also known as HOMA−%S [85]) correlates with whole body insulin sensitivity [81] and the inverse of HOMA-IR has also been used as an index of hepatic insulin sensitivity [91]. It has been suggested that HOMA and the inverse of HOMA are essentially indices of hepatic insulin sensitivity, as opposed to peripheral insulin sensitivity, because in the fasting state, glucose homeostasis is mostly dependent on hepatic insulin sensitivity [91]. In fact, a commonly used index of hepatic insulin sensitivity is either the product of (termed the hepatic insulin resistance index) or the inverse of the product of basal EGP (using tracer methods) and fasting plasma insulin [91–93].

The calculation of QUICKI is similar to that of the HOMA-IR,

$$\mathrm{QUICKI} = 1/[\log(\mathrm{FPI} \times \mathrm{FPG})]$$

and it is considered a mathematical derivation of HOMA-IR [85, 94]. Log transformations can be applied to data that do not have normal distributions, so that the linear correlations with hyperinsulinemic clamp-derived measures of insulin sensitivity can become stronger [79, 94]. The superiority of QUICKI vs. HOMA−%S as an index of insulin sensitivity, however, is debatable [79, 85]. QUICKI correlates with whole body insulin sensitivity measured during the hyperinsulinemic clamp in populations with different insulin sensitivities [81, 94]. The inclusion of fasting plasma free fatty acid (FFA) or glycerol concentrations in the QUICKI formula has been shown to increase the strength of this correlation [95]. QUICKI showed a stronger correlation with hyperinsulinemic euglycemic clamp estimates of whole body insulin sensitivity than HOMA-IR in healthy adult individuals, in patients with T2DM, and in children [81, 96, 97]. In a population of obese postmenopausal women, however, HOMA−%S and QUICKI were comparable (r's ≈ 0.4) [98].

In rats, HOMA−%S and QUICKI correlate ($r > 0.6$) with the index of insulin sensitivity SI_{clamp}, which is defined as Ginf divided by the product of the glucose concentration and the change in insulin concentration relative to baseline during the hyperinsulinemic euglycemic clamp [99]. Similar results were obtained in mice, where r's ≈ 0.45 for both HOMA−%S and QUICKI [84].

Insulin Tolerance Test

In humans, the insulin tolerance test (ITT) is performed after an overnight fast and it entails the i.v. administration of an insulin bolus, such as 0.1 U/kg body weight, as well as the measurement of plasma or blood glucose concentrations up to 15 min afterwards [100–102]. This ITT, also known as the short ITT, is a substitute for an older version of the ITT, which involved measuring glucose for 30–40 min following insulin administration [100, 103]. Since counterregulatory hormones have been found to be elevated after 15 min following the insulin bolus, making the test shorter is a way of avoiding these confounding variables [100].

A widely used equation for ITT-derived indices of insulin sensitivity is based on first order kinetics of glucose disappearance, where the log of plasma or blood glucose concentration changes linearly with time within the 3–15 min time frame; K_{itt}, the rate constant for glucose disappearance, is an ITT-derived index of insulin sensitivity that equals the slope of this graph multiplied by −100 and it has the units % per min [100–102]. K_{itt} can also be expressed as $K_{itt}=69.3/t_{1/2}$, where $t_{1/2}$ represents the time when the plasma glucose concentration at 3 min has decreased by half [100–102]. Others have used slightly different ITT-derived indices of insulin sensitivity, such as the slope of the blood glucose concentration vs. time graph in the 3–15 min time frame [104]. The ITT gives a cumulative measure of insulin-mediated glucose disposal and suppression of EGP in a dynamic setting [105]. Bonora et al. [100] have shown that counterregulatory mechanisms to insulin-stimulated glucose decrease that involve glucagon, catecholamines, growth hormone, and cortisol are not activated in the 15 min time frame of the ITT. Hypoglycemia during the ITT, however, has been documented and the use of 0.05 U of insulin per kg body weight, which is half of the insulin dosage typically used in the ITT, does not consistently avoid hypoglycemia [102, 104, 106]. Furthermore, some [102, 106], but not all studies [101, 104], suggest that ITT reproducibility is worse when using the lower vs. the higher dose of insulin. ITT-derived indices of insulin sensitivity correlate with whole body insulin sensitivity (M/I index, where M is [8] and I is clamp insulin) determined with the hyperinsulinemic euglycemic clamp in subjects with various degrees of insulin sensitivity; $r=0.811$ in Bonora et al. [100], $r=0.81$ for healthy subjects in Gelding et al. [104], and $r=0.86$ for healthy subjects and $r=0.81$ for T2DM subjects in Akinmokun et al. [105]. The correlation between K_{itt} and HOMA-%S is poor in T2DM subjects, where $r=0.44$ [107] and the correlation between K_{itt} and HOMA-IR appears to be only slightly stronger in healthy subjects, where $r=-0.57$ [108]. This suggests that ITT-derived indices of insulin sensitivity and HOMA likely reflect different facets of insulin sensitivity, with the former reflecting hepatic and peripheral insulin sensitivity and HOMA reflecting more hepatic insulin sensitivity [107].

Since ITT is easy to perform and entails minimal blood loss, especially when repeated measures are required in the same animal, it is often used to assess insulin sensitivity in rodents and when its results are compared between treatment groups or genotypes, the significance may mirror that obtained with the hyperinsulinemic euglycemic clamp [109–111]. Surprisingly, however, direct comparisons of

ITT-derived indices of insulin sensitivity with the hyperinsulinemic euglycemic clamp, to assess validity, are lacking in rodent studies. The ITT in mice is usually preceded by a 3–6 h fasting period [79, 109, 111, 112] and it typically involves i.p. administration of an insulin bolus (0.75–2 U per kg body weight), that is followed by blood glucose measurements at time intervals until 30–120 min [109, 111–113]. Analysis of ITT results involve comparing K_{itt}, comparing blood glucose concentrations over time, or comparing the area under the curve (AUC) [110, 111, 113, 114]. Concerns about counterregulatory responses to hypoglycemia have been raised in ITTs performed in rodents [115], as ITTs in rodents usually last longer than in humans.

Oral Glucose Tolerance Test and Intraperitoneal Glucose Tolerance Test

The oral glucose tolerance test (OGTT), which indicates whether glucose homeostasis, and not insulin sensitivity per se, is altered has been used in the assessment of insulin sensitivity [116]. The OGTT involves ingestion of 75 g of glucose in water and the plasma glucose concentration at 2 h can be diagnostic of T2DM [117, 118]. Various indices of insulin sensitivity have been obtained from OGTT results, which are based on slightly different principles [91, 119–121]. In particular, calculations derived from fasting and OGTT glucose as well as insulin concentrations have yielded robust correlations with clamp-derived whole body insulin sensitivity [91]. OGTT-derived indices of insulin sensitivity correlate as well or better than HOMA with clamp-derived measures of insulin sensitivity. This is expected due to additional information about the glucose system provided by OGTT stimulation. The OGTT-derived composite index of hepatic and peripheral insulin sensitivity developed by Matsuda et al. [91], appears to correlate as well as HOMA-%S with whole body insulin sensitivity derived from the clamp ($r=0.732$ and $r=0.691$, respectively). Soonthornpun et al. [119] have put forward an OGTT-derived index of peripheral insulin sensitivity that correlates as well as the composite index with whole body insulin sensitivity in healthy subjects ($r=0.869$ and $r=0.734$, respectively), and is superior to HOMA−%S and QUICKI ($r=0.404$ and $r=0.434$, respectively). The core principle of this index is that glucose disposal depends on the difference between the plasma glucose concentration during the OGTT without insulin (an estimate) and the actual AUC for glucose during the OGTT; the latter consists of glucose that is not taken up by tissues and EGP [119]. Separate indices of hepatic and peripheral insulin sensitivity, obtained from OGTT data, were found to correlate with the hepatic insulin resistance index ($r=0.64$) and whole body insulin sensitivity from the euglycemic clamp ($r=0.78$), respectively, in subjects without diabetes [93]. The OGTT-derived hepatic insulin sensitivity index equals the product of the AUC for glucose and insulin during the initial 30 min of the OGTT because insulin and glucose exert their inhibitory effects on EGP mostly during that time frame [93]. In turn, the index of peripheral insulin sensitivity equals the rate of change in plasma glucose concentration (starting at the maximal glucose concentration until its minimum, a time period which is assumed to coincide with already suppressed EGP) divided by the average plasma insulin concentration [93].

OGTTs are also performed in rodents and conclusions from the OGTT in rodents are usually drawn from AUC for glucose and insulin, and individual glucose and insulin measurements [83, 114, 122, 123]. Although rather poor correlations ($r \leq 0.6$) have been found between the latter indices and euglycemic clamp-derived estimates of insulin sensitivity in humans [34], Tran et al. [83] have found good correlations for the AUC for insulin and for the ratio of glucose to insulin, where the magnitude of r's ≈ 0.7, in rats given a high dose OGTT.

Intraperitoneal glucose tolerance tests (IPGTTs), which involve injection of a glucose solution bolus intraperitoneally and collection of blood samples at time intervals for about 120 min, are routinely used in rodent studies to assess glucose homeostasis [124, 125]. The interpretation of IPGTTs is based on comparisons of blood or plasma glucose and plasma insulin concentrations and the AUC for insulin and glucose over that time period [124, 125]. Similar to OGTTs, it is difficult to discern insulin sensitivity from secretion in IPGTTs [79].

Frequently Sampled Intravenous Glucose Tolerance Test

The frequently sampled intravenous glucose tolerance test (FSIVGTT)-minimal model method is commonly used in the estimation of insulin sensitivity when a less invasive protocol than a hyperinsulinemic euglycemic clamp is required, for example, in children and pregnant women. In the FSIVGTT, following an overnight fast, an i.v. glucose bolus is administered (300 mg/kg body weight over a short period of time) and blood samples are obtained during the subsequent time period, usually 3–4 h [126–128]. A computer program, MINMOD, is then used to analyze the plasma glucose and insulin concentrations during the FSIVGTT and determine the insulin sensitivity index (S_I) [126, 127]. More specifically, MINMOD gives the user estimates of parameters for equations originating from a minimal model [126, 129]. The model is based on various tenets, including glucose kinetics being represented by a single compartment, the difference between net hepatic balance and peripheral glucose uptake determines the rate at which glucose changes, and insulin acts on glucose metabolism at the level of the liver and periphery [126, 129, 130]. The precision and validity of S_I depends upon a robust increase in plasma insulin, specifically at a point when plasma glucose concentration is lowering, such that glucose effectiveness can be separated from insulin sensitivity [79, 127, 128, 131, 132]. Therefore, tolbutamide (a sulfonylurea) and exogenous insulin have been administered intravenously during the FSIVGTT, typically at 20 min. In healthy subjects, the decrease in plasma glucose during the insulin-modified FSIVGTT has been found to stimulate counterregulatory hormones, thereby diminishing S_I and, hence, hypoglycemia should be limited during FSIVGTTs, potentially via glucose infusion [133].

Among healthy patients without diabetes, S_I's from tolbutamide- and insulin-modified FSIVGTTs have been found to correlate equally well (r's ≈ 0.7) with clamp-derived whole body insulin sensitivity, although the magnitude of S_I's differs between FSIVGTTs [134]. A weaker correlation was found in another study, with S_I derived from insulin-modified FSIVGTT, among non-diabetic subjects ($r \approx 0.5$–0.6) [28]. Among patients with T2DM, the strength of the correlation between S_I derived from insulin-modified FSIVGTT and measures of insulin sensitivity obtained with the clamp, can vary widely, with Coates et al. [132] obtaining a value of $r \approx 0.7$, while Saad et al. [28] obtained an r value ≈ 0.4. Moreover, in a population with different levels of insulin sensitivity, S_I from insulin-modified FSIVGTT correlated worse than QUICKI with SI_{clamp} [94].

Recent additional alterations to the original methodology and analysis of FSIVGTT include collection of less blood samples to minimize invasiveness and use of computer programs other than MINMOD [128, 135]. The use of tracers during FSIVGTTs, known as "hot FSIVGTTs," has resulted in larger and better estimates of S_I and it has permitted the calculation of hepatic insulin sensitivity [134, 136–138]; however, the addition of tracer increases the cost and invasiveness of the FSIVGTT.

IVGTT-minimal model has been used to calculate S_I in rodents, but the minimal model has not always been applied to IVGTT data in rodent studies [139–141]. Instead, AUC for plasma glucose and insulin, and plasma glucose and insulin concentrations have been utilized to interpret IVGTT results. In mice, analysis of IVGTT results using the minimal model has been shown to yield S_I's that correlate robustly ($r = 0.964$) with whole body insulin sensitivity, as assessed with the hyperinsulinemic euglycemic clamp [142]. Furthermore, Pacini et al. [143] have recently devised a formula for calculating insulin sensitivity (CS_I) based on IVGTT data in mice, which bypasses the need for analysis with the minimal model and that shows a good correlation with S_I ($r \approx 0.9$) and is similar in magnitude to S_I.

Insulin Suppression Test

The basic concept of the insulin suppression test (IST) is that plasma glucose concentrations become an index of insulin sensitivity when glucose and insulin are infused at a constant rate, in the context of inhibition of insulin secretion [79, 144, 145]. Inhibition of insulin secretion was initially achieved by i.v. administration of epinephrine and propanolol, but more recently somatostatin or the somatostatin analogue octreotide, both of which blunt insulin as well as glucagon secretion, have been used [146–149]. Typical protocols involve the parallel, constant i.v. infusion of somatostatin (≈ 5 μg min^{-1}) or octreotide (0.27 μg m^{-2} min^{-1}), insulin (25 mU m^{-2} min^{-1} or 32 mU m^{-2} min^{-1}), and glucose (240 mg m^{-2} min^{-1} or 267 mg m^{-2} min^{-1}) for 180 min, after an overnight fast [145, 150, 151]. The steady state is defined as the period 150–180 min, when blood samples are taken every 10 min, and the steady state plasma glucose concentrations (SSPG) are the index of insulin sensitivity, since steady state plasma insulin concentrations (SSPI) do not differ greatly in a study population [145, 150, 151]. Since EGP is totally suppressed during the IST in normal subjects because of hyperinsulinemia and hyperglycemia [25], SSPG is indicative of insulin-induced glucose utilization, such that higher SSPG usually implies peripheral insulin resistance [79, 144, 146]. Robust correlations ($r=0.93$) have been shown between SSPG and whole body insulin sensitivity determined with the hyperinsulinemic euglycemic clamp [152]. The IST protocols used in rats and mice are analogous to those in humans [153–155].

Hyperglycemic Clamp

The hyperglycemic clamp, which involves elevating and maintaining plasma glucose at a specific concentration, is the gold standard technique to determine β cell function in vivo [8, 156, 157]. Nevertheless, an inverse relationship exists between insulin sensitivity and insulin secretion [158] and indices of insulin sensitivity can be calculated from the hyperglycemic clamp, which depend on the glucose infusion rate and plasma insulin concentrations achieved during the hyperglycemic clamp [156, 157, 159]. Calculation of these indices in subjects with different insulin levels during the hyperglycemic clamp is based on the assumption of linearity of the insulin–glucose system, which is only valid for small differences [8]. However, a good correlation ($r=0.84$) between and similar magnitude for hyperglycemic clamp-derived and hyperinsulinemic euglycemic clamp-derived indices of insulin sensitivity have been found in humans [160]. The insulin levels attained during the hyperglycemic clamp plus hyperglycemia per se may be sufficient to completely suppress EGP [25, 161]. Therefore, the index of insulin sensitivity during hyperglycemic clamps mainly or only reflects glucose utilization.

Selection of an Appropriate Index of Insulin Sensitivity

Various factors, including invasiveness of the technique for the study population, financial resources, time, technical ability, and whether insulin sensitivity is a main study endpoint should be considered when selecting an index of insulin sensitivity. It is important to note that the strength of the correlation of a given index with estimates obtained from the hyperinsulinemic euglycemic clamp may differ in different populations and even in different rodent strains. The correlations between clamp variables and indices of insulin sensitivity are generally stronger in humans than in mice [84]; this may depend on specific aspects of the methodology used in mice, such as length of fasting time, which can affect insulin sensitivity [162].

The Insulin Signaling Cascade

Assessment of insulin sensitivity after a hyperinsulinemic euglycemic clamp or insulin bolus also includes assessment of the insulin signaling cascade status, especially in animals [15]. The insulin receptor, upon binding to insulin, autophosphorylates and phosphorylates insulin receptor substrates (IRS), which are the main substrates of the insulin receptor that lead to the metabolic effects of insulin [163]. Although there are six isoforms of IRS, whole-body gene knockout (KO) studies in mice

(IRS-1 through 4) indicate that IRS-1 and -2 are the main IRS isoforms involved in the regulation of glucose homeostasis [164–168]. Among insulin sensitive tissues, IRS-3 gene expression occurs in the liver and adipose tissue, but not skeletal muscle and brain [169], while IRS-4 gene expression occurs in skeletal muscle, liver, and brain, but IRS-4 protein is not found in appreciable amounts in tissues [170]. Neither whole-body glucose homeostasis nor insulin signaling in adipose tissue, the main location of IRS-3 expression, is altered in IRS-3 KO mice [166]. Interestingly, however, double IRS-1/IRS-3 KO mice have lipoatrophic diabetes, indicating that both IRS-1 and IRS-3 are involved in adipose tissue development [171]. There is a slight impairment in glucose homeostasis in IRS-4 KO mice, as determined by OGTT, but the fact that double IRS-1/IRS-4 KO mice have the same phenotype as IRS-1 KO mice suggests that IRS-1 is more important for glucose homeostasis and insulin sensitivity [167, 171].

Both IRS-1 and -2 are expressed in insulin sensitive tissues, namely skeletal muscle, liver, and adipose tissue [172, 173]. IRS-1 KO mice are characterized by insulin resistance in skeletal muscle, but they have normal fasting blood glucose concentrations and do not develop diabetes [164, 174]. IRS-2 KO mice, however, are characterized by type 2-like diabetes, which is associated with extensive hepatic insulin resistance [165, 175] and diminished β cell mass [175], although the extent of impaired peripheral insulin sensitivity is debatable [165, 175]. These KO mice studies indicate that IRS-2 plays a more prominent role in hepatic insulin sensitivity than IRS-1 [3, 165, 174, 175] and this is further substantiated by studies in double heterozygous KO mice, whose genes for the insulin receptor and IRS-1 or IRS-2 have been knocked out [176]. However, a recent study using RNA interference (RNAi) showed that both IRS-1 and IRS-2 mediate the action of insulin in the liver, but while IRS-1 is mainly associated with glucose metabolism, IRS-2 mainly mediates insulin-stimulated lipid metabolism [177]. Indeed, liver-specific IRS-2 KO mice do not have impaired insulin-mediated suppression of EGP [178], although Dong et al. [179] have found these mice to develop fasting hyperglycemia with age. The roles of IRS-5 and -6 in the metabolic effects induced by insulin remain to be completely elucidated [168].

IRS-1 and -2 contain pleckstrin-homology (PH) and phosphotyrosine-binding (PTB) domains (reviewed in [173] and [7]). The PH domain of IRS-1 and IRS-2 interacts with membrane phospholipids, namely 3-phosphorylated phosphoinositides [180]. The PTB domains permit the binding of IRS-1 and -2 to tyrosine-phosphorylated motifs on the insulin receptor [181–183]. IRS-2 also binds to the insulin receptor via another IRS-2 region when specific tyrosine residues on the insulin receptor are phosphorylated [181, 182].

IRS proteins are typically described as docking proteins because they provide a link between the activated insulin receptor and downstream effectors, such as phosphatidylinositol 3-kinase (PI3K). PI3K represents a vital component in the pathway of insulin's effect on glucose metabolism [7, 184, 185] and its activity is often an indicator of insulin sensitivity at the tissue level [185, 186]. PI3K is activated by binding to phosphotyrosine residues of IRS proteins via Src-homology-2 (SH2) domains of its regulatory subunit [187–190]. PI3K phosphorylates inositol phospholipids at the 3 position and phosphatidylinositol-3,4,5-triphosphate (PIP_3) is among its products [189, 190]. PI3K is a heterodimer composed of a catalytic subunit and a regulatory subunit; the catalytic subunits consist of p110α, p110β, and p110δ, while the regulatory subunits, often called p85, are p85α, p85β, p55γ, p55α, and p50α [188]. While mice null for the regulatory subunits of PI3K have been found to have improved insulin signaling and insulin sensitivity [191–194], heterozygous null mice for α and β isoforms of the catalytic subunit show impaired components of the insulin signaling cascade and glucose intolerance [195]. Furthermore, liver-specific KO of p85α in mice augments insulin-mediated suppression of EGP [196]. Although at first glance these results are conflictive, they can be reconciled because: (1) a low ratio of p110-bound to free p85 subunit may adversely affect insulin sensitivity [188, 195], and (2) p85 activates c-jun N-terminal kinase (JNK) [197] and phosphatase and tensin homolog deleted on chromosome 10 (PTEM) [196], both of which impair insulin sensitivity.

Akt, a serine/threonine kinase also referred to as protein kinase B (PKB), is downstream of PI3K and is generally considered to be essential in insulin-mediated glucose metabolism [7, 185, 198–200]. Akt activation requires direct binding of PIP_3 to the PH domain of Akt and subsequent phosphorylation of Akt's Ser 473 and Thr 308 [201, 202]. Phosphoinositide-dependent kinase 1 (PDK1), which requires PIP_3 for activation, phosphorylates Thr 308 [201, 202], while Ser 473 is phosphorylated by PDK2, which includes the subunits mammalian target of rapamycin (mTOR) and rapamycin insensitive companion of mTOR (rictor), a complex as mTORC2 [203–205]. Three isoforms of Akt have been identified, namely Akt1, Akt2, and Akt3 (also known as PKBα, PKBβ, and PKBγ, respectively) [206], and studies in KO mice appear to indicate that only Akt2 is involved in mediating the effects of insulin on glucose metabolism [206–211]. Other studies, however, suggest that the relative importance of Akt isoforms with respect to insulin sensitivity depends on the species and tissue being analyzed [212, 213].

Insulin resistance is defined as blunted insulin action at a given insulin concentration [214]. Abnormalities in the levels and function of intermediaries of insulin signaling have been found in human and animal states of insulin resistance, which include obesity and T2DM, and these impairments can be triggered by plasma/tissue cytokines and fat (discussed in Sect. "Modulators of Insulin-Mediated Glucose Metabolism"). Serine phosphorylation of IRS-1, which is a common mechanism of induction of insulin resistance by cytokines and fat [15, 215], reduces tyrosine phosphorylation of IRS-1 and augments IRS-1 degradation, thereby blunting insulin signaling [216–219]. Suppressors of cytokine signaling (SOCS), whose protein expression is increased by cytokines, inhibit IRS tyrosine phosphorylation and increase IRS degradation [220–222]. As an example, a genetic model of obesity and T2DM, the *ob/ob* mouse, shows diminished protein expression of IRS-1 and -2 in liver and skeletal muscle [223]. Moreover, insulin-stimulated IRS tyrosine phosphorylation is blunted and insulin-stimulated IRS-associated PI3K activity is reduced in both tissues [223]. The extent of insulin-stimulated Akt Ser 473 phosphorylation is also impaired in *ob/ob* mice [224]. In addition, another model of insulin resistance, the high fat diet-fed rodent, is characterized by elevated skeletal muscle Ser 307 phosphorylation of IRS-1 and SOCS-3 protein levels [225]. Since SOCS-3 has been found to associate with the insulin receptor and IRS-1, SOCS-3 may inhibit insulin signaling via steric hindrance [225]. Adipose tissue from *ob/ob* mice and high fat diet-fed mice shows elevated IRS-1 serine phosphorylation [226, 227].

Obese individuals have diminished adipocyte IRS-1 gene expression [228]. In adipocytes from T2DM subjects, IRS-1 protein levels are reduced [229] and insulin-stimulated IRS tyrosine phosphorylation is impaired [230]. In addition, the skeletal muscle of obese subjects and patients with T2DM has been found to have reduced protein levels and insulin-induced tyrosine phosphorylation of the insulin receptor and IRS-1 [186, 231–233], decreased insulin-induced PI3K activity associated with IRS-1 [186, 231, 232, 234], and elevated protein levels of PI3K regulatory subunits that are accompanied by a reduction in insulin-stimulated IRS-1-associated p85 and p110 [186]. Insulin-mediated Akt activity and phosphorylation at Ser 473 and Thr 308 is blunted in skeletal muscle of T2DM patients [235]. Similarly, insulin-stimulated IRS-1-associated PI3K activity, Akt activity, and Akt Ser phosphorylation are reduced in adipocytes of T2DM subjects [236, 237]. Augmented IRS-1 Ser 307 phosphorylation has also been shown in skeletal muscle of obese and T2DM subjects [186]. SOCS-3 mRNA is augmented in the skeletal muscle of T2DM subjects and in the adipose tissue of obese subjects [238]. There is, however, some discrepancy over the relative importance of impairments in proximal insulin signaling in skeletal muscle of T2DM patients [239]. For example, in some studies, insulin-stimulated Akt activity has been found not to be altered, despite reduced PI3K activity, in muscle of T2DM [240] and impaired skeletal muscle IRS expression in T2DM has not been found in other studies [233].

Taken together (also see sections below), the literature data indicate that insulin resistance of carbohydrate metabolism mostly involves impairments in the PI3K pathway, and not the insulin-stimulated Ras-mitogen-activated protein kinase (MAPK) pathway [241]. This is because the Ras-MAPK pathway is mostly independent of IRS proteins. Briefly, in the Ras-MAPK pathway activation of the GTPase Ras requires exchange of GTP for GDP and this is achieved via son of sevenless (Sos), a guanine nucleotide exchange factor; Sos is bound to growth-factor-receptor-bound protein-2 (Grb2), a protein that binds to insulin receptor-phosphorylated Src-homology-2-containing protein (Shc) and Grb2-associated binder-1 (Gab1) [7, 241–245]. Grb2 can also bind to IRS-1 phosphotyrosine residues [246]. Ras activates Raf and a phosphorylation cascade follows, where Raf activates MAPK-kinases (MEKs), which in turn activate the MAPKs extracellular signal-regulated kinase (ERK) 1/2 [7, 241, 242]. The end result of the Ras-MAPK pathway is modulation of cell survival, cell differentiation, and mitogenesis [241, 247]. The Ras-MAPK pathway can be activated by factors other than insulin and inappropriate activation of the Ras-MAPK pathway is involved in the pathogenesis of cancer [242, 248, 249].

The PI3K pathway can also stimulate survival and growth [205]. Activation of components of the PI3K pathway is associated with cancer and, therefore, its attenuation is a proposed treatment for cancer [205]. One of the components downstream of PI3K is mTORC1, a complex consisting of mTOR, the regulatory associated protein of mTOR (raptor), and mLST8; binding of the proline-rich Akt substrate 40 kDa (PRAS40) inhibits the complex [205, 250]. mTORC1 can be activated by

Akt and mTORC1 activation augments protein synthesis via S6 kinase (S6K1, also referred to as p70S6K) activation and eukaryotic initiation factor 4E-binding protein (4E-BP1) inhibition [205, 250, 251]. mTORC1, however, represents a convergent point of various pathways, since it is also activated by amino acids [252], it can be activated by ERK1/2 from the Ras-MAPK pathway [250, 253], and it is inhibited by AMP-activated protein kinase (AMPK), an energy sensor that is activated during low energy states by LKB1, a tumor suppressor [254]. In turn, insulin activation of S6K1 or ERK1/2 induces IRS-1 serine phosphorylation [216, 255–257], which blunts insulin signaling. The cross-talk between PI3K and Ras-MAPK pathways in the context of negative regulation of insulin action is further addressed in the sections below.

Tissue-Specific Mechanisms of Insulin-Mediated Glucose Metabolism

Liver

In healthy humans, alterations in EGP require minimal alterations in circulating insulin, thereby placing the liver as a central tissue in the regulation of glucose homeostasis by insulin [258]. The liver is at the crossroads of glucose metabolism: it takes up, utilizes, stores, and produces glucose. The glucose transporter GLUT2 permits the movement of glucose across the cell membrane of hepatocytes down its concentration gradient via facilitated diffusion [259]. GLUT2 is characterized by a high K_m, thereby preventing its saturation at physiological glucose concentrations [259]. Once glucose molecules enter hepatocytes, regulation of glucose metabolism by insulin occurs at the level of glucokinase, an enzyme that converts glucose to glucose 6-phosphate, which can be used in glycolysis and glycogenesis [23, 260]. Conversion of glucose to glucose 6-phosphate maintains a concentration gradient for glucose across the cell membrane, permitting the entry of glucose into hepatocytes, as in the postprandial period. Insulin stimulates the gene expression of glucokinase, a process that remains to be completely elucidated, but requires the transcription factor sterol regulatory element binding protein-1c (SREBP-1c) [261, 262]. The importance of glucokinase in glucose metabolism is reinforced by the hyperglycemia of liver-specific glucokinase KO mice [263].

Insulin simultaneously affects the function of the main enzymes responsible for glycogen metabolism: glycogen synthase, which promotes glycogenesis, and glycogen phosphorylase, which promotes glycogenolysis [23]. Insulin inhibits glycogen synthase kinase 3 (GSK3) through Akt activation; specifically, Akt directly phosphorylates Ser 21 of GSK3α and Ser 9 of GSK3β (reviewed in [264]). Once inactivated, GSK3 is unable to phosphorylate and inhibit glycogen synthase [264, 265]. Interestingly, GSK3 has also been shown to downregulate insulin signaling by phosphorylating IRS proteins on serine residues [266]. Studies investigating glucose metabolism in KO mice suggest that of the two GSK3 isoforms (α and β), GSK3α is the most important isoform in the liver, while GSK3β is the most important isoform in skeletal muscle [267, 268].

Inhibition of glycogen phosphorylase by insulin is also mediated by Akt and it limits glycogen breakdown [269, 270]. Moreover, insulin-induced glycogen phosphorylase inactivation causes glycogen synthase activation [269]. A potential mediator of this effect is glycogen-associated form of protein phosphatase-1 (PP1), which binds to glycogen-targeting subunits [271, 272]. Since PP1 is inhibited allosterically by the active form of glycogen phosphorylase and PP1 can activate glycogen synthase, inactivation of glycogen phosphorylase would limit PP1 inhibition and permit PP1 to act on glycogen synthase [271, 273–275]. Evidence for direct regulation of PP1 by insulin comes from studies in streptozotocin-induced diabetes in rodents. Streptozotocin-induced diabetes decreases the expression of the glycogen-targeting subunits to which PP1 binds, but these levels are increased by insulin administration [276].

Hepatic glucose output is the result of glycogenolysis and GNG. In conditions where hepatic insulin sensitivity is normal and glycogen is not depleted, hepatic autoregulation maintains hepatic glucose output constant by concurrent alterations in glycogenolysis and GNG (Reviewed in [277]). The mechanisms of hepatic autoregulation include production of glucose 6-phosphate from GNG to stimulate glycogen synthase [277]. The proportion of glucose production from GNG augments as fasting time increases [45] and control of GNG occurs at the level of phosphoenolpyruvate carboxykinase (PEPCK) and glucose 6-phosphatase (G6Pase) [23]. PEPCK, which converts oxaloacetate to phosphoenolpyruvate, is rate-limiting for GNG [278] and G6Pase, which converts glucose 6-phosphate to glucose, catalyzes the last reaction of GNG and glycogenolysis [279].

Insulin diminishes PEPCK and G6Pase gene expression [279, 280] through various mechanisms. Expression of PEPCK and G6Pase is mediated by the binding of the transcription factor forkhead box-containing protein of the O subfamily (FOXO)-1 to its coactivator peroxisome proliferator-activated receptor-γ coactivator-1α (PGC-1α) [281–284]. Insulin, via Akt-dependent phosphorylation, inhibits FOXO1 and PGC-1α function [285–288]. Specifically, Akt-mediated phosphorylation of FOXO1 prevents it from binding DNA [287] and PGC-1α [283], causes FOXO1 to translocate from the nucleus to the cytoplasm [287, 289, 290], and promotes its degradation [291]. Insulin also diminishes the transcriptional activity of PGC-1α via Akt-mediated phosphorylation [288] and it appears to reduce the transcription of PGC-1α, partially through FOXO1 inhibition [292, 293]. FOXO1 simultaneously inhibits glucokinase expression and promotes G6Pase expression via its interaction with the transcription factor hepatocyte nuclear factor-4 (HNF-4); while FOXO1 represses HNF-4's stimulatory action on the glucokinase gene, it enhances HNF-4 action to promote G6Pase expression [294]. Insulin control of G6Pase gene expression, however, may not be completely dependent on Akt and FOXO1 signaling [279]. Moreover, insulin can suppress gluconeogenic enzyme expression via phosphorylation (Akt-mediated) and ensuing degradation of transducer of regulated cAMP responsive elements (CRE) binding protein activity 2 (TORC2), a coactivator that binds to the transcription factor CRE binding protein (CREB) [295, 296].

The previous discussion focused on the direct effects of insulin on hepatic glucose metabolism, but many investigators, including us, have shown that insulin can also suppress glucose production by the liver indirectly [297, 298]. In humans, the relative contribution of the direct and indirect effects of insulin on EGP suppression has been studied by comparing the effects of (1) portal insulin, which was elevated by tolbutamide administration, (2) "full-rate" peripheral insulin, which was infused via a peripheral vein at the same rate as the insulin secretion in (1), and (3) "half-rate" peripheral insulin, which involved half the insulin infusion rate of (2) so that peripheral insulin concentrations equaled those in (1); this protocol was performed in the presence of euglycemia and it involved tracer methodology [297]. It was found that "full-rate" peripheral insulin causes a greater suppression in EGP than portal insulin, which in turn causes a greater suppression in EGP than "half-rate" peripheral insulin [297]. Hence, these results show that insulin acts directly and indirectly on the liver to suppress EGP and that at a given insulin dosage, insulin suppresses EGP to a greater extent if delivered peripherally than if delivered portally [297]. Since the "full-rate" peripheral insulin and portal insulin diminish peripheral glucagon and FFAs [297], Intralipid plus heparin (to elevate plasma FFAs) and/or glucagon have also been administered to investigate the role of these alterations on insulin-mediated EGP suppression. The results indicate that while glucagon boosts the direct effect of insulin by sensitizing the liver to insulin action, the decreases in glucagon and FFAs represent mechanisms of peripheral (indirect) effects of insulin on EGP [298–300]. The relative contribution of direct and indirect effects of insulin on EGP is inconsistent across studies, potentially due to different methodological approaches [301, 302], and it depends upon glycemia [303]. It has been shown that the direct effect of insulin to suppress liver EGP is blunted in T2DM [304].

In the last decade, the role of the CNS, particularly the hypothalamus, in controlling hepatic insulin sensitivity has gained attention. Insulin activates hypothalamic ATP-sensitive potassium channels, resulting in signal relay to the liver via the vagus nerve and ultimately, suppression of hepatic PEPCK and G6Pase gene expression as well as EGP [305–309]. In the liver, a molecular link between vagal neural input and suppression of glucose production appears to be the transcription factor signal transducer and activator of transcription-3 (STAT3) [309–311].

Skeletal Muscle

Insulin increases glucose uptake in skeletal muscle by stimulating the translocation of the glucose transporter GLUT4 to the cell membrane [200]. Glucose then enters skeletal muscle by facilitated diffusion. GLUT4 translocation to the cell membrane depends on a series of events, from movement of GLUT4-containing vesicles to the cell membrane to their fusion with the cell membrane [312]. Insulin-induced GLUT4 translocation is mediated by multiple parallel pathways, including pathways involving Akt and atypical protein kinase Cs (aPKCs) [7, 313]. Akt has been shown to mediate GLUT4 translocation by phosphorylating and thereby inhibiting Akt substrate of 160 kDa (AS160) [7, 200, 312, 314]. Specifically, AS160 inactivation permits the process of vesicle fusion with the cell membrane [315]. The activation of aPKCs, by

PDK1 phosphorylation of aPKCs, can mediate insulin-induced GLUT4 translocation [316, 317]. In vivo, muscle-specific GLUT4 KO mice are characterized by blunted insulin-mediated glucose uptake in skeletal muscle and peripheral glucose disposal as well as hyperglycemia [39]. The key role of insulin-stimulated GLUT4 translocation in skeletal muscle for insulin sensitivity and glucose homeostasis is further reinforced in ex vivo analyses of skeletal muscle from obese and T2DM subjects demonstrating blunted insulin-mediated glucose uptake and aPKC activation [186, 233, 235]. Glucose transport and GLUT4 translocation are rate-limiting steps in insulin-mediated skeletal muscle glucose disposal [318–320]. Consequently, diminished insulin-mediated glycogen synthesis and glucose oxidation have been found in skeletal muscle in insulin resistant states like T2DM [319, 321]. Defects in the components of the glycogenic and glucose oxidative pathways, which are also regulated by insulin [322, 323], have also been found. Subjects with T2DM show reduced skeletal muscle glycogen synthase and pyruvate dehydrogenase activities [321, 324] as well as increased GSK3 protein expression and activity [325]. The effects of GSK3, however, are not limited to the control of glycogen synthesis [268]. GSK3 also downregulates insulin signaling via serine phosphorylation of IRS-1 [227] and accordingly, GSK3 inhibitor administration to obese Zucker rats augments whole body insulin sensitivity and in skeletal muscle, tyrosine phosphorylation of IRS-1 [326].

Insulin resistance is typically associated with lipid accumulation in skeletal muscle [327–330]. In states of energy excess, when FFAs, glucose, and insulin are elevated, intracellular malonyl-CoA increases, which inhibits carnitine palmitoyltransferase-1 (CPT-1), thereby reducing FFA transport into the mitochondria [277, 328, 331]. Hence, there is a shift in the metabolism of FFAs from β oxidation in the mitochondria to esterification in the cytoplasm, where fatty acid metabolites such as long-chain fatty acyl-CoA (LCFA-CoA), diacylglycerol (DAG), and triglycerides build up [277, 331, 332]. Among these metabolites, LCFA-CoAs and DAG especially have a prominent role in inducing insulin resistance in skeletal muscle and the liver because they can activate PKC isoforms, which in turn can blunt insulin signaling, including insulin-stimulated glucose transport in skeletal muscle and suppression of EGP (see Sect. "Modulators of Insulin-Mediated Glucose Metabolism") [277, 333, 334]. In addition to energy excess in both skeletal muscle and liver, mitochondrial dysfunction, specifically reduced β oxidation, has been put forward as a cause of the intracellular lipid accumulation and the ensuing insulin resistance [333]. In insulin resistant subjects, skeletal muscle mitochondrial oxidative phosphorylation is diminished [330, 335]. However, whether this is a cause or effect of insulin resistance is unclear [336]. Moreover, long-chain acyl-CoA dehydrogenase (LCAD) is an enzyme of β oxidation and LCAD KO mice demonstrate hepatic steatosis (hepatic lipid accumulation) and hepatic insulin resistance [337]. Interestingly, LCAD KO mice also show insulin-stimulated increases in hepatic DAG and PKC-ε activity [337]. The debate over whether and how mitochondrial dysfunction causes insulin resistance in skeletal muscle has been intensifying recently [338]. In rodents, skeletal muscle β oxidation has been found to be increased in obesity, while mice that are null for malonyl-CoA decarboxylase (MCD) (an enzyme that decreases malonyl-CoA levels and increases β oxidation) show improved glucose tolerance when fed a high fat diet in the context of augmented LCFA-CoAs in skeletal muscle [339]. The authors suggest that in obesity while β oxidation is impaired in the liver, it is increased in skeletal muscle, where metabolites of elevated mitochondrial β oxidation may, somehow, mediate insulin resistance [339].

Adipose Tissue

Similar to skeletal muscle, insulin induces membrane translocation of GLUT4 in adipocytes, and this process has been found to involve various mediators, including PI3K and aPKCs; Akt is involved in at least some of the steps resulting in insulin-induced GLUT4 localization to the cell membrane [184, 213, 340–343]. Independently of the PI3K pathway, the TC10 pathway has also been found to mediate insulin-induced GLUT4 translocation in adipocytes [342, 344, 345]. The TC10 pathway is associated with lipid raft domains on the cell membrane. A complex of Casitas b-lineage lymphoma proto-oncogene (Cbl) and Cbl-associated protein (CAP) associates with adaptor protein containing PH and SH2 domains (APS), which is an IRS, so that the insulin receptor phosphorylates Cbl [342, 344]. Phosphorylated Cbl then interacts with a complex consisting of CrkII and C3G, which is a guanylnucleotide exchange factor; C3G then activates TC10, a GTPase, but the ensuing steps leading to GLUT4 translocation are unknown [342, 344]. Interestingly, adipose tissue-specific GLUT4 KO mice are characterized not only by diminished adipose tissue insulin-induced glucose uptake, but also by blunted insulin-stimulated glucose uptake in skeletal muscle and insulin-mediated EGP suppression [346]. One interpretation of these results is that although the quantitative contribution of adipose tissue to insulin-stimulated peripheral glucose disposal is minor compared to skeletal muscle, dysregulation of adipose tissue insulin sensitivity can induce insulin resistance in other tissues, potentially via cytokines [346]. Indeed, adipose tissue is not an inert organ; through lipolysis, it contributes to increased plasma FFAs and it is also a source of cytokines that can modulate insulin sensitivity in other tissues (Reviewed in [347] and [348]). Adipose tissue-derived cytokines, such as tumor necrosis factor α (TNF-α) and interleukin 6 (IL-6), are augmented in obesity and correlate positively with insulin resistance [349–351]. Other adipose tissue-derived hormones, such as adiponectin, are decreased and are associated with diminished insulin sensitivity [349, 352, 353]. The effects of certain adipokines on insulin sensitivity, however, may depend on chronicity of exposure, as IL-6 only impairs insulin sensitivity in rodents after prolonged exposure [354]. The mediators of cytokine-induced and fat-induced insulin resistance often overlap and cytokines themselves may mediate fat-induced insulin resistance [355]. The effects of elevated plasma FFAs on insulin sensitivity are addressed in the section below.

Modulators of Insulin-Mediated Glucose Metabolism

Cytokines and fat accumulation are important initiators of insulin resistance, although their relative contribution is complex. One approach used by us and others to study the mechanisms of fat-induced insulin resistance in vivo is i.v. administration of lipid emulsions to elevate plasma FFA concentrations and thereby mimic the increased circulating FFA levels found in obesity [15, 356]. Mediators of fat-induced insulin resistance include PKC, inflammatory kinase IκBα kinase β (IKKβ), JNK, oxidative stress, and p38 MAPK. They induce insulin resistance by downregulating insulin signaling and/or by promoting gluconeogenic enzyme gene expression.

Protein Kinase C

PKC refers to a group of serine/threonine kinases that can be subdivided into classical, novel, and atypical isoforms [357]. Classical PKCs (βII), which are Ca^{2+} and DAG-dependent, and novel PKCs (θ, δ, ε), which are DAG-dependent, translocate from the cytosol to the cell membrane when activated [357–361]. Lipid infusion in rats augments skeletal muscle PKC-θ activation, which is accompanied by decreases in skeletal muscle insulin-mediated glucose disposal, PI3K, and IRS-1 tyrosine phosphorylation [360]. In rodents fed a high fat diet, both skeletal muscle PKC-θ and PKC-ε are activated [357]. Importantly, PKC-θ KO mice do not show impaired skeletal muscle insulin sensitivity when challenged with lipid infusions [356].

The PKC isoforms activated in humans differ from those in rodents: Itani et al. [361] showed that Intralipid infusion causes skeletal muscle PKC-βII and PKC-δ activation. PKCs may impair insulin signaling indirectly, for instance via IKKβ and JNK1 [361–365], or directly: in vitro experiments indicate that PKC isoforms can directly phosphorylate the insulin receptor and IRS-1 on Ser/Thr residues, thereby diminishing the insulin receptor and IRS-1's ability to undergo tyrosine phosphorylation and stimulate PI3K activity [366, 367]. As to hepatic insulin resistance, our group [368] and others [369] showed that lipid infusion causes an increase in the activation of PKC-δ in the liver. A short-term high fat diet in rats leads to hepatic PKC-ε activation that is associated with impaired insulin-mediated suppression of EGP and diminished tyrosine phosphorylation of IRS-1 and IRS-2 [362]. PKC-ε knockdown improves insulin's suppressive effect on EGP and IRS-2 tyrosine phosphorylation [334].

IκBα Kinase β

Insulin resistance is intricately associated with inflammation. IKKβ is a subunit of the IKK complex and it phosphorylates IκBα, thereby targeting it for degradation and freeing nuclear factor κB (NFκB), a transcription factor that increases the expression of various cytokines, including IL-6 and TNF-α [364, 370, 371]. Clinical studies have used a family of non-steroidal anti-inflammatory agents that inhibit IKKβ and NFκB [347, 372–374], namely aspirin, sodium salicylate, and salsalate, to show that they decrease blood glucose and increase insulin sensitivity in T2DM [375, 376]. In a pivotal study, Kim et al. [377] showed that IKKβ plays a causative role in lipid-induced insulin resistance: (1) treatment with salicylate, an IKKβ inhibitor, overcame lipid-induced whole body and skeletal muscle insulin resistance in rats and (2) whole body and skeletal muscle glucose uptake were not affected by lipid infusion in IKKβ KO (heterozygous) mice. We have found that inhibition of the inflammatory kinase IKKβ with sodium salicylate prevents hepatic insulin resistance in vivo as well as hepatic phosphorylation of IRS-1 Ser 307 caused by plasma FFA elevation [15]. However, a daily dose of 4.5 g of sodium salicylate for one week did not prevent fat-induced insulin resistance in humans [378]. Models of obesity are characterized by increases in hepatic IKKβ and NFκB activities [371] and in high fat feeding, liver-specific IKKβ-null mice show improved hepatic insulin sensitivity [379]. IKK adversely affects insulin signaling by phoshorylating serine residues of IRS-1, including Ser 307 [380]. The IKKβ/NFκB pathway also induces SOCS gene expression [371]. In binding to the insulin receptor, SOCS proteins inhibit IRS-1 and -2 tyrosine phosphorylation; SOCS proteins also increase IRS degradation [220, 222, 381]. FFAs can stimulate IKKβ activation through toll-like receptors (TLRs), PKCs, and oxidative stress [364, 382–385].

c-Jun N-Terminal Kinase

FFAs also induce JNK activation [355, 386]. Among the JNK isoforms, JNK1 is more important than JNK2 in the pathogenesis of insulin resistance [387]. Administration of JNK-inhibitory peptide diminished EGP and improved glucose utilization in *db/db* mice [388]. Hepatic downregulation of JNK and JNK1 improved hepatic insulin sensitivity in *db/db* mice [389] and prevented hepatic insulin resistance in mice fed a high fat diet [390]. JNK phosphorylates IRS-1 on Ser 307, which inhibits its tyrosine phosphorylation [217]. Furthermore, JNK may phosphorylate IRS-2 on Thr 348 [386].

Although FFAs can activate JNK via PKC and oxidative stress [365, 382, 385, 391, 392], FFAs can also induce JNK activation via TLRs [384] and endoplasmic reticulum (ER) stress has emerged as a trigger for JNK and IKK activation [393, 394]. ER stress occurs when the ER shows elevated amounts of misfolded or unfolded proteins and recently, obesity has been shown to stimulate ER stress [393]. Oxidative stress has been shown to both cause and result in ER stress [395–397].

Oxidative Stress

Oxidative stress is an imbalance in reactive oxygen species (ROS), such as free radicals or compounds that can generate free radicals, relative to antioxidant capabilities and results in adverse alterations to proteins, lipids, and DNA [370, 385, 398]. FFAs induce ROS production through various pathways, including electron transport chain and PKC-mediated activation of NADPH oxidase, an enzyme that produces superoxide anion from molecular oxygen [385, 392, 398, 399]. ROS induce the activation of stress and inflammatory kinases, such as JNK and IKKβ [364, 365, 385, 391], which phosphorylate serine 307 of IRS-1 [217, 380], and p38 MAPK [385]. Moreover, oxidative stress has been found to decrease insulin-stimulated IRS-1 tyrosine phosphorylation [400, 401].

Oxidative stress diminishes insulin-mediated glucose uptake in adipocytes [401, 402] and muscle cells [403] and antioxidant treatment reverses this impairment [402, 403]. Oxidative stress also promotes FOXO1 nuclear localization via JNK [404] and this process requires JNK-mediated phosphorylation of FOXO [405]. In muscle, oxidative stress augments PGC-1α protein levels and nuclear localization [406, 407] while in hepatocytes, JNK mediates the increase in PGC-1α transcription caused by oxidative stress [391].

p38 Mitogen-Activated Protein Kinase

FFAs activate p38 MAPK, a serine/threonine kinase [408], in hepatocytes [409, 410] as well as other cell types [411–413] and p38 MAPK activation is enhanced in adipocytes [229] and skeletal muscle [414] obtained from T2DM subjects. In primary hepatocytes, increases in GNG caused by 4 h of oleate exposure are mediated by p38 MAPK [409]. In the same study, treatment of primary hepatocytes with FFAs stimulates p38 MAPK-mediated transcription of PEPCK [409] and the underlying mechanism involves p38 MAPK-mediated phosphorylation of the coactivator PGC-1α and the transcription factor CREB [282, 409]. p38 MAPK also increases PGC-1α transcription [409] and can phosphorylate FOXO1 on serine residues [415]. Prolonged (16 h) exposure of primary hepatocytes to oleate results in impairments of insulin-induced Akt activation and insulin-induced suppression of GNG through p38 MAPK [410]. These adverse affects of oleate on insulin action appear to be due to p38 MAPK-mediated increases in protein content of PTEN [410], which dephosphorylates PIP_3 and thereby dampens insulin signal transduction [416]. PTEN protein stabilization via serine/threonine phosphorylation likely underlies its augmented levels in these studies [410], but p38 MAPK also stimulates PTEN transcription in endothelial cells treated with palmitate [412]. Moreover, p38 MAPK has been shown to increase IRS-1 serine phosphorylation [417, 418] and reduce IRS-1 tyrosine phosphorylation [410]. PKC-δ has been shown to be upstream and necessary for p38 MAPK activation resulting from FFA exposure in hepatocytes [409].

Other Modulators of Insulin Sensitivity

Binding of insulin to its receptor promotes not only insulin signaling, but also negative feedback regulation of insulin signaling. For example, insulin activates S6K1, but S6K1 can subsequently phosphorylate IRS-1 on various residues, including Ser 307, which reduces tyrosine phosphorylation of IRS-1 by the insulin receptor and consequently, insulin signaling is dampened [216, 256, 257]. S6K1 null mice show improved insulin sensitivity when challenged with a high fat diet [256]. Moreover, S6K negatively regulates AMPK [419], which itself inhibits S6K via mTORC1. In S6K null skeletal muscle cells, AMPK activity is increased, lipid accumulation is reduced, and β oxidation is increased [419], thereby linking AMPK and S6K to insulin sensitivity via intracellular lipids.

Commonalities Between Insulin Resistance and Cancer

Insulin resistance is a risk factor for cancer [420], although it is unclear whether they share a common mechanism, for example, energy excess, inflammation, and AMPK suppression [421–424], or cancer is promoted by the compensatory hyperinsulinemia of insulin resistance. Cancer is usually characterized by overactivation of PI3K-mTOR and Ras-MAPK pathways [205, 425, 426] This would support a role for hyperinsulinemia in promoting cancer in insulin resistant.

Hyperinsulinemia is an underlying feature of insulin resistance and may result from decreased clearance and /or increased insulin secretion. The liver is the main site of insulin clearance and FFAs have been shown to diminish hepatic insulin clearance, thereby promoting hyperinsulinemia in the periphery [427]. The β cell responds to insulin resistance by increasing insulin secretion and the resulting hyperinsulinemia becomes part of a vicious cycle wherein hyperinsulinemia may exacerbate insulin resistance [428–430]. Insulin resistance is mostly related to blunted signuling through the PI3K pathway [241]. It has been suggested that even if hyperinsulinemia ameliorates insulin signaling through the PI3K pathway, albeit temporarily, this would come at the expense of over-stimulation of the Ras-MAPK pathway [421, 431]. In addition, hyperinsulinemia makes cells more sensitive to growth factors that also stimulate the Ras-MAPK pathway, because insulin activates farnesyltransferase, which results in increased translocation of Ras to the membrane [249, 432, 433]. Hence, hyperinsulinemia has the potential to promote cancer. However, it cannot be excluded that lack of insulin action per se may cause cancer via hyperglycemia and perhaps inflammation, since insulin has potent anti-inflammatory effects [434, 435].

Research in the twenty-first century continues the work initiated in the previous century to unveil the mechanisms of insulin action in healthy and pathophysiological states [271]. Although insulin action has been mostly investigated in the context of obesity and T2DM thus far, more studies are increasingly being done to understand the role of insulin and insulin resistance in other disorders, such as cancer [436].

Acknowledgments A.G. was supported by research grants from the Canadian Diabetes Association (GA-02062131-AG) and the Canadian Institutes of Health Research (CIHR) (MOP-89929) and (MOP-69018).

References

1. Tayek JA (1992) A review of cancer cachexia and abnormal glucose metabolism in humans with cancer. J Am Coll Nutr 11:445–456
2. Cersosimo E, Pisters PW, Pesola G, Rogatko A, Vydelingum NA, Bajorunas D, Brennan MF (1991) The effect of graded doses of insulin on peripheral glucose uptake and lactate release in cancer cachexia. Surgery 109:459–467
3. Kahn CR (2003) Knockout mice challenge our concepts of glucose homeostasis and the pathogenesis of diabetes. Exp Diabesity Res 4:169–182

4. Kasuga M, Karlsson FA, Kahn CR (1982) Insulin stimulates the phosphorylation of the 95,000-dalton subunit of its own receptor. Science 215:185–187
5. Petruzzelli LM, Ganguly S, Smith CJ, Cobb MH, Rubin CS, Rosen OM (1982) Insulin activates a tyrosine-specific protein kinase in extracts of 3T3-L1 adipocytes and human placenta. Proc Natl Acad Sci USA 79:6792–6796
6. Ish-Shalom D, Christoffersen CT, Vorwerk P, Sacerdoti-Sierra N, Shymko RM, Naor D, De MP (1997) Mitogenic properties of insulin and insulin analogues mediated by the insulin receptor. Diabetologia 40(Suppl):S25–31
7. Taniguchi CM, Emanuelli B, Kahn CR (2006) Critical nodes in signalling pathways: insights into insulin action. Nat Rev Mol Cell Biol 7:85–96
8. DeFronzo RA, Tobin JD, Andres R (1979) Glucose clamp technique: a method for quantifying insulin secretion and resistance. Am J Physiol 237:E214–E223
9. "euglycemia" (2007) Concise medical dictionary [article online]. www.oxfordreference.com. Accessed 12 May 2009
10. "clamp" (2009) Oxford English dictionary [article online]. http://dictionary.oed.com. Accessed 12 May 2009
11. "eu" (2007) Concise medical dictionary [article online]. www.oxfordreference.com. Accessed 12 May 2009
12. "iso" (2007) Concise medical dictionary [article online]. www.oxfordreference.com. Accessed 12 May 2009
13. Boden G, Chen X, Iqbal N (1998) Acute lowering of plasma fatty acids lowers basal insulin secretion in diabetic and nondiabetic subjects. Diabetes 47:1609–1612
14. Boden G, Chen X (1995) Effects of fat on glucose uptake and utilization in patients with non-insulin-dependent diabetes. J Clin Investig 96:1261–1268
15. Park E, Wong V, Guan X, Oprescu AI, Giacca A (2007) Salicylate prevents hepatic insulin resistance caused by short-term elevation of free fatty acids in vivo. J Endocrinol 195:323–331
16. Finegood DT, Bergman RN, Vranic M (1987) Estimation of endogenous glucose production during hyperinsulinemic-euglycemic glucose clamps. Comparison of unlabeled and labeled exogenous glucose infusates. Diabetes 36:914–924
17. Banerji MA, Lebovitz HE (1989) Insulin-sensitive and insulin-resistant variants in NIDDM. Diabetes 38:784–792
18. Staehr P, Hother-Nielsen O, Levin K, Holst JJ, Beck-Nielsen H (2001) Assessment of hepatic insulin action in obese type 2 diabetic patients. Diabetes 50:1363–1370
19. Stumvoll M, Chintalapudi U, Perriello G, Welle S, Gutierrez O, Gerich J (1995) Uptake and release of glucose by the human kidney. Postabsorptive rates and responses to epinephrine. J Clin Investig 96:2528–2533
20. Cersosimo E, Garlick P, Ferretti J (2000) Regulation of splanchnic and renal substrate supply by insulin in humans. Metabolism 49:676–683
21. Cersosimo E, Garlick P, Ferretti J (1999) Insulin regulation of renal glucose metabolism in humans. Am J Physiol 276:E78–E84
22. Previs SF, Brunengraber H (1998) Methods for measuring gluconeogenesis in vivo. Curr Opin Clin Nutr Metab Care 1:461–465
23. Devlin TM (2002) Textbook of biochemistry with clinical correlations. Wiley, New York
24. Baron AD, Brechtel G, Wallace P, Edelman SV (1988) Rates and tissue sites of non-insulin- and insulin-mediated glucose uptake in humans. Am J Physiol 255:E769–E774
25. DeFronzo RA, Ferrannini E, Hendler R, Felig P, Wahren J (1983) Regulation of splanchnic and peripheral glucose uptake by insulin and hyperglycemia in man. Diabetes 32:35–45
26. Wolfe RR, Chinkes DL (2005) Isotope tracers in metabolic research: principles and practice of kinetic analysis. Hoboken, New Jersey, Wiley-Liss
27. Steele R (1959) Influences of glucose loading and of injected insulin on hepatic glucose output. Ann NY Acad Sci 82:420–430

28. Saad MF, Anderson RL, Laws A, Watanabe RM, Kades WW, Chen YD, Sands RE, Pei D, Savage PJ, Bergman RN (1994) A comparison between the minimal model and the glucose clamp in the assessment of insulin sensitivity across the spectrum of glucose tolerance. Insulin resistance atherosclerosis study. Diabetes 43:1114–1121
29. Brackenridge A, Pearson ER, Shojaee-Moradie F, Hattersley AT, Russell-Jones D, Umpleby AM (2006) Contrasting insulin sensitivity of endogenous glucose production rate in subjects with hepatocyte nuclear factor-1beta and -1alpha mutations. Diabetes 55:405–411
30. Gastaldelli A, Cusi K, Pettiti M, Hardies J, Miyazaki Y, Berria R, Buzzigoli E, Sironi AM, Cersosimo E, Ferrannini E, DeFronzo RA (2007) Relationship between hepatic/visceral fat and hepatic insulin resistance in nondiabetic and type 2 diabetic subjects. Gastroenterology 133:496–506
31. Tayek JA, Bergner EA, Lee WP (1991) Correction of glucose carbon recycling for the determination of 'true' hepatic glucose production rates by (1-13C1)glucose. Biol Mass Spectrom 20:186–190
32. Lam TK, van de Werve G, Giacca A (2003) Free fatty acids increase basal hepatic glucose production and induce hepatic insulin resistance at different sites. Am J Physiol 284: E281–E290
33. Kolterman OG, Gray RS, Griffin J, Burstein P, Insel J, Scarlett JA, Olefsky JM (1981) Receptor and postreceptor defects contribute to the insulin resistance in noninsulin-dependent diabetes mellitus. J Clin Investig 68:957–969
34. Stumvoll M, Mitrakou A, Pimenta W, Jenssen T, Yki-Jarvinen H, Van HT, Renn W, Gerich J (2000) Use of the oral glucose tolerance test to assess insulin release and insulin sensitivity. Diabetes Care 23:295–301
35. Gastaldelli A, Miyazaki Y, Pettiti M, Buzzigoli E, Mahankali S, Ferrannini E, DeFronzo RA (2004) Separate contribution of diabetes, total fat mass, and fat topography to glucose production, gluconeogenesis, and glycogenolysis. J Clin Endocrinol Metab 89:3914–3921
36. Chevalier S, Burgess SC, Malloy CR, Gougeon R, Marliss EB, Morais JA (2006) The greater contribution of gluconeogenesis to glucose production in obesity is related to increased whole-body protein catabolism. Diabetes 55:675–681
37. Chevalier S, Marliss EB, Morais JA, Lamarche M, Gougeon R (2005) The influence of sex on the protein anabolic response to insulin. Metabolism 54:1529–1535
38. Del PS, Bonadonna RC, Bonora E, Gulli G, Solini A, Shank M, DeFronzo RA (1993) Characterization of cellular defects of insulin action in type 2 (non-insulin-dependent) diabetes mellitus. J Clin Investig 91:484–494
39. Kim JK, Zisman A, Fillmore JJ, Peroni OD, Kotani K, Perret P, Zong H, Dong J, Kahn CR, Kahn BB, Shulman GI (2001) Glucose toxicity and the development of diabetes in mice with muscle-specific inactivation of GLUT4. J Clin Investig 108:153–160
40. Wong V, Stavar L, Szeto L, Uffelman K, Wang CH, Fantus IG, Lewis GF (2006) Atorvastatin induces insulin sensitization in Zucker lean and fatty rats. Atherosclerosis 184:348–355
41. Colwell DR, Higgins JA, Denyer GS (1996) Incorporation of 2-deoxy-D-glucose into glycogen. Implications for measurement of tissue-specific glucose uptake and utilisation. Int J Biochem Cell Biol 28:115–121
42. Youn JH, Kim JK, Buchanan TA (1994) Time courses of changes in hepatic and skeletal muscle insulin action and GLUT4 protein in skeletal muscle after STZ injection. Diabetes 43:564–571
43. Adkins A, Basu R, Persson M, Dicke B, Shah P, Vella A, Schwenk WF, Rizza R (2003) Higher insulin concentrations are required to suppress gluconeogenesis than glycogenolysis in nondiabetic humans. Diabetes 52:2213–2220
44. Rothman DL, Magnusson I, Katz LD, Shulman RG, Shulman GI (1991) Quantitation of hepatic glycogenolysis and gluconeogenesis in fasting humans with 13C NMR. Science 254:573–576
45. Landau BR, Wahren J, Chandramouli V, Schumann WC, Ekberg K, Kalhan SC (1996) Contributions of gluconeogenesis to glucose production in the fasted state. J Clin Investig 98:378–385

46. Hellerstein MK, Neese RA, Linfoot P, Christiansen M, Turner S, Letscher A (1997) Hepatic gluconeogenic fluxes and glycogen turnover during fasting in humans. A stable isotope study. J Clin Investig 100:1305–1319
47. Bock G, Schumann WC, Basu R, Burgess SC, Yan Z, Chandramouli V, Rizza RA, Landau BR (2008) Evidence that processes other than gluconeogenesis may influence the ratio of deuterium on the fifth and third carbons of glucose: implications for the use of $2H_2O$ to measure gluconeogenesis in humans. Diabetes 57:50–55
48. Basu R, Chandramouli V, Dicke B, Landau BR, Rizza RA (2008) Plasma C5 glucose-to-$2H_2O$ ratio does not provide an accurate assessment of gluconeogenesis during hyperinsulinemic-euglycemic clamps in either nondiabetic or diabetic humans. Diabetes 57:1800–1804
49. Ackermans MT, Pereira Arias AM, Bisschop PH, Endert E, Sauerwein HP, Romijn JA (2001) The quantification of gluconeogenesis in healthy men by $(2)H_2O$ and [2-(13)C]glycerol yields different results: rates of gluconeogenesis in healthy men measured with $(2)H_2O$ are higher than those measured with [2-(13)C]glycerol. J Clin Endocrinol Metab 86:2220–2226
50. Landau BR (1999) Quantifying the contribution of gluconeogenesis to glucose production in fasted human subjects using stable isotopes. Proc Nutr Soc 58:963–972
51. Hetenyi G Jr (1982) Correction for the metabolic exchange of 14C for 12C atoms in the pathway of gluconeogenesis in vivo. Fed Proc 41:104–109
52. Hellerstein MK, Neese RA (1992) Mass isotopomer distribution analysis: a technique for measuring biosynthesis and turnover of polymers. Am J Physiol 263:E998–E1001
53. Chinkes DL, Aarsland A, Rosenblatt J, Wolfe RR (1996) Comparison of mass isotopomer dilution methods used to compute VLDL production in vivo. Am J Physiol 271:E373–E383
54. Landau BR, Fernandez CA, Previs SF, Ekberg K, Chandramouli V, Wahren J, Kalhan SC, Brunengraber H (1995) A limitation in the use of mass isotopomer distributions to measure gluconeogenesis in fasting humans. Am J Physiol 269:E18–E26
55. Previs SF, Fernandez CA, Yang D, Soloviev MV, David F, Brunengraber H (1995) Limitations of the mass isotopomer distribution analysis of glucose to study gluconeogenesis. Substrate cycling between glycerol and triose phosphates in liver. J Biol Chem 270:19806–19815
56. Previs SF, Cline GW, Shulman GI (1999) A critical evaluation of mass isotopomer distribution analysis of gluconeogenesis in vivo. Am J Physiol 277:E154–E160
57. Peroni O, Large V, Beylot M (1995) Measuring gluconeogenesis with [2-13C]glycerol and mass isotopomer distribution analysis of glucose. Am J Physiol 269:E516–E523
58. Tayek JA, Katz J (1996) Glucose production, recycling, and gluconeogenesis in normals and diabetics: a mass isotopomer [U-13C]glucose study. Am J Physiol 270:E709–E717
59. Kelleher JK (1999) Estimating gluconeogenesis with [U-13C]glucose: molecular condensation requires a molecular approach. Am J Physiol 277:E395–E400
60. Tayek JA, Katz J (1997) Glucose production, recycling, Cori cycle, and gluconeogenesis in humans: relationship to serum cortisol. Am J Physiol 272:E476–E484
61. Landau BR, Wahren J, Ekberg K, Previs SF, Yang D, Brunengraber H (1998) Limitations in estimating gluconeogenesis and Cori cycling from mass isotopomer distributions using [U-13C6]glucose. Am J Physiol 274:E954–E961
62. Katz J, Tayek JA (1999) Recycling of glucose and determination of the Cori Cycle and gluconeogenesis. Am J Physiol 277:E401–E407
63. Radziuk J, Lee WP (1999) Measurement of gluconeogenesis and mass isotopomer analysis based on [U-(13)C]glucose. Am J Physiol 277:E199–E207
64. Katz J, Tayek JA (1998) Gluconeogenesis and the Cori cycle in 12-, 20-, and 40-h-fasted humans. Am J Physiol 275:E537–E542
65. Mao CS, Bassilian S, Lim SK, Lee WN (2002) Underestimation of gluconeogenesis by the [U-(13)C(6)]glucose method: effect of lack of isotope equilibrium. Am J Physiol Endocrinol Metab 282:E376–E385
66. Haymond MW, Sunehag AL (2000) The reciprocal pool model for the measurement of gluconeogenesis by use of [U-(13)C]glucose. Am J Physiol Endocrinol Metab 278:E140–E145

67. Allick G, van der Crabben SN, Ackermans MT, Endert E, Sauerwein HP (2006) Measurement of gluconeogenesis by deuterated water: the effect of equilibration time and fasting period. Am J Physiol Endocrinol Metab 290:E1212–E1217
68. Jin ES, Jones JG, Merritt M, Burgess SC, Malloy CR, Sherry AD (2004) Glucose production, gluconeogenesis, and hepatic tricarboxylic acid cycle fluxes measured by nuclear magnetic resonance analysis of a single glucose derivative. Anal Biochem 327:149–155
69. Jones JG, Solomon MA, Cole SM, Sherry AD, Malloy CR (2001) An integrated (2)H and (13)C NMR study of gluconeogenesis and TCA cycle flux in humans. Am J Physiol Endocrinol Metab 281:E848–E856
70. Landau BR, Wahren J, Chandramouli V, Schumann WC, Ekberg K, Kalhan SC (1995) Use of $2H_2O$ for estimating rates of gluconeogenesis. Application to the fasted state. J Clin Investig 95:172–178
71. Jones JG, Carvalho RA, Sherry AD, Malloy CR (2000) Quantitation of gluconeogenesis by (2)H nuclear magnetic resonance analysis of plasma glucose following ingestion of (2)H(2)O. Anal Biochem 277:121–126
72. Basu R, Chandramouli V, Schumann W, Basu A, Landau BR, Rizza RA (2009) Additional evidence that transaldolase exchange, isotope discrimination during the triose-isomerase reaction, or both occur in humans: effects of type 2 diabetes. Diabetes 57:1539–1543
73. Giaccari A, Rossetti L (1989) Isocratic high-performance liquid chromatographic determination of the concentration and specific radioactivity of phosphoenolpyruvate and uridine diphosphate glucose in tissue extracts. J Chromatogr B Biomed Appl 497:69–78
74. Rossetti L, Massillon D, Barzilai N, Vuguin P, Chen W, Hawkins M, Wu J, Wang J (1997) Short term effects of leptin on hepatic gluconeogenesis and in vivo insulin action. J Biol Chem 272:27758–27763
75. Rossetti L, Giaccari A, Barzilai N, Howard K, Sebel G, Hu M (1993) Mechanism by which hyperglycemia inhibits hepatic glucose production in conscious rats. Implications for the pathophysiology of fasting hyperglycemia in diabetes. J Clin Investig 92:1126–1134
76. Massillon D, Chen W, Hawkins M, Liu R, Barzilai N, Rossetti L (1995) Quantitation of hepatic glucose fluxes and pathways of hepatic glycogen synthesis in conscious mice. Am J Physiol 269:E1037–E1043
77. Goldstein RE, Rossetti L, Palmer BA, Liu R, Massillon D, Scott M, Neal D, Williams P, Peeler B, Cherrington AD (2002) Effects of fasting and glucocorticoids on hepatic gluconeogenesis assessed using two independent methods in vivo. Am J Physiol Endocrinol Metab 283:E946–E957
78. Goldstein RE, Wasserman DH, McGuinness OP, Lacy DB, Cherrington AD, Abumrad NN (1993) Effects of chronic elevation in plasma cortisol on hepatic carbohydrate metabolism. Am J Physiol 264:E119–E127
79. Muniyappa R, Lee S, Chen H, Quon MJ (2008) Current approaches for assessing insulin sensitivity and resistance in vivo: advantages, limitations, and appropriate usage. Am J Physiol Endocrinol Metab 294:E15–E26
80. Choukem SP, Gautier JF (2008) How to measure hepatic insulin resistance? Diab Metab 34:E664–E673
81. Yokoyama H, Emoto M, Fujiwara S, Motoyama K, Morioka T, Komatsu M, Tahara H, Shoji T, Okuno Y, Nishizawa Y (2003) Quantitative insulin sensitivity check index and the reciprocal index of homeostasis model assessment in normal range weight and moderately obese type 2 diabetic patients. Diabetes Care 26:2426–2432
82. Laakso M (1993) How good a marker is insulin level for insulin resistance? Am J Epidemiol 137:959–965
83. Tran TT, Gupta N, Goh T, Naigamwalla D, Chia MC, Koohestani N, Mehrotra S, Keown-Eyssen G, Giacca A, Bruce WR (2003) Direct measure of insulin sensitivity with the hyperinsulinemic-euglycemic clamp and surrogate measures of insulin sensitivity with the oral glucose tolerance test: correlations with aberrant crypt foci promotion in rats. Cancer Epidemiol Biomark Prev 12:47–56

84. Lee S, Muniyappa R, Yan X, Chen H, Yue LQ, Hong EG, Kim JK, Quon MJ (2008) Comparison between surrogate indexes of insulin sensitivity and resistance and hyperinsulinemic euglycemic clamp estimates in mice. Am J Physiol Endocrinol Metab 294:E261–E270
85. Wallace TM, Levy JC, Matthews DR (2004) Use and abuse of HOMA modeling. Diabetes Care 27:1487–1495
86. Turner RC, Holman RR, Matthews D, Hockaday TD, Peto J (1979) Insulin deficiency and insulin resistance interaction in diabetes: estimation of their relative contribution by feedback analysis from basal plasma insulin and glucose concentrations. Metabolism 28:1086–1096
87. Matthews DR, Hosker JP, Rudenski AS, Naylor BA, Treacher DF, Turner RC (1985) Homeostasis model assessment: insulin resistance and beta-cell function from fasting plasma glucose and insulin concentrations in man. Diabetologia 28:412–419
88. Hosker JP, Matthews DR, Rudenski AS, Burnett MA, Darling P, Bown EG, Turner RC (1985) Continuous infusion of glucose with model assessment: measurement of insulin resistance and beta-cell function in man. Diabetologia 28:401–411
89. Bonora E, Targher G, Alberiche M, Bonadonna RC, Saggiani F, Zenere MB, Monauni T, Muggeo M (2000) Homeostasis model assessment closely mirrors the glucose clamp technique in the assessment of insulin sensitivity: studies in subjects with various degrees of glucose tolerance and insulin sensitivity. Diabetes Care 23:57–63
90. Tripathy D, Almgren P, Tuomi T, Groop L (2004) Contribution of insulin-stimulated glucose uptake and basal hepatic insulin sensitivity to surrogate measures of insulin sensitivity. Diabetes Care 27:2204–2210
91. Matsuda M, DeFronzo RA (1999) Insulin sensitivity indices obtained from oral glucose tolerance testing: comparison with the euglycemic insulin clamp. Diabetes Care 22: 1462–1470
92. Abdul-Ghani MA, Matsuda M, DeFronzo RA (2008) Strong association between insulin resistance in liver and skeletal muscle in non-diabetic subjects. Diabet Med 25:1289–1294
93. Abdul-Ghani MA, Matsuda M, Balas B, DeFronzo RA (2007) Muscle and liver insulin resistance indexes derived from the oral glucose tolerance test. Diabetes Care 30:89–94
94. Katz A, Nambi SS, Mather K, Baron AD, Follmann DA, Sullivan G, Quon MJ (2000) Quantitative insulin sensitivity check index: a simple, accurate method for assessing insulin sensitivity in humans. J Clin Endocrinol Metab 85:2402–2410
95. Rabasa-Lhoret R, Bastard JP, Jan V, Ducluzeau PH, Andreelli F, Guebre F, Bruzeau J, Louche-Pellissier C, Maltrepierre C, Peyrat J, Chagne J, Vidal H, Laville M (2003) Modified quantitative insulin sensitivity check index is better correlated to hyperinsulinemic glucose clamp than other fasting-based index of insulin sensitivity in different insulin-resistant states. J Clin Endocrinol Metab 88:4917–4923
96. Yokoyama H, Emoto M, Fujiwara S, Motoyama K, Morioka T, Komatsu M, Tahara H, Koyama H, Shoji T, Inaba M, Nishizawa Y (2004) Quantitative insulin sensitivity check index and the reciprocal index of homeostasis model assessment are useful indexes of insulin resistance in type 2 diabetic patients with wide range of fasting plasma glucose. J Clin Endocrinol Metab 89:1481–1484
97. Uwaifo GI, Fallon EM, Chin J, Elberg J, Parikh SJ, Yanovski JA (2002) Indices of insulin action, disposal, and secretion derived from fasting samples and clamps in normal glucose-tolerant black and white children. Diabetes Care 25:2081–2087
98. Malita FM, Karelis AD, St-Pierre DH, Garrel D, Bastard JP, Tardif A, Prud'homme D, Rabasa-Lhoret R (2006) Surrogate indexes vs. euglycaemic-hyperinsulinemic clamp as an indicator of insulin resistance and cardiovascular risk factors in overweight and obese postmenopausal women. Diabetes Metab 32:251–255
99. Cacho J, Sevillano J, de Castro J, Herrera E, Ramos MP (2008) Validation of simple indexes to assess insulin sensitivity during pregnancy in Wistar and Sprague-Dawley rats. Am J Physiol Endocrinol Metab 295:E1269–E1276

100. Bonora E, Moghetti P, Zancanaro C, Cigolini M, Querena M, Cacciatori V, Corgnati A, Muggeo M (1989) Estimates of in vivo insulin action in man: comparison of insulin tolerance tests with euglycemic and hyperglycemic glucose clamp studies. J Clin Endocrinol Metab 68:374–378
101. Hirst S, Phillips DI, Vines SK, Clark PM, Hales CN (1993) Reproducibility of the short insulin tolerance test. Diabet Med 10:839–842
102. Chen CC, Wang TY, Hsu SY, Chen RH, Chang CT, Chen SJ (1998) Is the short insulin tolerance test safe and reproducible? Diabet Med 15:924–927
103. Reaven GM (1983) Insulin resistance in noninsulin-dependent diabetes mellitus. Does it exist and can it be measured? Am J Med 74:3–17
104. Gelding SV, Robinson S, Lowe S, Niththyananthan R, Johnston DG (1994) Validation of the low dose short insulin tolerance test for evaluation of insulin sensitivity. Clin Endocrinol 40:611–615
105. Akinmokun A, Selby PL, Ramaiya K, Alberti KG (1992) The short insulin tolerance test for determination of insulin sensitivity: a comparison with the euglycaemic clamp. Diabet Med 9:432–437
106. Young RP, Critchley JA, Anderson PJ, Lau MS, Lee KK, Chan JC (1996) The short insulin tolerance test: feasibility study using venous sampling. Diabet Med 13:429–433
107. Inchiostro S (2005) Measurement of insulin sensitivity in Type 2 diabetes mellitus: comparison between KITT and HOMA-%S indices and evaluation of their relationship with the components of the insulin resistance syndrome. Diabet Med 22:39–44
108. Phillips DI, Clark PM, Hales CN, Osmond C (1994) Understanding oral glucose tolerance: comparison of glucose or insulin measurements during the oral glucose tolerance test with specific measurements of insulin resistance and insulin secretion. Diabet Med 11:286–292
109. Xu E, Dubois MJ, Leung N, Charbonneau A, Turbide C, Avramoglu RK, DeMarte L, Elchebly M, Streichert T, Levy E, Beauchemin N, Marette A (2009) Targeted disruption of carcinoembryonic antigen-related cell adhesion molecule 1 promotes diet-induced hepatic steatosis and insulin resistance. Endocrinology 150:3503–3512
110. Minami A, Iseki M, Kishi K, Wang M, Ogura M, Furukawa N, Hayashi S, Yamada M, Obata T, Takeshita Y, Nakaya Y, Bando Y, Izumi K, Moodie SA, Kajiura F, Matsumoto M, Takatsu K, Takaki S, Ebina Y (2003) Increased insulin sensitivity and hypoinsulinemia in APS knockout mice. Diabetes 52:2657–2665
111. Cariou B, van Harmelen K, Duran-Sandoval D, van Dijk TH, Grefhorst A, Abdelkarim M, Caron S, Torpier G, Fruchart JC, Gonzalez FJ, Kuipers F, Staels B (2006) The farnesoid X receptor modulates adiposity and peripheral insulin sensitivity in mice. J Biol Chem 281:11039–11049
112. Carvalho E, Kotani K, Peroni OD, Kahn BB (2005) Adipose-specific overexpression of GLUT4 reverses insulin resistance and diabetes in mice lacking GLUT4 selectively in muscle. Am J Physiol Endocrinol Metab 289:E551–E561
113. Araujo EP, De Souza CT, Ueno M, Cintra DE, Bertolo MB, Carvalheira JB, Saad MJ, Velloso LA (2007) Infliximab restores glucose homeostasis in an animal model of diet-induced obesity and diabetes. Endocrinology 148:5991–5997
114. Mulder H, Sorhede-Winzell M, Contreras JA, Fex M, Strom K, Ploug T, Galbo H, Arner P, Lundberg C, Sundler F, Ahren B, Holm C (2003) Hormone-sensitive lipase null mice exhibit signs of impaired insulin sensitivity whereas insulin secretion is intact. J Biol Chem 278: 36380–36388
115. Ahren B, Pacini G (2006) A novel approach to assess insulin sensitivity reveals no increased insulin sensitivity in mice with a dominant-negative mutant hepatocyte nuclear factor-1alpha. Am J Physiol Regul Integr Comp Physiol 291:R131–R137
116. Kahn SE (2003) The relative contributions of insulin resistance and beta-cell dysfunction to the pathophysiology of Type 2 diabetes. Diabetologia 46:3–19
117. American Diabetes Association (2009) Executive summary: standards of medical care in diabetes – 2009. Diabetes Care 32(Suppl 1):S6–S12
118. Canadian Diabetes Association Clinical Practice Guidelines Expert Committee (2008) Canadian Diabetes Association 2008 clinical practice guidelines for the prevention and management of diabetes in Canada. Can J Diabetes 32:S1–S201

119. Soonthornpun S, Setasuban W, Thamprasit A, Chayanunnukul W, Rattarasarn C, Geater A (2003) Novel insulin sensitivity index derived from oral glucose tolerance test. J Clin Endocrinol Metab 88:1019–1023
120. Kazama Y, Takamura T, Sakurai M, Shindo H, Ohkubo E, Aida K, Harii N, Taki K, Kaneshige M, Tanaka S, Shimura H, Endo T, Kobayashi T (2008) New insulin sensitivity index from the oral glucose tolerance test. Diab Res Clin Pract 79:24–30
121. Avignon A, Boegner C, Mariano-Goulart D, Colette C, Monnier L (1999) Assessment of insulin sensitivity from plasma insulin and glucose in the fasting or post oral glucose-load state. Int J Obes Relat Metab Disord 23:512–517
122. Tao R, Ye F, He Y, Tian J, Liu G, Ji T, Su Y (2009) Improvement of high-fat-diet-induced metabolic syndrome by a compound from Balanophora polyandra Griff in mice. Eur J Pharmacol 616:328–333
123. Nakaya Y, Minami A, Harada N, Sakamoto S, Niwa Y, Ohnaka M (2000) Taurine improves insulin sensitivity in the Otsuka Long-Evans Tokushima Fatty rat, a model of spontaneous type 2 diabetes. Am J Clin Nutr 71:54–58
124. Yao XH, Gregoire Nyomba BL (2007) Abnormal glucose homeostasis in adult female rat offspring after intrauterine ethanol exposure. Am J Physiol Regul Integr Comp Physiol 292:R1926–R1933
125. Parlevliet ET, Heijboer AC, Schroder-van der Elst JP, Havekes LM, Romijn JA, Pijl H, Corssmit EP (2008) Oxyntomodulin ameliorates glucose intolerance in mice fed a high-fat diet. Am J Physiol Endocrinol Metab 294:E142–E147
126. Pacini G, Bergman RN (1986) MINMOD: a computer program to calculate insulin sensitivity and pancreatic responsivity from the frequently sampled intravenous glucose tolerance test. Comput Meth Programs Biomed 23:113–122
127. Pacini G, Tonolo G, Sambataro M, Maioli M, Ciccarese M, Brocco E, Avogaro A, Nosadini R (1998) Insulin sensitivity and glucose effectiveness: minimal model analysis of regular and insulin-modified FSIGT. Am J Physiol 274:E592–E599
128. Mehring GH, Coates PA, Brunel PC, Luzio SD, Owens DR (2002) Insulin sensitivity in type 2 diabetes: univariate and multivariate techniques to derive estimates of insulin sensitivity from the insulin modified intravenous glucose tolerance test (FSIGT). Comput Meth Programs Biomed 68:161–176
129. Bergman RN, Ider YZ, Bowden CR, Cobelli C (1979) Quantitative estimation of insulin sensitivity. Am J Physiol 236:E667–E677
130. Bergman RN, Phillips LS, Cobelli C (1981) Physiologic evaluation of factors controlling glucose tolerance in man: measurement of insulin sensitivity and beta-cell glucose sensitivity from the response to intravenous glucose. J Clin Investig 68:1456–1467
131. Yang YJ, Youn JH, Bergman RN (1987) Modified protocols improve insulin sensitivity estimation using the minimal model. Am J Physiol 253:E595–E602
132. Coates PA, Luzio SD, Brunel P, Owens DR (1995) Comparison of estimates of insulin sensitivity from minimal model analysis of the insulin-modified frequently sampled intravenous glucose tolerance test and the isoglycemic hyperinsulinemic clamp in subjects with NIDDM. Diabetes 44:631–635
133. Brehm A, Thomaseth K, Bernroider E, Nowotny P, Waldhausl W, Pacini G, Roden M (2006) The role of endocrine counterregulation for estimating insulin sensitivity from intravenous glucose tolerance tests. J Clin Endocrinol Metab 91:2272–2278
134. Saad MF, Steil GM, Kades WW, Ayad MF, Elsewafy WA, Boyadjian R, Jinagouda SD, Bergman RN (1997) Differences between the tolbutamide-boosted and the insulin-modified minimal model protocols. Diabetes 46:1167–1171
135. Sumner AE, Luercio MF, Frempong BA, Ricks M, Sen S, Kushner H, Tulloch-Reid MK (2009) Validity of the reduced-sample insulin modified frequently-sampled intravenous glucose tolerance test using the nonlinear regression approach. Metabolism 58:220–225
136. Caumo A, Vicini P, Zachwieja JJ, Avogaro A, Yarasheski K, Bier DM, Cobelli C (1999) Undermodeling affects minimal model indexes: insights from a two-compartment model. Am J Physiol 276:E1171–E1193

137. Hoffman RP, Vicini P, Cobelli C (2002) Comparison of insulin sensitivity and glucose effectiveness determined by the one- and two-compartment-labeled minimal model in late prepubertal children and early adolescents. Metabolism 51:1582–1586
138. Krudys KM, Dodds MG, Nissen SM, Vicini P (2005) Integrated model of hepatic and peripheral glucose regulation for estimation of endogenous glucose production during the hot IVGTT. Am J Physiol Endocrinol Metab 288:E1038–E1046
139. Tokuyama K, Suzuki M (1998) Intravenous glucose tolerance test-derived glucose effectiveness in endurance-trained rats. Metabolism 47:190–194
140. Pawlak DB, Bryson JM, Denyer GS, Brand-Miller JC (2001) High glycemic index starch promotes hypersecretion of insulin and higher body fat in rats without affecting insulin sensitivity. J Nutr 131:99–104
141. O'Rourke CM, Davis JA, Saltiel AR, Cornicelli JA (1997) Metabolic effects of troglitazone in the Goto-Kakizaki rat, a non-obese and normolipidemic rodent model of non-insulin-dependent diabetes mellitus. Metabolism 46:192–198
142. Pacini G, Thomaseth K, Ahren B (2001) Contribution to glucose tolerance of insulin-independent vs. insulin-dependent mechanisms in mice. Am J Physiol Endocrinol Metab 281:E693–E703
143. Pacini G, Ahren M, Ahren B (2009) Reappraisal of the intravenous glucose tolerance index for a simple assessment of insulin sensitivity in mice. Am J Physiol Regul Integr Comp Physiol 296:R1316–R1324
144. Pei D, Jones CN, Bhargava R, Chen YD, Reaven GM (1994) Evaluation of octreotide to assess insulin-mediated glucose disposal by the insulin suppression test. Diabetologia 37:843–845
145. Kim SH, Reaven GM (2008) Isolated impaired fasting glucose and peripheral insulin sensitivity: not a simple relationship. Diabetes Care 31:347–352
146. Shen SW, Reaven GM, Farquhar JW (1970) Comparison of impedance to insulin-mediated glucose uptake in normal subjects and in subjects with latent diabetes. J Clin Investig 49:2151–2160
147. Hwu CM, Kwok CF, Chiang SC, Wang PY, Hsiao LC, Lee SH, Lin SH, Ho LT (2001) A comparison of insulin suppression tests performed with somatostatin and octreotide with particular reference to tolerability. Diab Res Clin Pract 51:187–193
148. Ikebuchi M, Suzuki M, Kageyama A, Hirose J, Yokota C, Ikeda K, Shinozaki K, Todo R, Harano Y (1996) Modified method using a somatostatin analogue, octreotide acetate (Sandostatin) to assess in vivo insulin sensitivity. Endocr J 43:125–130
149. Weir GC, Bonner-Weir S (1990) Islets of Langerhans: the puzzle of intraislet interactions and their relevance to diabetes. J Clin Investig 85:983–987
150. Maheux P, Azhar S, Kern PA, Chen YD, Reuven GM (1997) Relationship between insulin-mediated glucose disposal and regulation of plasma and adipose tissue lipoprotein lipase. Diabetologia 40:850–858
151. Facchini F, Humphreys MH, Jeppesen J, Reaven GM (1999) Measurements of insulin-mediated glucose disposal are stable over time. J Clin Endocrinol Metab 84:1567–1569
152. Greenfield MS, Doberne L, Kraemer F, Tobey T, Reaven G (1981) Assessment of insulin resistance with the insulin suppression test and the euglycemic clamp. Diabetes 30:387–392
153. Rodnick KJ, Mondon CE, Haskell WL, Azhar S, Reaven GM (1990) Differences in insulin-induced glucose uptake and enzyme activity in running rats. J Appl Physiol 68:513–519
154. Maegawa H, Kobayashi M, Ishibashi O, Takata Y, Shigeta Y (1986) Effect of diet change on insulin action: difference between muscles and adipocytes. Am J Physiol 251:E616–E623
155. Maegawa H, Hasegawa M, Sugai S, Obata T, Ugi S, Morino K, Egawa K, Fujita T, Sakamoto T, Nishio Y, Kojima H, Haneda M, Yasuda H, Kikkawa R, Kashiwagi A (1999) Expression of a dominant negative SHP-2 in transgenic mice induces insulin resistance. J Biol Chem 274:30236–30243
156. Uwaifo GI, Parikh SJ, Keil M, Elberg J, Chin J, Yanovski JA (2002) Comparison of insulin sensitivity, clearance, and secretion estimates using euglycemic and hyperglycemic clamps in children. J Clin Endocrinol Metab 87:2899–2905

157. Carpentier A, Zinman B, Leung N, Giacca A, Hanley AJ, Harris SB, Hegele RA, Lewis GF (2003) Free fatty acid-mediated impairment of glucose-stimulated insulin secretion in non-diabetic Oji-Cree individuals from the Sandy Lake community of Ontario, Canada: a population at very high risk for developing type 2 diabetes. Diabetes 52:1485–1495
158. Mari A, Ahren B, Pacini G (2005) Assessment of insulin secretion in relation to insulin resistance. Curr Opin Clin Nutr Metab Care 8:529–533
159. Goh TT, Mason TM, Gupta N, So A, Lam TK, Lam L, Lewis GF, Mari A, Giacca A (2007) Lipid-induced beta-cell dysfunction in vivo in models of progressive beta-cell failure. Am J Physiol Endocrinol Metab 292:E549–E560
160. Mitrakou A, Vuorinen-Markkola H, Raptis G, Toft I, Mokan M, Strumph P, Pimenta W, Veneman T, Jenssen T, Bolli G (1992) Simultaneous assessment of insulin secretion and insulin sensitivity using a hyperglycemia clamp. J Clin Endocrinol Metab 75:379–382
161. Elahi D, Meneilly GS, Minaker KL, Andersen DK, Rowe JW (1989) Escape of hepatic glucose production during hyperglycemic clamp. Am J Physiol 257:E704–E711
162. Ayala JE, Bracy DP, McGuinness OP, Wasserman DH (2006) Considerations in the design of hyperinsulinemic-euglycemic clamps in the conscious mouse. Diabetes 55:390–397
163. Xu B, Bird VG, Miller WT (1995) Substrate specificities of the insulin and insulin-like growth factor 1 receptor tyrosine kinase catalytic domains. J Biol Chem 270: 29825–29830
164. Araki E, Lipes MA, Patti ME, Bruning JC, Haag B III, Johnson RS, Kahn CR (1994) Alternative pathway of insulin signalling in mice with targeted disruption of the IRS-1 gene. Nature 372:186–190
165. Withers DJ, Gutierrez JS, Towery H, Burks DJ, Ren JM, Previs S, Zhang Y, Bernal D, Pons S, Shulman GI, Bonner-Weir S, White MF (1998) Disruption of IRS-2 causes type 2 diabetes in mice. Nature 391:900–904
166. Liu SC, Wang Q, Lienhard GE, Keller SR (1999) Insulin receptor substrate 3 is not essential for growth or glucose homeostasis. J Biol Chem 274:18093–18099
167. Fantin VR, Wang Q, Lienhard GE, Keller SR (2000) Mice lacking insulin receptor substrate 4 exhibit mild defects in growth, reproduction, and glucose homeostasis. Am J Physiol Endocrinol Metab 278:E127–E133
168. Cai D, Dhe-Paganon S, Melendez PA, Lee J, Shoelson SE (2003) Two new substrates in insulin signaling, IRS5/DOK4 and IRS6/DOK5. J Biol Chem 278:25323–25330
169. Sciacchitano S, Taylor SI (1997) Cloning, tissue expression, and chromosomal localization of the mouse IRS-3 gene. Endocrinology 138:4931–4940
170. Fantin VR, Lavan BE, Wang Q, Jenkins NA, Gilbert DJ, Copeland NG, Keller SR, Lienhard GE (1999) Cloning, tissue expression, and chromosomal location of the mouse insulin receptor substrate 4 gene. Endocrinology 140:1329–1337
171. Laustsen PG, Michael MD, Crute BE, Cohen SE, Ueki K, Kulkarni RN, Keller SR, Lienhard GE, Kahn CR (2002) Lipoatrophic diabetes in Irs1(-/-)/Irs3(-/-) double knockout mice. Genes Dev 16:3213–3222
172. Goren HJ, Kulkarni RN, Kahn CR (2004) Glucose homeostasis and tissue transcript content of insulin signaling intermediates in four inbred strains of mice: C57BL/6, C57BLKS/6, DBA/2, and 129X1. Endocrinology 145:3307–3323
173. Thirone AC, Huang C, Klip A (2006) Tissue-specific roles of IRS proteins in insulin signaling and glucose transport. Trends Endocrinol Metab 17:72–78
174. Yamauchi T, Tobe K, Tamemoto H, Ueki K, Kaburagi Y, Yamamoto-Honda R, Takahashi Y, Yoshizawa F, Aizawa S, Akanuma Y, Sonenberg N, Yazaki Y, Kadowaki T (1996) Insulin signalling and insulin actions in the muscles and livers of insulin-resistant, insulin receptor substrate 1-deficient mice. Mol Cell Biol 16:3074–3084
175. Kubota N, Tobe K, Terauchi Y, Eto K, Yamauchi T, Suzuki R, Tsubamoto Y, Komeda K, Nakano R, Miki H, Satoh S, Sekihara H, Sciacchitano S, Lesniak M, Aizawa S, Nagai R, Kimura S, Akanuma Y, Taylor SI, Kadowaki T (2000) Disruption of insulin receptor substrate 2 causes type 2 diabetes because of liver insulin resistance and lack of compensatory beta-cell hyperplasia. Diabetes 49:1880–1889

176. Kido Y, Burks DJ, Withers D, Bruning JC, Kahn CR, White MF, Accili D (2000) Tissue-specific insulin resistance in mice with mutations in the insulin receptor, IRS-1, and IRS-2. J Clin Investig 105:199–205
177. Taniguchi CM, Ueki K, Kahn R (2005) Complementary roles of IRS-1 and IRS-2 in the hepatic regulation of metabolism. J Clin Invest 115:718–727
178. Simmgen M, Knauf C, Lopez M, Choudhury AI, Charalambous M, Cantley J, Bedford DC, Claret M, Iglesias MA, Heffron H, Cani PD, Vidal-Puig A, Burcelin R, Withers DJ (2006) Liver-specific deletion of insulin receptor substrate 2 does not impair hepatic glucose and lipid metabolism in mice. Diabetologia 49:552–561
179. Dong X, Park S, Lin X, Copps K, Yi X, White MF (2006) Irs1 and Irs2 signaling is essential for hepatic glucose homeostasis and systemic growth. J Clin Investig 116:101–114
180. Razzini G, Ingrosso A, Brancaccio A, Sciacchitano S, Esposito DL, Falasca M (2000) Different subcellular localization and phosphoinositides binding of insulin receptor substrate protein pleckstrin homology domains. Mol Endocrinol 14:823–836
181. Sawka-Verhelle D, Tartare-Deckert S, White MF, Van OE (1996) Insulin receptor substrate-2 binds to the insulin receptor through its phosphotyrosine-binding domain and through a newly identified domain comprising amino acids 591-786. J Biol Chem 271:5980–5983
182. He W, Craparo A, Zhu Y, O'Neill TJ, Wang LM, Pierce JH, Gustafson TA (1996) Interaction of insulin receptor substrate-2 (IRS-2) with the insulin and insulin-like growth factor I receptors. Evidence for two distinct phosphotyrosine-dependent interaction domains within IRS-2. J Biol Chem 271:11641–11645
183. Wolf G, Trub T, Ottinger E, Groninga L, Lynch A, White MF, Miyazaki M, Lee J, Shoelson SE (1995) PTB domains of IRS-1 and Shc have distinct but overlapping binding specificities. J Biol Chem 270:27407–27410
184. Cheatham B, Vlahos CJ, Cheatham L, Wang L, Blenis J, Kahn CR (1994) Phosphatidylinositol 3-kinase activation is required for insulin stimulation of pp 70 S6 kinase, DNA synthesis, and glucose transporter translocation. Mol Cell Biol 14:4902–4911
185. Taniguchi CM, Kondo T, Sajan M, Luo J, Bronson R, Asano T, Farese R, Cantley LC, Kahn CR (2006) Divergent regulation of hepatic glucose and lipid metabolism by phosphoinositide 3-kinase via Akt and PKClambda/zeta. Cell Metab 3:343–353
186. Bandyopadhyay GK, Yu JG, Ofrecio J, Olefsky JM (2005) Increased p85/55/50 expression and decreased phosphotidylinositol 3-kinase activity in insulin-resistant human skeletal muscle. Diabetes 54:2351–2359
187. Myers MG Jr, Backer JM, Sun XJ, Shoelson S, Hu P, Schlessinger J, Yoakim M, Schaffhausen B, White MF (1992) IRS-1 activates phosphatidylinositol 3'-kinase by associating with src homology 2 domains of p85. Proc Natl Acad Sci USA 89:10350–10354
188. Geering B, Cutillas PR, Nock G, Gharbi SI, Vanhaesebroeck B (2007) Class IA phosphoinositide 3-kinases are obligate p85-p110 heterodimers. Proc Natl Acad Sci USA 104:7809–7814
189. Vanhaesebroeck B, Leevers SJ, Panayotou G, Waterfield MD (1997) Phosphoinositide 3-kinases: a conserved family of signal transducers. Trends Biochem Sci 22:267–272
190. Shepherd PR, Withers DJ, Siddle K (1998) Phosphoinositide 3-kinase: the key switch mechanism in insulin signalling. Biochem J 333:471–490
191. Terauchi Y, Tsuji Y, Satoh S, Minoura H, Murakami K, Okuno A, Inukai K, Asano T, Kaburagi Y, Ueki K, Nakajima H, Hanafusa T, Matsuzawa Y, Sekihara H, Yin Y, Barrett JC, Oda H, Ishikawa T, Akanuma Y, Komuro I, Suzuki M, Yamamura K, Kodama T, Suzuki H, Yamamura K, Kodama T, Suzuki H, Koyasu S, Aizawa S, Tobe K, Fukui Y, Yazaki Y, Kadowaki T (1999) Increased insulin sensitivity and hypoglycaemia in mice lacking the p85 alpha subunit of phosphoinositide 3-kinase. Nat Genet 21:230–235
192. Chen D, Mauvais-Jarvis F, Bluher M, Fisher SJ, Jozsi A, Goodyear LJ, Ueki K, Kahn CR (2004) p50alpha/p55alpha phosphoinositide 3-kinase knockout mice exhibit enhanced insulin sensitivity. Mol Cell Biol 24:320–329
193. Ueki K, Yballe CM, Brachmann SM, Vicent D, Watt JM, Kahn CR, Cantley LC (2002) Increased insulin sensitivity in mice lacking p85beta subunit of phosphoinositide 3-kinase. Proc Natl Acad Sci USA 99:419–424

194. Aoki K, Matsui J, Kubota N, Nakajima H, Iwamoto K, Takamoto I, Tsuji Y, Ohno A, Mori S, Tokuyama K, Murakami K, Asano T, Aizawa S, Tobe K, Kadowaki T, Terauchi Y (2009) Role of the liver in glucose homeostasis in PI 3-kinase p85alpha-deficient mice. Am J Physiol 296:E842–E853
195. Brachmann SM, Ueki K, Engelman JA, Kahn RC, Cantley LC (2005) Phosphoinositide 3-kinase catalytic subunit deletion and regulatory subunit deletion have opposite effects on insulin sensitivity in mice. Mol Cell Biol 25:1596–1607
196. Taniguchi CM, Tran TT, Kondo T, Luo J, Ueki K, Cantley LC, Kahn CR (2006) Phosphoinositide 3-kinase regulatory subunit p85alpha suppresses insulin action via positive regulation of PTEN. Proc Natl Acad Sci USA 103:12093–12097
197. Taniguchi CM, Aleman JO, Ueki K, Luo J, Asano T, Kaneto H, Stephanopoulos G, Cantley LC, Kahn CR (2007) The p85alpha regulatory subunit of phosphoinositide 3-kinase potentiates c-Jun N-terminal kinase-mediated insulin resistance. Mol Cell Biol 27:2830–2840
198. Logie L, Ruiz-Alcaraz AJ, Keane M, Woods YL, Bain J, Marquez R, Alessi DR, Sutherland C (2007) Characterization of a protein kinase B inhibitor in vitro and in insulin-treated liver cells. Diabetes 56:2218–2227
199. Tanti JF, Grillo S, Gremeaux T, Coffer PJ, Van OE, Le Marchand-Brustel Y (1997) Potential role of protein kinase B in glucose transporter 4 translocation in adipocytes. Endocrinology 138:2005–2010
200. Wang Q, Somwar R, Bilan PJ, Liu Z, Jin J, Woodgett JR, Klip A (1999) Protein kinase B/Akt participates in GLUT4 translocation by insulin in L6 myoblasts. Mol Cell Biol 19: 4008–4018
201. Scheid MP, Marignani PA, Woodgett JR (2002) Multiple phosphoinositide 3-kinase-dependent steps in activation of protein kinase B. Mol Cell Biol 22:6247–6260
202. Stokoe D, Stephens LR, Copeland T, Gaffney PR, Reese CB, Painter GF, Holmes AB, McCormick F, Hawkins PT (1997) Dual role of phosphatidylinositol-3,4,5-trisphosphate in the activation of protein kinase B. Science 277:567–570
203. Sarbassov DD, Guertin DA, Ali SM, Sabatini DM (2005) Phosphorylation and regulation of Akt/PKB by the rictor-mTOR complex. Science 307:1098–1101
204. Jacinto E, Facchinetti V, Liu D, Soto N, Wei S, Jung SY, Huang Q, Qin J, Su B (2006) SIN1/MIP1 maintains rictor-mTOR complex integrity and regulates Akt phosphorylation and substrate specificity. Cell 127:125–137
205. Liu P, Heng H, Roberts TM, Hao JJ (2009) Targeting the phosphoinositide 3-kinase pathway in cancer. Nat Rev Drug Discov 8:627–644
206. Bae SS, Cho H, Mu J, Birnbaum MJ (2003) Isoform-specific regulation of insulin-dependent glucose uptake by Akt/protein kinase B. J Biol Chem 278:49530–49536
207. Cho H, Mu J, Kim JK, Thorvaldsen JL, Chu Q, Crenshaw EB III, Kaestner KH, Bartolomei MS, Shulman GI, Birnbaum MJ (2001) Insulin resistance and a diabetes mellitus-like syndrome in mice lacking the protein kinase Akt2 (PKB beta). Science 292:1728–1731
208. Garofalo RS, Orena SJ, Rafidi K, Torchia AJ, Stock JL, Hildebrandt AL, Coskran T, Black SC, Brees DJ, Wicks JR, McNeish JD, Coleman KG (2003) Severe diabetes, age-dependent loss of adipose tissue, and mild growth deficiency in mice lacking Akt2/PKB beta. J Clin Investig 112:197–208
209. Tschopp O, Yang ZZ, Brodbeck D, Dummler BA, Hemmings-Mieszczak M, Watanabe T, Michaelis T, Frahm J, Hemmings BA (2005) Essential role of protein kinase B gamma (PKB gamma/Akt3) in postnatal brain development but not in glucose homeostasis. Development 132:2943–2954
210. Cho H, Thorvaldsen JL, Chu Q, Feng F, Birnbaum MJ (2001) Akt1/PKBalpha is required for normal growth but dispensable for maintenance of glucose homeostasis in mice. J Biol Chem 276:38349–38352
211. Dummler B, Tschopp O, Hynx D, Yang ZZ, Dirnhofer S, Hemmings BA (2006) Life with a single isoform of Akt: mice lacking Akt2 and Akt3 are viable but display impaired glucose homeostasis and growth deficiencies. Mol Cell Biol 26:8042–8051

212. Brozinick JT Jr, Roberts BR, Dohm GL (2003) Defective signaling through Akt-2 and -3 but not Akt-1 in insulin-resistant human skeletal muscle: potential role in insulin resistance. Diabetes 52:935–941
213. Kim YB, Peroni OD, Franke TF, Kahn BB (2000) Divergent regulation of Akt1 and Akt2 isoforms in insulin target tissues of obese Zucker rats. Diabetes 49:847–856
214. Kahn CR (1978) Insulin resistance, insulin insensitivity, and insulin unresponsiveness: a necessary distinction. Metabolism 27(12 Suppl 2):1893–1902
215. Ozes ON, Akca H, Mayo LD, Gustin JA, Maehama T, Dixon JE, Donner DB (2001) A phosphatidylinositol 3-kinase/Akt/mTOR pathway mediates and PTEN antagonizes tumor necrosis factor inhibition of insulin signaling through insulin receptor substrate-1. Proc Natl Acad Sci USA 98:4640–4645
216. Paz K, Hemi R, LeRoith D, Karasik A, Elhanany E, Kanety H, Zick Y (1997) A molecular basis for insulin resistance. Elevated serine/threonine phosphorylation of IRS-1 and IRS-2 inhibits their binding to the juxtamembrane region of the insulin receptor and impairs their ability to undergo insulin-induced tyrosine phosphorylation. J Biol Chem 272: 29911–29918
217. Aguirre V, Uchida T, Yenush L, Davis R, White MF (2000) The c-Jun NH(2)-terminal kinase promotes insulin resistance during association with insulin receptor substrate-1 and phosphorylation of Ser(307). J Biol Chem 275:9047–9054
218. Greene MW, Sakaue H, Wang L, Alessi DR, Roth RA (2003) Modulation of insulin-stimulated degradation of human insulin receptor substrate-1 by Serine 312 phosphorylation. J Biol Chem 278:8199–8211
219. Zhang J, Gao Z, Yin J, Quon MJ, Ye J (2008) S6K directly phosphorylates IRS-1 on Ser-270 to promote insulin resistance in response to TNF-(alpha) signaling through IKK2. J Biol Chem 283:35375–35382
220. Emanuelli B, Peraldi P, Filloux C, Chavey C, Freidinger K, Hilton DJ, Hotamisligil GS, Van OE (2001) SOCS-3 inhibits insulin signaling and is up-regulated in response to tumor necrosis factor-alpha in the adipose tissue of obese mice. J Biol Chem 276:47944–47949
221. Ueki K, Kondo T, Kahn CR (2004) Suppressor of cytokine signaling 1 (SOCS-1) and SOCS-3 cause insulin resistance through inhibition of tyrosine phosphorylation of insulin receptor substrate proteins by discrete mechanisms. Mol Cell Biol 24:5434–5446
222. Rui L, Yuan M, Frantz D, Shoelson S, White MF (2002) SOCS-1 and SOCS-3 block insulin signaling by ubiquitin-mediated degradation of IRS1 and IRS2. J Biol Chem 277: 42394–42398
223. Kerouz NJ, Horsch D, Pons S, Kahn CR (1997) Differential regulation of insulin receptor substrates-1 and -2 (IRS-1 and IRS-2) and phosphatidylinositol 3-kinase isoforms in liver and muscle of the obese diabetic (ob/ob) mouse. J Clin Investig 100:3164–3172
224. Gum RJ, Gaede LL, Koterski SL, Heindel M, Clampit JE, Zinker BA, Trevillyan JM, Ulrich RG, Jirousek MR, Rondinone CM (2003) Reduction of protein tyrosine phosphatase 1B increases insulin-dependent signaling in ob/ob mice. Diabetes 52:21–28
225. Yaspelkis BB III, Kvasha IA, Figueroa TY (2009) High-fat feeding increases insulin receptor and IRS-1 coimmunoprecipitation with SOCS-3, IKKalpha/beta phosphorylation and decreases PI-3 kinase activity in muscle. Am J Physiol Regul Integr Comp Physiol 296:R1709–R1715
226. Liberman Z, Plotkin B, Tennenbaum T, Eldar-Finkelman H (2008) Coordinated phosphorylation of insulin receptor substrate-1 by glycogen synthase kinase-3 and protein kinase C betaII in the diabetic fat tissue. Am J Physiol Endocrinol Metab 294:E1169–E1177
227. Liberman Z, Eldar-Finkelman H (2005) Serine 332 phosphorylation of insulin receptor substrate-1 by glycogen synthase kinase-3 attenuates insulin signaling. J Biol Chem 280: 4422–4428
228. Kovacs P, Hanson RL, Lee YH, Yang X, Kobes S, Permana PA, Bogardus C, Baier LJ (2003) The role of insulin receptor substrate-1 gene (IRS1) in type 2 diabetes in Pima Indians. Diabetes 52:3005–3009

229. Carlson CJ, Koterski S, Sciotti RJ, Poccard GB, Rondinone CM (2003) Enhanced basal activation of mitogen-activated protein kinases in adipocytes from type 2 diabetes: potential role of p38 in the downregulation of GLUT4 expression. Diabetes 52:634–641
230. Danielsson A, Ost A, Lystedt E, Kjolhede P, Gustavsson J, Nystrom FH, Stralfors P (2005) Insulin resistance in human adipocytes occurs downstream of IRS1 after surgical cell isolation but at the level of phosphorylation of IRS1 in type 2 diabetes. FEBS J 272:141–151
231. Goodyear LJ, Giorgino F, Sherman LA, Carey J, Smith RJ, Dohm GL (1995) Insulin receptor phosphorylation, insulin receptor substrate-1 phosphorylation, and phosphatidylinositol 3-kinase activity are decreased in intact skeletal muscle strips from obese subjects. J Clin Investig 95:2195–2204
232. Bjornholm M, Kawano Y, Lehtihet M, Zierath JR (1997) Insulin receptor substrate-1 phosphorylation and phosphatidylinositol 3-kinase activity in skeletal muscle from NIDDM subjects after in vivo insulin stimulation. Diabetes 46:524–527
233. Krook A, Bjornholm M, Galuska D, Jiang XJ, Fahlman R, Myers MG Jr, Wallberg-Henriksson H, Zierath JR (2000) Characterization of signal transduction and glucose transport in skeletal muscle from type 2 diabetic patients. Diabetes 49:284–292
234. Beeson M, Sajan MP, Dizon M, Grebenev D, Gomez-Daspet J, Miura A, Kanoh Y, Powe J, Bandyopadhyay G, Standaert ML, Farese RV (2003) Activation of protein kinase C-zeta by insulin and phosphatidylinositol-3,4,5-(PO4)3 is defective in muscle in type 2 diabetes and impaired glucose tolerance: amelioration by rosiglitazone and exercise. Diabetes 52:1926–1934
235. Casaubon L, Sajan MP, Rivas J, Powe JL, Standaert ML, Farese RV (2006) Contrasting insulin dose-dependent defects in activation of atypical protein kinase C and protein kinase B/Akt in muscles of obese diabetic humans. Diabetologia 49:3000–3008
236. Rondinone CM, Carvalho E, Wesslau C, Smith UP (1999) Impaired glucose transport and protein kinase B activation by insulin, but not okadaic acid, in adipocytes from subjects with Type II diabetes mellitus. Diabetologia 42:819–825
237. Rondinone CM, Wang LM, Lonnroth P, Wesslau C, Pierce JH, Smith U (1997) Insulin receptor substrate (IRS) 1 is reduced and IRS-2 is the main docking protein for phosphatidylinositol 3-kinase in adipocytes from subjects with non-insulin-dependent diabetes mellitus. Proc Natl Acad Sci USA 94:4171–4175
238. Rieusset J, Bouzakri K, Chevillotte E, Ricard N, Jacquet D, Bastard JP, Laville M, Vidal H (2004) Suppressor of cytokine signaling 3 expression and insulin resistance in skeletal muscle of obese and type 2 diabetic patients. Diabetes 53:2232–2241
239. Smith U (2002) Impaired ('diabetic') insulin signaling and action occur in fat cells long before glucose intolerance – is insulin resistance initiated in the adipose tissue? Int J Obes Relat Metab Disord 26:897–904
240. Kim YB, Nikoulina SE, Ciaraldi TP, Henry RR, Kahn BB (1999) Normal insulin-dependent activation of Akt/protein kinase B, with diminished activation of phosphoinositide 3-kinase, in muscle in type 2 diabetes. J Clin Investig 104:733–741
241. Avruch J (1998) Insulin signal transduction through protein kinase cascades. Mol Cell Biochem 182:31–48
242. Matozaki T, Murata Y, Saito Y, Okazawa H, Ohnishi H (2009) Protein tyrosine phosphatase SHP-2: a proto-oncogene product that promotes Ras activation. Cancer Sci 100(10):1786–1793
243. Li N, Batzer A, Daly R, Yajnik V, Skolnik E, Chardin P, Bar-Sagi D, Margolis B, Schlessinger J (1993) Guanine-nucleotide-releasing factor hSos1 binds to Grb2 and links receptor tyrosine kinases to Ras signalling. Nature 363:85–88
244. Ravichandran KS, Lorenz U, Shoelson SE, Burakoff SJ (1995) Interaction of Shc with Grb2 regulates association of Grb2 with mSOS. Mol Cell Biol 15:593–600
245. Holgado-Madruga M, Emlet DR, Moscatello DK, Godwin AK, Wong AJ (1996) A Grb2-associated docking protein in EGF- and insulin-receptor signalling. Nature 379:560–564
246. Baltensperger K, Kozma LM, Cherniack AD, Klarlund JK, Chawla A, Banerjee U, Czech MP (1993) Binding of the Ras activator son of sevenless to insulin receptor substrate-1 signaling complexes. Science 260:1950–1952

247. Bonni A, Brunet A, West AE, Datta SR, Takasu MA, Greenberg ME (1999) Cell survival promoted by the Ras-MAPK signaling pathway by transcription-dependent and -independent mechanisms. Science 286:1358–1362
248. Dunn KL, Espino PS, Drobic B, He S, Davie JR (2005) The Ras-MAPK signal transduction pathway, cancer and chromatin remodeling. Biochem Cell Biol 83:1–14
249. Roberts PJ, Der CJ (2007) Targeting the Raf-MEK-ERK mitogen-activated protein kinase cascade for the treatment of cancer. Oncogene 26:3291–3310
250. Ma XM, Blenis J (2009) Molecular mechanisms of mTOR-mediated translational control. Nat Rev Mol Cell Biol 10:307–318
251. Hay N, Sonenberg N (2004) Upstream and downstream of mTOR. Genes Dev 18: 1926–1945
252. Avruch J, Long X, Ortiz-Vega S, Rapley J, Papageorgiou A, Dai N (2009) Amino acid regulation of TOR complex 1. Am J Physiol Endocrinol Metab 296:E592–E602
253. Anjum R, Blenis J (2008) The RSK family of kinases: emerging roles in cellular signalling. Nat Rev Mol Cell Biol 9:747–758
254. Memmott RM, Dennis PA (2009) Akt-dependent and -independent mechanisms of mTOR regulation in cancer. Cell Signal 21:656–664
255. Bouzakri K, Roques M, Gual P, Espinosa S, Guebre-Egziabher F, Riou JP, Laville M, Le Marchand-Brustel Y, Tanti JF, Vidal H (2003) Reduced activation of phosphatidylinositol-3 kinase and increased serine 636 phosphorylation of insulin receptor substrate-1 in primary culture of skeletal muscle cells from patients with type 2 diabetes. Diabetes 52:1319–1325
256. Um SH, Frigerio F, Watanabe M, Picard F, Joaquin M, Sticker M, Fumagalli S, Allegrini PR, Kozma SC, Auwerx J, Thomas G (2004) Absence of S6K1 protects against age- and diet-induced obesity while enhancing insulin sensitivity. Nature 431:200–205
257. Tremblay F, Gagnon A, Veilleux A, Sorisky A, Marette A (2005) Activation of the mammalian target of rapamycin pathway acutely inhibits insulin signaling to Akt and glucose transport in 3T3-L1 and human adipocytes. Endocrinology 146:1328–1337
258. Katz H, Butler P, Homan M, Zerman A, Caumo A, Cobelli C, Rizza R (1993) Hepatic and extrahepatic insulin action in humans: measurement in the absence of non-steady-state error. Am J Physiol 264:E561–E566
259. Olson AL, Pessin JE (1996) Structure, function, and regulation of the mammalian facilitative glucose transporter gene family. Annu Rev Nutr 16:235–256
260. Dentin R, Pegorier JP, Benhamed F, Foufelle F, Ferre P, Fauveau V, Magnuson MA, Girard J, Postic C (2004) Hepatic glucokinase is required for the synergistic action of ChREBP and SREBP-1c on glycolytic and lipogenic gene expression. J Biol Chem 279:20314–20326
261. Sibrowski W, Seitz HJ (1984) Rapid action of insulin and cyclic AMP in the regulation of functional messenger RNA coding for glucokinase in rat liver. J Biol Chem 259:343–346
262. Kim SY, Kim HI, Kim TH, Im SS, Park SK, Lee IK, Kim KS, Ahn YH (2004) SREBP-1c mediates the insulin-dependent hepatic glucokinase expression. J Biol Chem 279: 30823–30829
263. Postic C, Shiota M, Niswender KD, Jetton TL, Chen Y, Moates JM, Shelton KD, Lindner J, Cherrington AD, Magnuson MA (1999) Dual roles for glucokinase in glucose homeostasis as determined by liver and pancreatic beta cell-specific gene knock-outs using Cre recombinase. J Biol Chem 274:305–315
264. Frame S, Cohen P (2001) GSK3 takes centre stage more than 20 years after its discovery. Biochem J 359:1–16
265. Imazu M, Strickland WG, Chrisman TD, Exton JH (1984) Phosphorylation and inactivation of liver glycogen synthase by liver protein kinases. J Biol Chem 259:1813–1821
266. Sharfi H, Eldar-Finkelman H (2008) Sequential phosphorylation of insulin receptor substrate-2 by glycogen synthase kinase-3 and c-Jun NH_2-terminal kinase plays a role in hepatic insulin signaling. Am J Physiol Endocrinol Metab 294:E307–E315
267. MacAulay K, Doble BW, Patel S, Hansotia T, Sinclair EM, Drucker DJ, Nagy A, Woodgett JR (2007) Glycogen synthase kinase 3alpha-specific regulation of murine hepatic glycogen metabolism. Cell Metab 6:329–337

268. Patel S, Doble BW, MacAulay K, Sinclair EM, Drucker DJ, Woodgett JR (2008) Tissue-specific role of glycogen synthase kinase 3beta in glucose homeostasis and insulin action. Mol Cell Biol 28:6314–6328
269. Aiston S, Coghlan MP, Agius L (2003) Inactivation of phosphorylase is a major component of the mechanism by which insulin stimulates hepatic glycogen synthesis. Eur J Biochem 270:2773–2781
270. Aiston S, Hampson LJ, Arden C, Iynedjian PB, Agius L (2006) The role of protein kinase B/Akt in insulin-induced inactivation of phosphorylase in rat hepatocytes. Diabetologia 49:174–182
271. Cohen P (2006) The twentieth century struggle to decipher insulin signalling. Nat Rev Mol Cell Biol 7:867–873
272. Munro S, Ceulemans H, Bollen M, Diplexcito J, Cohen PT (2005) A novel glycogen-targeting subunit of protein phosphatase 1 that is regulated by insulin and shows differential tissue distribution in humans and rodents. FEBS J 272:1478–1489
273. Alemany S, Cohen P (1986) Phosphorylase a is an allosteric inhibitor of the glycogen and microsomal forms of rat hepatic protein phosphatase-1. FEBS Lett 198:194–202
274. Moorhead G, MacKintosh C, Morrice N, Cohen P (1995) Purification of the hepatic glycogen-associated form of protein phosphatase-1 by microcystin-Sepharose affinity chromatography. FEBS Lett 362:101–105
275. Bollen M, Keppens S, Stalmans W (1998) Specific features of glycogen metabolism in the liver. Biochem J 336:19–31
276. Doherty MJ, Cadefau J, Stalmans W, Bollen M, Cohen PT (1998) Loss of the hepatic glycogen-binding subunit (GL) of protein phosphatase 1 underlies deficient glycogen synthesis in insulin-dependent diabetic rats and in adrenalectomized starved rats. Biochem J 333: 253–257
277. Lam TK, Carpentier A, Lewis GF, van de Werve G, Fantus IG, Giacca A (2003) Mechanisms of the free fatty acid-induced increase in hepatic glucose production. Am J Physiol Endocrinol Metab 284:E863–E873
278. O'Brien RM, Granner DK (1996) Regulation of gene expression by insulin. Physiol Rev 76:1109–1161
279. Schmoll D, Walker KS, Alessi DR, Grempler R, Burchell A, Guo S, Walther R, Unterman TG (2000) Regulation of glucose-6-phosphatase gene expression by protein kinase Balpha and the forkhead transcription factor FKHR. Evidence for insulin response unit-dependent and -independent effects of insulin on promoter activity. J Biol Chem 275:36324–36333
280. Gabbay RA, Sutherland C, Gnudi L, Kahn BB, O'Brien RM, Granner DK, Flier JS (1996) Insulin regulation of phosphoenolpyruvate carboxykinase gene expression does not require activation of the Ras/mitogen-activated protein kinase signaling pathway. J Biol Chem 271:1890–1897
281. Accili D (2004) Lilly lecture 2003: the struggle for mastery in insulin action: from triumvirate to republic. Diabetes 53:1633–1642
282. Puigserver P, Spiegelman BM (2003) Peroxisome proliferator-activated receptor-gamma coactivator 1 alpha (PGC-1 alpha): transcriptional coactivator and metabolic regulator. Endocr Rev 24:78–90
283. Puigserver P, Rhee J, Donovan J, Walkey CJ, Yoon JC, Oriente F, Kitamura Y, Altomonte J, Dong H, Accili D, Spiegelman BM (2003) Insulin-regulated hepatic gluconeogenesis through FOXO1-PGC-1alpha interaction. Nature 423:550–555
284. Zhang W, Patil S, Chauhan B, Guo S, Powell DR, Le J, Klotsas A, Matika R, Xiao X, Franks R, Heidenreich KA, Sajan MP, Farese RV, Stolz DB, Tso P, Koo SH, Montminy M, Unterman TG (2006) FoxO1 regulates multiple metabolic pathways in the liver: effects on gluconeogenic, glycolytic, and lipogenic gene expression. J Biol Chem 281:10105–10117
285. Rena G, Guo S, Cichy SC, Unterman TG, Cohen P (1999) Phosphorylation of the transcription factor forkhead family member FKHR by protein kinase B. J Biol Chem 274:17179–17183
286. Guo S, Rena G, Cichy S, He X, Cohen P, Unterman T (1999) Phosphorylation of serine 256 by protein kinase B disrupts transactivation by FKHR and mediates effects of insulin on

insulin-like growth factor-binding protein-1 promoter activity through a conserved insulin response sequence. J Biol Chem 274:17184–17192
287. Zhang X, Gan L, Pan H, Guo S, He X, Olson ST, Mesecar A, Adam S, Unterman TG (2002) Phosphorylation of serine 256 suppresses transactivation by FKHR (FOXO1) by multiple mechanisms. Direct and indirect effects on nuclear/cytoplasmic shuttling and DNA binding. J Biol Chem 277:45276–45284
288. Li X, Monks B, Ge Q, Birnbaum MJ (2007) Akt/PKB regulates hepatic metabolism by directly inhibiting PGC-1alpha transcription coactivator. Nature 447:1012–1016
289. Greer EL, Brunet A (2005) FOXO transcription factors at the interface between longevity and tumor suppression. Oncogene 24:7410–7425
290. Zhao X, Gan L, Pan H, Kan D, Majeski M, Adam SA, Unterman TG (2004) Multiple elements regulate nuclear/cytoplasmic shuttling of FOXO1: characterization of phosphorylation- and 14-3-3-dependent and -independent mechanisms. Biochem J 378:3–49
291. Matsuzaki H, Daitoku H, Hatta M, Tanaka K, Fukamizu A (2003) Insulin-induced phosphorylation of FKHR (Foxo1) targets to proteasomal degradation. Proc Natl Acad Sci USA 100:11285–11290
292. Yoon JC, Puigserver P, Chen G, Donovan J, Wu Z, Rhee J, Adelmant G, Stafford J, Kahn CR, Granner DK, Newgard CB, Spiegelman BM (2001) Control of hepatic gluconeogenesis through the transcriptional coactivator PGC-1. Nature 413:131–138
293. Daitoku H, Yamagata K, Matsuzaki H, Hatta M, Fukamizu A (2003) Regulation of PGC-1 promoter activity by protein kinase B and the forkhead transcription factor FKHR. Diabetes 52:642–649
294. Hirota K, Sakamaki J, Ishida J, Shimamoto Y, Nishihara S, Kodama N, Ohta K, Yamamoto M, Tanimoto K, Fukamizu A (2008) A combination of HNF-4 and Foxo1 is required for reciprocal transcriptional regulation of glucokinase and glucose-6-phosphatase genes in response to fasting and feeding. J Biol Chem 283:32432–32441
295. Dentin R, Liu Y, Koo SH, Hedrick S, Vargas T, Heredia J, Yates J III, Montminy M (2007) Insulin modulates gluconeogenesis by inhibition of the coactivator TORC2. Nature 449:366–369
296. Koo SH, Flechner L, Qi L, Zhang X, Screaton RA, Jeffries S, Hedrick S, Xu W, Boussouar F, Brindle P, Takemori H, Montminy M (2005) The CREB coactivator TORC2 is a key regulator of fasting glucose metabolism. Nature 437:1109–1111
297. Lewis GF, Zinman B, Groenewoud Y, Vranic M, Giacca A (1996) Hepatic glucose production is regulated both by direct hepatic and extrahepatic effects of insulin in humans. Diabetes 45:454–462
298. Lewis GF, Vranic M, Harley P, Giacca A (1997) Fatty acids mediate the acute extrahepatic effects of insulin on hepatic glucose production in humans. Diabetes 46:1111–1119
299. Lewis GF, Vranic M, Giacca A (1997) Glucagon enhances the direct suppressive effect of insulin on hepatic glucose production in humans. Am J Physiol 272:E371–E378
300. Lewis GF, Vranic M, Giacca A (1998) Role of free fatty acids and glucagon in the peripheral effect of insulin on glucose production in humans. Am J Physiol 275:E177–E186
301. McCall RH, Wiesenthal SR, Shi ZQ, Polonsky K, Giacca A (1998) Insulin acutely suppresses glucose production by both peripheral and hepatic effects in normal dogs. Am J Physiol 274:E346–E356
302. Edgerton DS, Lautz M, Scott M, Everett CA, Stettler KM, Neal DW, Chu CA, Cherrington AD (2006) Insulin's direct effects on the liver dominate the control of hepatic glucose production. J Clin Investig 116:521–527
303. Gupta N, Sandhu H, Goh T, Shah K, Wiesenthal SR, Yoshii H, Chong V, Lam TK, Haber CA, Williams W, Tchipashvili V, Giacca A (2002) Insulin inhibits glucose production by a direct effect in diabetic depancreatized dogs during euglycemia. Am J Physiol Endocrinol Metab 283:E1002–E1007
304. Lewis GF, Carpentier A, Vranic M, Giacca A (1999) Resistance to insulin's acute direct hepatic effect in suppressing steady-state glucose production in individuals with type 2 diabetes. Diabetes 48:570–576

305. Pocai A, Lam TK, Gutierrez-Juarez R, Obici S, Schwartz GJ, Bryan J, Guilar-Bryan L, Rossetti L (2005) Hypothalamic K(ATP) channels control hepatic glucose production. Nature 434:1026–1031
306. Obici S, Zhang BB, Karkanias G, Rossetti L (2002) Hypothalamic insulin signaling is required for inhibition of glucose production. Nat Med 8:1376–1382
307. Spanswick D, Smith MA, Mirshamsi S, Routh VH, Ashford ML (2000) Insulin activates ATP-sensitive K+ channels in hypothalamic neurons of lean, but not obese rats. Nat Neurosci 3:757–758
308. Obici S, Feng Z, Karkanias G, Baskin DG, Rossetti L (2002) Decreasing hypothalamic insulin receptors causes hyperphagia and insulin resistance in rats. Nat Neurosci 5:566–572
309. Buettner C, Camacho RC (2008) Hypothalamic control of hepatic glucose production and its potential role in insulin resistance. Endocrinol Metab Clin North Am 37:825–840
310. Inoue H, Ogawa W, Asakawa A, Okamoto Y, Nishizawa A, Matsumoto M, Teshigawara K, Matsuki Y, Watanabe E, Hiramatsu R, Notohara K, Katayose K, Okamura H, Kahn CR, Noda T, Takeda K, Akira S, Inui A, Kasuga M (2006) Role of hepatic STAT3 in brain-insulin action on hepatic glucose production. Cell Metab 3:267–275
311. Inoue H, Ogawa W, Ozaki M, Haga S, Matsumoto M, Furukawa K, Hashimoto N, Kido Y, Mori T, Sakaue H, Teshigawara K, Jin S, Iguchi H, Hiramatsu R, LeRoith D, Takeda K, Akira S, Kasuga M (2004) Role of STAT-3 in regulation of hepatic gluconeogenic genes and carbohydrate metabolism in vivo. Nat Med 10:168–174
312. Sakamoto K, Holman GD (2008) Emerging role for AS160/TBC1D4 and TBC1D1 in the regulation of GLUT4 traffic. Am J Physiol Endocrinol Metab 295:E29–E37
313. Isakoff SJ, Taha C, Rose E, Marcusohn J, Klip A, Skolnik EY (1995) The inability of phosphatidylinositol 3-kinase activation to stimulate GLUT4 translocation indicates additional signaling pathways are required for insulin-stimulated glucose uptake. Proc Natl Acad Sci USA 92:10247–10251
314. Sano H, Kane S, Sano E, Miinea CP, Asara JM, Lane WS, Garner CW, Lienhard GE (2003) Insulin-stimulated phosphorylation of a Rab GTPase-activating protein regulates GLUT4 translocation. J Biol Chem 278:14599–14602
315. Randhawa VK, Ishikura S, Talior-Volodarsky I, Cheng AW, Patel N, Hartwig JH, Klip A (2008) GLUT4 vesicle recruitment and fusion are differentially regulated by Rac, AS160, and Rab8A in muscle cells. J Biol Chem 283:27208–27219
316. Bandyopadhyay G, Standaert ML, Sajan MP, Karnitz LM, Cong L, Quon MJ, Farese RV (1999) Dependence of insulin-stimulated glucose transporter 4 translocation on 3-phosphoinositide-dependent protein kinase-1 and its target threonine-410 in the activation loop of protein kinase C-zeta. Mol Endocrinol 13:1766–1772
317. Bandyopadhyay G, Kanoh Y, Sajan MP, Standaert ML, Farese RV (2000) Effects of adenoviral gene transfer of wild-type, constitutively active, and kinase-defective protein kinase C-lambda on insulin-stimulated glucose transport in L6 myotubes. Endocrinology 141:4120–4127
318. Garvey WT, Maianu L, Zhu JH, Brechtel-Hook G, Wallace P, Baron AD (1998) Evidence for defects in the trafficking and translocation of GLUT4 glucose transporters in skeletal muscle as a cause of human insulin resistance. J Clin Investig 101:2377–2386
319. Cline GW, Petersen KF, Krssak M, Shen J, Hundal RS, Trajanoski Z, Inzucchi S, Dresner A, Rothman DL, Shulman GI (1999) Impaired glucose transport as a cause of decreased insulin-stimulated muscle glycogen synthesis in type 2 diabetes. N Engl J Med 341:240–246
320. Ren JM, Marshall BA, Mueckler MM, McCaleb M, Amatruda JM, Shulman GI (1995) Overexpression of Glut4 protein in muscle increases basal and insulin-stimulated whole body glucose disposal in conscious mice. J Clin Investig 95:429–432
321. Kelley DE, Mokan M, Mandarino LJ (1992) Intracellular defects in glucose metabolism in obese patients with NIDDM. Diabetes 41:698–706
322. Kim YI, Lee FN, Choi WS, Lee S, Youn JH (2006) Insulin regulation of skeletal muscle PDK4 mRNA expression is impaired in acute insulin-resistant states. Diabetes 55: 2311–2317

323. Bouskila M, Hirshman MF, Jensen J, Goodyear LJ, Sakamoto K (2008) Insulin promotes glycogen synthesis in the absence of GSK3 phosphorylation in skeletal muscle. Am J Physiol Endocrinol Metab 294:E28–E35
324. Vaag A, Alford F, Henriksen FL, Christopher M, Beck-Nielsen H (1995) Multiple defects of both hepatic and peripheral intracellular glucose processing contribute to the hyperglycaemia of NIDDM. Diabetologia 38:326–336
325. Nikoulina SE, Ciaraldi TP, Mudaliar S, Mohideen P, Carter L, Henry RR (2000) Potential role of glycogen synthase kinase-3 in skeletal muscle insulin resistance of type 2 diabetes. Diabetes 49:263–271
326. Dokken BB, Henriksen EJ (2006) Chronic selective glycogen synthase kinase-3 inhibition enhances glucose disposal and muscle insulin action in prediabetic obese Zucker rats. Am J Physiol Endocrinol Metab 291:E207–E213
327. Krssak M, Falk PK, Dresner A, DiPietro L, Vogel SM, Rothman DL, Roden M, Shulman GI (1999) Intramyocellular lipid concentrations are correlated with insulin sensitivity in humans: a 1H NMR spectroscopy study. Diabetologia 42:113–116
328. Dobbins RL, Szczepaniak LS, Bentley B, Esser V, Myhill J, McGarry JD (2001) Prolonged inhibition of muscle carnitine palmitoyltransferase-1 promotes intramyocellular lipid accumulation and insulin resistance in rats. Diabetes 50:123–130
329. Petersen KF, Befroy D, Dufour S, Dziura J, Ariyan C, Rothman DL, DiPietro L, Cline GW, Shulman GI (2003) Mitochondrial dysfunction in the elderly: possible role in insulin resistance. Science 300:1140–1142
330. Petersen KF, Dufour S, Befroy D, Garcia R, Shulman GI (2004) Impaired mitochondrial activity in the insulin-resistant offspring of patients with type 2 diabetes. N Engl J Med 350:664–671
331. Rasmussen BB, Holmback UC, Volpi E, Morio-Liondore B, Paddon-Jones D, Wolfe RR (2002) Malonyl coenzyme A and the regulation of functional carnitine palmitoyltransferase-1 activity and fat oxidation in human skeletal muscle. J Clin Investig 110:1687–1693
332. Gaster M, Beck-Nielsen H (2006) Triacylglycerol accumulation is not primarily affected in myotubes established from type 2 diabetic subjects. Biochim Biophys Acta 1761:100–110
333. Morino K, Petersen KF, Shulman GI (2006) Molecular mechanisms of insulin resistance in humans and their potential links with mitochondrial dysfunction. Diabetes 55(Suppl 2): S9–S15
334. Samuel VT, Liu ZX, Wang A, Beddow SA, Geisler JG, Kahn M, Zhang XM, Monia BP, Bhanot S, Shulman GI (2007) Inhibition of protein kinase Cepsilon prevents hepatic insulin resistance in nonalcoholic fatty liver disease. J Clin Investig 117:739–745
335. Befroy DE, Petersen KF, Dufour S, Mason GF, de Graaf RA, Rothman DL, Shulman GI (2007) Impaired mitochondrial substrate oxidation in muscle of insulin-resistant offspring of type 2 diabetic patients. Diabetes 56:1376–1381
336. Turner N, Heilbronn LK (2008) Is mitochondrial dysfunction a cause of insulin resistance? Trends Endocrinol Metab 19:324–330
337. Zhang D, Liu ZX, Choi CS, Tian L, Kibbey R, Dong J, Cline GW, Wood PA, Shulman GI (2007) Mitochondrial dysfunction due to long-chain Acyl-CoA dehydrogenase deficiency causes hepatic steatosis and hepatic insulin resistance. Proc Natl Acad Sci USA 104:17075–17080
338. Galgani JE, Moro C, Ravussin E (2008) Metabolic flexibility and insulin resistance. Am J Physiol Endocrinol Metab 295:E1009–E1017
339. Koves TR, Ussher JR, Noland RC, Slentz D, Mosedale M, Ilkayeva O, Bain J, Stevens R, Dyck JR, Newgard CB, Lopaschuk GD, Muoio DM (2008) Mitochondrial overload and incomplete fatty acid oxidation contribute to skeletal muscle insulin resistance. Cell Metab 7:45–56
340. Bandyopadhyay G, Standaert ML, Kikkawa U, Ono Y, Moscat J, Farese RV (1999) Effects of transiently expressed atypical (zeta, lambda), conventional (alpha, beta) and novel (delta, epsilon) protein kinase C isoforms on insulin-stimulated translocation of epitope-tagged GLUT4 glucose transporters in rat adipocytes: specific interchangeable effects of protein kinases C-zeta and C-lambda. Biochem J 337:461–470

341. Ducluzeau PH, Fletcher LM, Vidal H, Laville M, Tavare JM (2002) Molecular mechanisms of insulin-stimulated glucose uptake in adipocytes. Diab Metab 28:85–92
342. Watson RT, Kanzaki M, Pessin JE (2004) Regulated membrane trafficking of the insulin-responsive glucose transporter 4 in adipocytes. Endocr Rev 25:177–204
343. Gonzalez E, McGraw TE (2006) Insulin signaling diverges into Akt-dependent and -independent signals to regulate the recruitment/docking and the fusion of GLUT4 vesicles to the plasma membrane. Mol Biol Cell 17:4484–4493
344. Chiang SH, Baumann CA, Kanzaki M, Thurmond DC, Watson RT, Neudauer CL, Macara IG, Pessin JE, Saltiel AR (2001) Insulin-stimulated GLUT4 translocation requires the CAP-dependent activation of TC10. Nature 410:944–948
345. Liu J, DeYoung SM, Hwang JB, O'Leary EE, Saltiel AR (2003) The roles of Cbl-b and c-Cbl in insulin-stimulated glucose transport. J Biol Chem 278:36754–36762
346. Abel ED, Peroni O, Kim JK, Kim YB, Boss O, Hadro E, Minnemann T, Shulman GI, Kahn BB (2001) Adipose-selective targeting of the GLUT4 gene impairs insulin action in muscle and liver. Nature 409:729–733
347. Shoelson SE, Lee J, Goldfine AB (2006) Inflammation and insulin resistance. J Clin Investig 116:1793–1801
348. Lewis GF, Carpentier A, Adeli K, Giacca A (2002) Disordered fat storage and mobilization in the pathogenesis of insulin resistance and type 2 diabetes. Endocr Rev 23:201–229
349. Kershaw EE, Flier JS (2004) Adipose tissue as an endocrine organ. J Clin Endocrinol Metab 89:2548–2556
350. Kern PA, Ranganathan S, Li C, Wood L, Ranganathan G (2001) Adipose tissue tumor necrosis factor and interleukin-6 expression in human obesity and insulin resistance. Am J Physiol Endocrinol Metab 280:E745–E751
351. Hotamisligil GS, Arner P, Caro JF, Atkinson RL, Spiegelman BM (1995) Increased adipose tissue expression of tumor necrosis factor-alpha in human obesity and insulin resistance. J Clin Investig 95:2409–2415
352. Weyer C, Funahashi T, Tanaka S, Hotta K, Matsuzawa Y, Pratley RE, Tataranni PA (2001) Hypoadiponectinemia in obesity and type 2 diabetes: close association with insulin resistance and hyperinsulinemia. J Clin Endocrinol Metab 86:1930–1935
353. Arita Y, Kihara S, Ouchi N, Takahashi M, Maeda K, Miyagawa J, Hotta K, Shimomura I, Nakamura T, Miyaoka K, Kuriyama H, Nishida M, Yamashita S, Okubo K, Matsubara K, Muraguchi M, Ohmoto Y, Funahashi T, Matsuzawa Y (1999) Paradoxical decrease of an adipose-specific protein, adiponectin, in obesity. Biochem Biophys Res Commun 257:79–83
354. Nieto-Vazquez I, Fernandez-Veledo S, de Alvero C, Lorenzo M (2008) Dual role of interleukin-6 in regulating insulin sensitivity in murine skeletal muscle. Diabetes 57:3211–3221
355. Nguyen MT, Satoh H, Favelyukis S, Babendure JL, Imamura T, Sbodio JI, Zalevsky J, Dahiyat BI, Chi NW, Olefsky JM (2005) JNK and tumor necrosis factor-alpha mediate free fatty acid-induced insulin resistance in 3T3-L1 adipocytes. J Biol Chem 280:35361–35371
356. Kim JK, Fillmore JJ, Sunshine MJ, Albrecht B, Higashimori T, Kim DW, Liu ZX, Soos TJ, Cline GW, O'Brien WR, Littman DR, Shulman GI (2004) PKC-theta knockout mice are protected from fat-induced insulin resistance. J Clin Investig 114:823–827
357. Schmitz-Peiffer C, Browne CL, Oakes ND, Watkinson A, Chisholm DJ, Kraegen EW, Biden TJ (1997) Alterations in the expression and cellular localization of protein kinase C isozymes epsilon and theta are associated with insulin resistance in skeletal muscle of the high-fat-fed rat. Diabetes 46:169–178
358. Perseghin G, Petersen K, Shulman GI (2003) Cellular mechanism of insulin resistance: potential links with inflammation. Int J Obes Relat Metab Disord 27(Suppl 3):S6–S11
359. Yu C, Chen Y, Cline GW, Zhang D, Zong H, Wang Y, Bergeron R, Kim JK, Cushman SW, Cooney GJ, Atcheson B, White MF, Kraegen EW, Shulman GI (2002) Mechanism by which fatty acids inhibit insulin activation of insulin receptor substrate-1 (IRS-1)-associated phosphatidylinositol 3-kinase activity in muscle. J Biol Chem 277:50230–50236
360. Griffin ME, Marcucci MJ, Cline GW, Bell K, Barucci N, Lee D, Goodyear LJ, Kraegen EW, White MF, Shulman GI (1999) Free fatty acid-induced insulin resistance is associated with

activation of protein kinase C theta and alterations in the insulin signaling cascade. Diabetes 48:1270–1274
361. Itani SI, Ruderman NB, Schmieder F, Boden G (2002) Lipid-induced insulin resistance in human muscle is associated with changes in diacylglycerol, protein kinase C, and IkappaB-alpha. Diabetes 51:2005–2011
362. Samuel VT, Liu ZX, Qu X, Elder BD, Bilz S, Befroy D, Romanelli AJ, Shulman GI (2004) Mechanism of hepatic insulin resistance in non-alcoholic fatty liver disease. J Biol Chem 279:32345–32353
363. Talior I, Tennenbaum T, Kuroki T, Eldar-Finkelman H (2005) PKC-delta-dependent activation of oxidative stress in adipocytes of obese and insulin-resistant mice: role for NADPH oxidase. Am J Physiol Endocrinol Metab 288:E405–E411
364. Kamata H, Manabe T, Oka S, Kamata K, Hirata H (2002) Hydrogen peroxide activates IkappaB kinases through phosphorylation of serine residues in the activation loops. FEBS Lett 519:231–237
365. Wang X, Martindale JL, Liu Y, Holbrook NJ (1998) The cellular response to oxidative stress: influences of mitogen-activated protein kinase signalling pathways on cell survival. Biochem J 333:291–300
366. Ravichandran LV, Esposito DL, Chen J, Quon MJ (2001) Protein kinase C-zeta phosphorylates insulin receptor substrate-1 and impairs its ability to activate phosphatidylinositol 3-kinase in response to insulin. J Biol Chem 276:3543–3549
367. Bollag GE, Roth RA, Beaudoin J, Mochly-Rosen D, Koshland DE Jr (1986) Protein kinase C directly phosphorylates the insulin receptor in vitro and reduces its protein-tyrosine kinase activity. Proc Natl Acad Sci USA 83:5822–5824
368. Lam TK, Yoshii H, Haber CA, Bogdanovic E, Lam L, Fantus IG, Giacca A (2002) Free fatty acid-induced hepatic insulin resistance: a potential role for protein kinase C-delta. Am J Physiol Endocrinol Metab 283:E682–E691
369. Boden G, She P, Mozzoli M, Cheung P, Gumireddy K, Reddy P, Xiang X, Luo Z, Ruderman N (2005) Free fatty acids produce insulin resistance and activate the proinflammatory nuclear factor-kappaB pathway in rat liver. Diabetes 54:3458–3465
370. Evans JL, Goldfine ID, Maddux BA, Grodsky GM (2003) Are oxidative stress-activated signaling pathways mediators of insulin resistance and beta-cell dysfunction? Diabetes 52:1–8
371. Cai D, Yuan M, Frantz DF, Melendez PA, Hansen L, Lee J, Shoelson SE (2005) Local and systemic insulin resistance resulting from hepatic activation of IKK-beta and NF-kappaB. Nat Med 11:183–190
372. Yin MJ, Yamamoto Y, Gaynor RB (1998) The anti-inflammatory agents aspirin and salicylate inhibit the activity of I(kappa)B kinase-beta. Nature 396:77–80
373. Kopp E, Ghosh S (1994) Inhibition of NF-kappa B by sodium salicylate and aspirin. Science 265:956–959
374. Fleischman A, Shoelson SE, Bernier R, Goldfine AB (2008) Salsalate improves glycemia and inflammatory parameters in obese young adults. Diabetes Care 31:289–294
375. Gilgore SG, Rupp JJ (1961) Response of blood glucose to intravenous salicylate. Metab Clin Exp 10:419–421
376. Hundal RS, Petersen KF, Mayerson AB, Randhawa PS, Inzucchi S, Shoelson SE, Shulman GI (2002) Mechanism by which high-dose aspirin improves glucose metabolism in type 2 diabetes. J Clin Investig 109:1321–1326
377. Kim JK, Kim YJ, Fillmore JJ, Chen Y, Moore I, Lee J, Yuan M, Li ZW, Karin M, Perret P, Shoelson SE, Shulman GI (2001) Prevention of fat-induced insulin resistance by salicylate. J Clin Investig 108:437–446
378. Xiao C, Giacca A, Lewis GF (2009) The effect of high-dose sodium salicylate on chronically elevated plasma nonesterified fatty acid-induced insulin resistance and Beta-cell dysfunction in overweight and obese nondiabetic men. Am J Physiol Endocrinol Metab 297:E1205–E1211
379. Arkan MC, Hevener AL, Greten FR, Maeda S, Li ZW, Long JM, Wynshaw-Boris A, Poli G, Olefsky J, Karin M (2005) IKK-beta links inflammation to obesity-induced insulin resistance. Nat Med 11:191–198

380. Gao Z, Hwang D, Bataille F, Lefevre M, York D, Quon MJ, Ye J (2002) Serine phosphorylation of insulin receptor substrate 1 by inhibitor kappa B kinase complex. J Biol Chem 277: 48115–48121
381. Ueki K, Kondo T, Kahn CR (2004) Suppressor of cytokine signaling 1 (SOCS-1) and SOCS-3 cause insulin resistance through inhibition of tyrosine phosphorylation of insulin receptor substrate proteins by discrete mechanisms. Mol Cell Biol 24:5434–5446
382. Seifert R, Schachtele C, Rosenthal W, Schultz G (1988) Activation of protein kinase C by cis- and trans-fatty acids and its potentiation by diacylglycerol. Biochem Biophys Res Commun 154:20–26
383. Ghosh S, Baltimore D (1990) Activation in vitro of NF-kappa B by phosphorylation of its inhibitor I kappa B. Nature 344:678–682
384. Shi H, Kokoeva MV, Inouye K, Tzameli I, Yin H, Flier JS (2006) TLR4 links innate immunity and fatty acid-induced insulin resistance. J Clin Investig 116:3015–3025
385. Evans JL, Goldfine ID, Maddux BA, Grodsky GM (2002) Oxidative stress and stress-activated signaling pathways: a unifying hypothesis of type 2 diabetes. Endocr Rev 23:599–622
386. Solinas G, Naugler W, Galimi F, Lee MS, Karin M (2006) Saturated fatty acids inhibit induction of insulin gene transcription by JNK-mediated phosphorylation of insulin-receptor substrates. Proc Natl Acad Sci USA 103:16454–16459
387. Hirosumi J, Tuncman G, Chang L, Gorgun CZ, Uysal KT, Maeda K, Karin M, Hotamisligil GS (2002) A central role for JNK in obesity and insulin resistance. Nature 420:333–336
388. Kaneto H, Nakatani Y, Miyatsuka T, Kawamori D, Matsuoka TA, Matsuhisa M, Kajimoto Y, Ichijo H, Yamasaki Y, Hori M (2004) Possible novel therapy for diabetes with cell-permeable JNK-inhibitory peptide. Nat Med 10:1128–1132
389. Nakatani Y, Kaneto H, Kawamori D, Hatazaki M, Miyatsuka T, Matsuoka TA, Kajimoto Y, Matsuhisa M, Yamasaki Y, Hori M (2004) Modulation of the JNK pathway in liver affects insulin resistance status. J Biol Chem 279:45803–45809
390. Yang R, Wilcox DM, Haasch DL, Jung PM, Nguyen PT, Voorbach MJ, Doktor S, Brodjian S, Bush EN, Lin E, Jacobson PB, Collins CA, Landschulz KT, Trevillyan JM, Rondinone CM, Surowy TK (2007) Liver-specific knockdown of JNK1 up-regulates proliferator-activated receptor gamma coactivator 1 beta and increases plasma triglyceride despite reduced glucose and insulin levels in diet-induced obese mice. J Biol Chem 282: 22765–22774
391. Kumashiro N, Tamura Y, Uchida T, Ogihara T, Fujitani Y, Hirose T, Mochizuki H, Kawamori R, Watada H (2008) Impact of oxidative stress and peroxisome proliferator-activated receptor gamma coactivator-1alpha in hepatic insulin resistance. Diabetes 57:2083–2091
392. Inoguchi T, Li P, Umeda F, Yu HY, Kakimoto M, Imamura M, Aoki T, Etoh T, Hashimoto T, Naruse M, Sano H, Utsumi H, Nawata H (2000) High glucose level and free fatty acid stimulate reactive oxygen species production through protein kinase C–dependent activation of NAD(P)H oxidase in cultured vascular cells. Diabetes 49:1939–1945
393. Ozcan U, Cao Q, Yilmaz E, Lee AH, Iwakoshi NN, Ozdelen E, Tuncman G, Gorgun C, Glimcher LH, Hotamisligil GS (2004) Endoplasmic reticulum stress links obesity, insulin action, and type 2 diabetes. Science 306:457–461
394. Hung JH, Su IJ, Lei HY, Wang HC, Lin WC, Chang WT, Huang W, Chang WC, Chang YS, Chen CC, Lai MD (2004) Endoplasmic reticulum stress stimulates the expression of cyclooxygenase-2 through activation of NF-kappaB and pp 38 mitogen-activated protein kinase. J Biol Chem 279:46384–46392
395. Harding HP, Zhang Y, Zeng H, Novoa I, Lu PD, Calfon M, Sadri N, Yun C, Popko B, Paules R, Stojdl DF, Bell JC, Hettmann T, Leiden JM, Ron D (2003) An integrated stress response regulates amino acid metabolism and resistance to oxidative stress. Mol Cell 11:619–633
396. Cardozo AK, Ortis F, Storling J, Feng YM, Rasschaert J, Tonnesen M, Van EF, Mandrup-Poulsen T, Herchuelz A, Eizirik DL (2005) Cytokines downregulate the sarcoendoplasmic reticulum pump Ca2+ ATPase 2b and deplete endoplasmic reticulum Ca2+, leading to induction of endoplasmic reticulum stress in pancreatic beta-cells. Diabetes 54:452–461

397. Hennige AM, Lembert N, Wahl MA, Ammon HP (2000) Oxidative stress increases potassium efflux from pancreatic islets by depletion of intracellular calcium stores. Free Radic Res 33:507–516
398. Finkel T, Holbrook NJ (2000) Oxidants, oxidative stress and the biology of ageing. Nature 408:239–247
399. Dang PM, Stensballe A, Boussetta T, Raad H, Dewas C, Kroviarski Y, Hayem G, Jensen ON, Gougerot-Pocidalo MA, El-Benna J (2006) A specific p47phox -serine phosphorylated by convergent MAPKs mediates neutrophil NADPH oxidase priming at inflammatory sites. J Clin Investig 116:2033–2043
400. Hansen LL, Ikeda Y, Olsen GS, Busch AK, Mosthaf L (1999) Insulin signaling is inhibited by micromolar concentrations of H(2)O(2). Evidence for a role of H(2)O(2) in tumor necrosis factor alpha-mediated insulin resistance. J Biol Chem 274:25078–25084
401. Tirosh A, Potashnik R, Bashan N, Rudich A (1999) Oxidative stress disrupts insulin-induced cellular redistribution of insulin receptor substrate-1 and phosphatidylinositol 3-kinase in 3T3-L1 adipocytes. A putative cellular mechanism for impaired protein kinase B activation and GLUT4 translocation. J Biol Chem 274:10595–10602
402. Houstis N, Rosen ED, Lander ES (2006) Reactive oxygen species have a causal role in multiple forms of insulin resistance. Nature 440:944–948
403. Maddux BA, See W, Lawrence JC Jr, Goldfine AL, Goldfine ID, Evans JL (2001) Protection against oxidative stress-induced insulin resistance in rat L6 muscle cells by mircomolar concentrations of alpha-lipoic acid. Diabetes 50:404–410
404. Kawamori D, Kaneto H, Nakatani Y, Matsuoka TA, Matsuhisa M, Hori M, Yamasaki Y (2006) The forkhead transcription factor Foxo1 bridges the JNK pathway and the transcription factor PDX-1 through its intracellular translocation. J Biol Chem 281:1091–1098
405. Essers MA, Weijzen S, de Vries-Smits AM, Saarloos I, de Ruiter ND, Bos JL, Burgering BM (2004) FOXO transcription factor activation by oxidative stress mediated by the small GTPase Ral and JNK. EMBO J 23:4802–4812
406. Suliman HB, Welty-Wolf KE, Carraway M, Tatro L, Piantadosi CA (2004) Lipopolysaccharide induces oxidative cardiac mitochondrial damage and biogenesis. Cardiovasc Res 64:279–288
407. Puigserver P, Rhee J, Lin J, Wu Z, Yoon JC, Zhang CY, Krauss S, Mootha VK, Lowell BB, Spiegelman BM (2001) Cytokine stimulation of energy expenditure through p38 MAP kinase activation of PPARgamma coactivator-1. Mol Cell 8:971–982
408. Kyriakis JM, Avruch J (1996) Sounding the alarm: protein kinase cascades activated by stress and inflammation. J Biol Chem 271:24313–24316
409. Collins QF, Xiong Y, Lupo EG Jr, Liu HY, Cao W (2006) p38 Mitogen-activated protein kinase mediates free fatty acid-induced gluconeogenesis in hepatocytes. J Biol Chem 281:24336–24344
410. Liu HY, Collins QF, Xiong Y, Moukdar F, Lupo EG Jr, Liu Z, Cao W (2007) Prolonged treatment of primary hepatocytes with oleate induces insulin resistance through p38 mitogen-activated protein kinase. J Biol Chem 282:14205–14212
411. Dersch K, Ichijo H, Bhakdi S, Husmann M (2005) Fatty acids liberated from low-density lipoprotein trigger endothelial apoptosis via mitogen-activated protein kinases. Cell Death Differ 12:1107–1114
412. Wang XL, Zhang L, Youker K, Zhang MX, Wang J, LeMaire SA, Coselli JS, Shen YH (2006) Free fatty acids inhibit insulin signaling-stimulated endothelial nitric oxide synthase activation through upregulating PTEN or inhibiting Akt kinase. Diabetes 55:2301–2310
413. Miller TA, LeBrasseur NK, Cote GM, Trucillo MP, Pimentel DR, Ido Y, Ruderman NB, Sawyer DB (2005) Oleate prevents palmitate-induced cytotoxic stress in cardiac myocytes. Biochem Biophys Res Commun 336:309–315
414. Koistinen HA, Chibalin AV, Zierath JR (2003) Aberrant p38 mitogen-activated protein kinase signalling in skeletal muscle from Type 2 diabetic patients. Diabetologia 46:1324–1328

415. Asada S, Daitoku H, Matsuzaki H, Saito T, Sudo T, Mukai H, Iwashita S, Kako K, Kishi T, Kasuya Y, Fukamizu A (2007) Mitogen-activated protein kinases, Erk and p38, phosphorylate and regulate Foxo1. Cell Signal 19:519–527
416. Maehama T, Taylor GS, Dixon JE (2001) PTEN and myotubularin: novel phosphoinositide phosphatases. Annu Rev Biochem 70:247–279
417. Li G, Barrett EJ, Barrett MO, Cao W, Liu Z (2007) Tumor necrosis factor-alpha induces insulin resistance in endothelial cells via a p38 mitogen-activated protein kinase-dependent pathway. Endocrinology 148:3356–3363
418. de Alvero C, Teruel T, Hernandez R, Lorenzo M (2004) Tumor necrosis factor alpha produces insulin resistance in skeletal muscle by activation of inhibitor kappaB kinase in a p38 MAPK-dependent manner. J Biol Chem 279:17070–17078
419. Aguilar V, Alliouachene S, Sotiropoulos A, Sobering A, Athea Y, Djouadi F, Miraux S, Thiaudiere E, Foretz M, Viollet B, Diolez P, Bastin J, Benit P, Rustin P, Carling D, Sandri M, Ventura-Clapier R, Pende M (2007) S6 kinase deletion suppresses muscle growth adaptations to nutrient availability by activating AMP kinase. Cell Metab 5:476–487
420. Vona-Davis L, Howard-McNatt M, Rose DP (2007) Adiposity, type 2 diabetes and the metabolic syndrome in breast cancer. Obes Rev 8:395–408
421. Godsland I (2010) Insulin resistance and hyperinsulinemia in the development and progression of cancer. Clin Sci 118:315–332
422. Taliaferro-Smith L, Nagalingam A, Zhong D, Zhou W, Saxena NK, Sharma D (2009) LKB1 is required for adiponectin-mediated modulation of AMPK-S6K axis and inhibition of migration and invasion of breast cancer cells. Oncogene 28:2621–2633
423. Ziemke F, Mantzoros CS (2010) Adiponectin in insulin resistance: lessons from translational research. Am J Clin Nutr 91:258S–261S
424. Wang C, Mao X, Wang L, Liu M, Wetzel MD, Guan KL, Dong LQ, Liu F (2007) Adiponectin sensitizes insulin signaling by reducing p70 S6 kinase-mediated serine phosphorylation of IRS-1. J Biol Chem 282:7991–7996
425. Grant S (2008) Cotargeting survival signaling pathways in cancer. J Clin Invest 118: 3003–3006
426. Jia S, Roberts TM, Zhao JJ (2009) Should individual PI3 kinase isoforms be targeted in cancer? Curr Opin Cell Biol 21:199–208
427. Wiesenthal SR, Sandhu H, McCall RH, Tchipashvili V, Yoshii H, Polonsky K, Shi ZQ, Lewis GF, Mari A, Giacca A (1999) Free fatty acids impair hepatic insulin extraction in vivo. Diabetes 48:766–774
428. DeFronzo RA (1992) Pathogenesis of type 2 (non-insulin dependent) diabetes mellitus: a balanced overview. Diabetologia 35:389–397
429. Semple RK, Sleigh A, Murgatroyd PR, Adams CA, Bluck L, Jackson S, Vottero A, Kanabar D, Charlton-Menys V, Durrington P, Soos MA, Carpenter TA, Lomas DJ, Cochran EK, Gorden P, O'Rahilly S, Savage DB (2009) Postreceptor insulin resistance contributes to human dyslipidemia and hepatic steatosis. J Clin Investig 119:315–322
430. George S, Rochford JJ, Wolfrum C, Gray SL, Schinner S, Wilson JC, Soos MA, Murgatroyd PR, Williams RM, Acerini CL, Dunger DB, Barford D, Umpleby AM, Wareham NJ, Davies HA, Schafer AJ, Stoffel M, O'Rahilly S, Barroso I (2004) A family with severe insulin resistance and diabetes due to a mutation in AKT2. Science 304:1325–1328
431. Montagnani M, Golovchenko I, Kim I, Koh GY, Goalstone ML, Mundhekar AN, Johansen M, Kucik DF, Quon MJ, Draznin B (2002) Inhibition of phosphatidylinositol 3-kinase enhances mitogenic actions of insulin in endothelial cells. J Biol Chem 277:1794–1799
432. Draznin B (2010) Mitogenic action of insulin: friend, foe or 'frenemy'? Diabetologia 53:229–233
433. Goalstone ML, Leitner JW, Wall K, Dolgonos L, Rother KI, Accili D, Draznin B (1998) Effect of insulin on farnesyltransferase. Specificity of insulin action and potentiation of nuclear effects of insulin-like growth factor-1, epidermal growth factor, and platelet-derived growth factor. J Biol Chem 273:23892–23896

434. Giovannucci E, Michaud D (2007) The role of obesity and related metabolic disturbances in cancers of the colon, prostate, and pancreas. Gastroenterology 132:2208–2225
435. Dandona P, Chaudhuri A, Mohanty P, Ghanim H (2007) Anti-inflammatory effects of insulin. Curr Opin Clin Nutr Metab Care 10:511–517
436. Tran TT, Naigamwalla D, Oprescu AI, Lam L, Keown-Eyssen G, Bruce WR, Giacca A (2006) Hyperinsulinemia, but not other factors associated with insulin resistance, acutely enhances colorectal epithelial proliferation in vivo. Endocrinology 147:1830–1837

Chapter 2
Insulin/IGF-1 Signaling Nodes and their Role in Carcinogenesis

Cullen M. Taniguchi and C. Ronald Kahn

Introduction

The dominant hormone regulating metabolic homeostasis and the switch between the anabolic and catabolic states is insulin. At the cellular level, the action of insulin and the closely related insulin-like growth factors (IGF)-1 and -2, are mediated through a complex network of diverging and converging events (reviewed in [1]). The insulin and IGF-1 receptors (IR and IGF-1R) are members of the family of receptor tyrosine kinases. Following hormone binding, these receptors undergo autophosphorylation, which activates the kinase toward other substrates termed the insulin receptor substrate (IRS) proteins. In contrast to most other tyrosine kinase receptors, it is the phosphorylated IRS proteins, rather than the receptors themselves, that link the action of these hormones to two main signaling pathways: the phosphatidylinositol 3-kinase (PI3K)-Akt pathway, which is responsible for most of the metabolic actions of insulin, and the Ras-MAP kinase pathway, which regulates expression of some genes and cooperates with the PI3K pathway to control cell growth and differentiation (reviewed in [2]) (Fig. 2.1).

Although this signaling pathway may appear to be a relatively simple cascade, its complexity become apparent when considering the number of gene and protein isoforms involved just in the activation of Akt and the generation of metabolic effects. For instance, the insulin receptor (IR) exists as two splice isoforms, which are usually co-expressed in cells with the highly-related IGF-1 receptor that can also

C.R. Kahn (✉)
Department of Medicine, Joslin Diabetes Center, Harvard Medical School, Boston, MA 02215, USA

Division of Signal Transduction, Department of Medicine, Beth Israel Deaconess Medical Center, Boston, MA, USA
e-mail: c.ronald.kahn@joslin.harvard.edu

I.G. Fantus (ed.), *Insulin Resistance and Cancer: Epidemiology, Cellular and Molecular Mechanisms and Clinical Implications*, Energy Balance and Cancer 1,
DOI 10.1007/978-1-4419-9911-5_2,

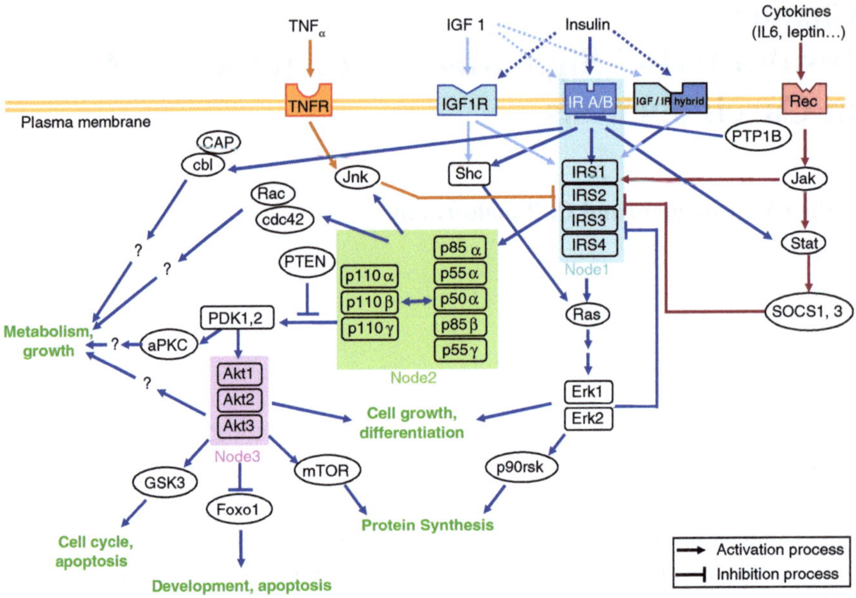

Fig. 2.1 Critical nodes in the insulin signaling network. We show here the concept of critical nodes in a signaling pathway using the insulin network (*dark blue arrows*) and the highly related IGF-1R signaling network (*light blue arrows*). Cytokines (TNFα, IL6, leptin) signaling pathways have been shown to interfere with the insulin signaling and are also represented on this figure (*orange* and *red arrows*). The three major nodes in this pathway are the insulin receptor coupled to IRS proteins (*light blue box*), PI 3-Kinase (*green box*), and Akt (*pink box*). *Dashed arrows* represent an activation process with less intensity. *Plain arrows* represent an activation process, *block arrows* represent an inhibition process, and *dashed arrows* represent activation process with less intensity

be activated by insulin. Furthermore, there are at least 11 known substrate proteins of the insulin and IGF-1 receptors, and these are capable of interacting with eight known forms of the PI3K regulatory subunit, which associate with three forms of the PI3K catalytic subunit that can generate PIP_3 leading to activation of the three known isoforms of Akt. Thus, in these first three steps in insulin action, the IR/IGF-1 system can generate over 1,000 possible interactions of signaling partnerships based on combinations of isoforms. This number increases further if we consider the spatiotemporal aspects of compartmentalization, kinetics, and other downstream components in the signaling network.

In addition, these three "critical nodes" of signal divergence, that is, the insulin and IGF-1 receptors and their substrates, the enzyme PI 3-kinase, and the various isoforms of Akt (Akt 1–3) and atypical protein kinase C (PKC) isoforms, such as PKCλ and PKCζ that serve as its targets, are highly regulated – both positively and negatively. This extensive regulation at these nodes facilitate the control of multiple processes by the insulin/IGF-1 pathways throughout the organism from metabolism to growth and lifespan [1]. Thus, it is important to understand these critical nodes and how oncogenic processes can usurp the normal functions of the insulin/IGF-1 axis to initiate and maintain the growth of cancers.

The central molecular defect in obesity and type 2 diabetes is the dysregulation of the insulin/IGF-1 axis. Interestingly, this dysfunction of insulin/IGF-1 signaling at the root of both obesity and type 2 diabetes now may have implications in cancer biology. Elevated body mass index (BMI) and type 2 diabetes are now recognized as general risk factors for cancer, and may afford as much as a twofold increase in the risk of all forms of cancer [3]. Indeed, the rising rate of obesity, and associated insulin resistance, in the population may be driving an increase in cancer risk, that now approaches the cancer risk garnered from smoking [4, 5]. Furthermore, several tumor types have been noted to grow faster in animal models of type 1 and type 2 diabetes [6, 7]. Thus, the link between insulin signaling and metabolic regulation is not only of experimental interest, it may very well have a general clinical and epidemiological impact.

The Insulin Receptor

The insulin receptor (IR) is a tetrameric protein consisting of two α- and two β-subunits and belongs to a subfamily of receptor tyrosine kinases that also includes the IGF-1 receptor and an orphan receptor called the insulin receptor-related receptor (IRR) [8, 9] (Fig. 2.2). Each of these receptors is the product of a separate gene in which the two subunits are derived from a single chain precursor or proreceptor that is processed by a furin-like enzyme to give a single α–β subunit complex [10]. The alpha subunit is the extracellular, ligand binding portion of the complex, while the beta subunit has tyrosine kinase activity. To form a functional receptor, two α–β dimers are disulfide linked to form a tetramer. Due to the homology of these receptors, functional heterotetramers can form between α–β dimers of the insulin receptor, the IGF-1 receptor, and IRR forming hybrid receptors (Fig. 2.2). The biologic relevance of these hybrid receptors is still not clearly understood.

The insulin/IGF-1 receptor behaves as a classical allosteric enzyme in which the α-subunit inhibits the tyrosine kinase activity intrinsic to the β-subunit. When the ligand binds to the extracellular domain of the α-subunit, the β-subunit is de-repressed, enabling the kinase activity of the β-subunit. The activated beta subunit can then trans-phosphorylate the adjoining beta subunit of the tetramer, causing a conformational change which further increases the kinase activity of the phosphorylated β-subunit. This increased activity of the insulin receptor leads to the phosphorylation of the IRSs and the commencement of further downstream signaling [11, 12]. De-repression of the β-subunit can also occur by removal of the α-subunit by proteolysis or genetic deletion, but these mechanisms do not have any clinical relevance [13, 14].

The activity of the insulin and IGF-1 receptors are tightly regulated, since unchecked activation of these molecules would lead to profound metabolic and growth consequences. Thus, there are several mechanisms of negative regulation. One class of regulatory proteins are tyrosine phosphatases, the most studied of which is protein tyrosine phosphatase-1B (PTP-1B). PTP-1B interacts directly with the IR to dephosphorylate key tyrosine residues involved in receptor activation, and knockouts of PTP1B show enhanced insulin sensitivity [15, 16]. Similarly, antisense and small molecule inhibitors of PTP-1B have shown remarkable efficacy in improving

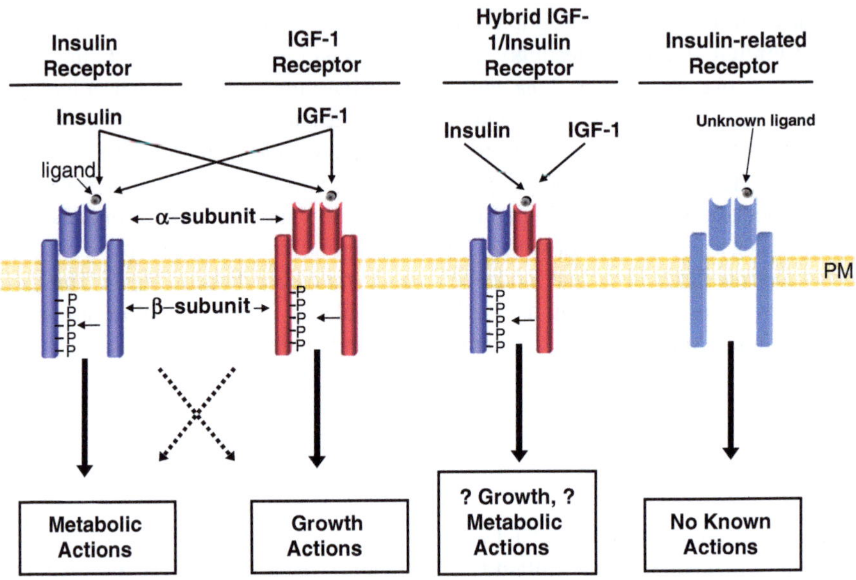

Fig. 2.2 The insulin receptor family. On the *left side* of the panel, insulin or IGF-1 (ligand denoted as a *sphere*) can bind to the extracellular portion of the receptor to induce a change in the beta-subunits, facilitating transphosphoryllation and activation. Due to high homology between receptors, the ligands can bind to both insulin and IGF-1 receptors, but with different affinities. In the *middle panel*, note that insulin and IGF-1 receptor can form heterotetramers by combining two different α–β dimers. The *right part* of the panel showed the insulin-related receptor, which has a similar structure, but unknown ligand and function

insulin sensitivity in vivo [17, 18] through improved insulin signaling [19]. Other proteins such as suppressors of cytokine signaling-1 and -3 (SOCS-1 and SOCS-3) [20–23], growth factor receptor binder 10 (Grb10) [24] and the molecule plasma cell membrane glycoprotein-1 (PC-1/ENPP1) [25] downregulate IR function by sterically blocking its interaction with the IRS proteins, or by modifying its kinase activity. The SOCS proteins are of particular importance, because they have been shown to be upregulated in states of insulin resistance, such as obesity, and, therefore, might contribute to the pathophysiology of insulin resistance [20, 23]. The SOCS proteins also regulate the JAK/STAT pathway, which is involved in multiple forms of cancers, chiefly those of the hematologic variety [26]. The IR is also subject to down-regulation at the protein level by ligand stimulated internalization and degradation [27]. This downregulation is a common feature of most insulin resistant, hyperinsulinemic states, including obesity and type 2 diabetes [28].

Insulin Receptor and Cancer

The precise role of the insulin receptor in oncogenesis is unclear, but it is known that for some tumors higher levels of insulin receptor expression correlate with worse outcomes.

For instance, breast cancer patients with tumors expressing high levels of IR had a significantly lower 5-year progression free survival compared to those expressed even moderate levels of IR [29]. Further multivariate analysis reveals IR expression to be strongest independent predictive factor in disease free survival.

The oncogenic effects of the insulin receptor may be most strongly related to one of its splice isoforms (see Fig. 2.2). During transcription of the IR proreceptor, the sequence which encodes the future α-subunit insulin receptor undergoes differential mRNA splicing into two isoforms that either contain (IR_B, +Ex11) or lack exon 11 (IR_A, −Ex11), which encodes 12 amino acids near the C-terminus of the α-subunit [30, 31]. The A and B isoforms of the insulin receptor are known to have differential expression patterns, where the A isoform (−Ex11) is expressed in fetal tissue and the adult cells of the central nervous system and hematopoeitic lineages. IR_B, on the other hand, is the predominant form expressed in adult liver, muscle and fat. While the precise physiological role of the two receptor isoforms remains unknown, the IR_B isoform exhibits greater autophosphorylation, internalization kinetics [32] and signaling capacity [33], whereas the IR_A isoform (−Ex11) exhibits somewhat higher affinity for insulin and IGF-II binding [34–36]. In addition the A isoform is increased in expression in cancers of the lung, colon, breast and thyroid. In addition, one study has suggested that the −Ex11 insulin receptor better activates the PI3K pathway [37]. Hybrid receptors between the IR and the IGF-1R may also be responsible for some of the tumorigenic phenotype, though it is unclear to what extent these hybrid receptors play.

The molecular mechanisms of IR and IGF-1R dysregulation in cancer are still unknown, but they may be linked to the well-known tumor suppressor p53 (*TRP53*). *TRP53* suppresses the expression of both the insulin and IGF-1 receptors [38] Thus, loss of p53 function by mutation, deletion or inactivation may lead to a significant and pathologic increase in IR/IGF-1R [39]. This is of particular relevance since TRP53 is the most commonly mutated gene in human cancer. Furthermore, the dysfunction of other p53 regulators, such as high mobility group A1 (HMGA1) may also cause a net upregulation of IR or IGF-1R expression [40].

Insulin Receptor Substrates

At least 11 intracellular substrates of the insulin and IGF-1 receptor kinases have been identified. Six of these belong to the family of IRS proteins and have been termed IRS-1–6 [41–45]. Other substrates of the insulin/IGF-1 receptors include Gab-1 [46], $p62^{dok}$ [47], Cbl [48] and the various isoforms of Shc [49].

The IRS proteins have three types of function domains. Near the N-terminus there are both pleckstrin homology (PH) and phosphotyrosine binding (PTB) domains that account for the high affinity of these substrates for the membrane lipids and the IR (Fig. 2.3). The center and C-terminal regions of the IRS proteins contain up to 20 potential tyrosine phosphorylation sites that serve as the most important functional domains. After phosphorylation by the insulin or IGF-1 receptor, these phosphotyrosines

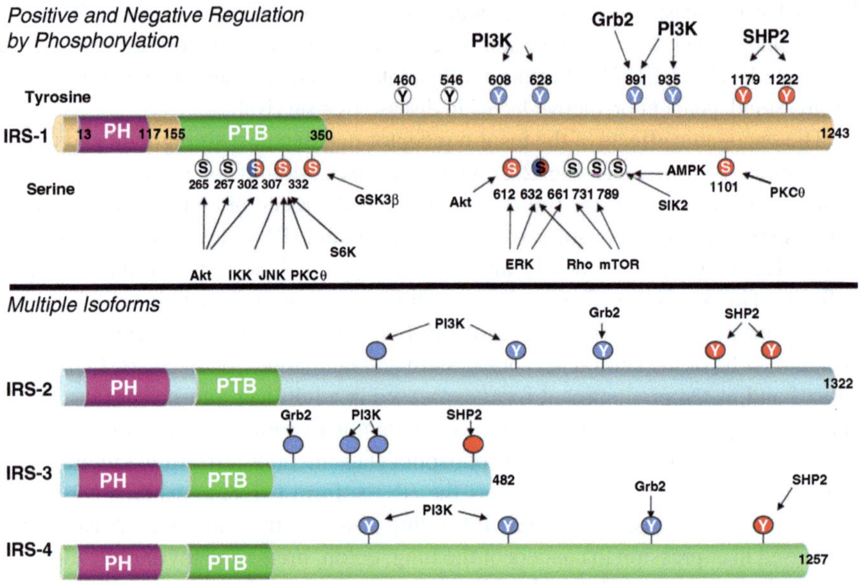

Fig. 2.3 Insulin receptor substrates as a critical node. The structures of the four IRS isoforms, IRS1-4, are represented. They all share a PH domain (*magenta*), a PTB domain (*green*) and multiple sites of phosphorylation on tyrosine and serine residues. On the *upper side* of the IRS diagrams are shown the positions of the tyrosine residues (Y) phosphorylated by the insulin receptor and the downstream signaling proteins that bind to this sites. On the *lower side* of the IRS diagrams are shown the positions of the serine residues (S) and the kinases responsible for their phosphorylation. *Blue circles* represent sites of positive regulation. *Red circles* represent sites of negative regulation. A combination of both colors show sites where the regulation has been shown to be positive or negative. White circles represent sites where the effect of phosphorylation is currently unknown

bind to intracellular molecules that contain Src-homology 2 (SH2) domains that continue the cascade of insulin/IGF-1 signaling. IRS-1 and -2 are widely distributed, whereas IRS-3 is largely limited to the adipocyte and brain, and IRS-4 is expressed primarily in embryonic tissues or cell lines. IRS-5 and IRS-6, on the other hand, appear to have very limited tissue expression and function in signaling [45]. Also, in humans, IRS-3 appears to be a pseudogene that produces no functional protein [50], so most studies in human adults have focused on IRS-1 and -2 only.

The SH2 proteins that bind to phosphorylated IRS proteins fall into two main categories. The best studied are adaptor molecules, such as the regulatory subunit of PI 3-kinase or the adaptor molecule Grb2, which associates with SOS to activate the Ras-MAP kinase pathway (reviewed in [51, 52]). The other category of proteins that bind to IRS proteins are enzymes, such as the phosphotyrosine phosphatase SHP2 [53] and cytoplasmic tyrosine kinases, such as Fyn [54]. There are also a few proteins that bind to phosphotyrosines in the IRS proteins and do not contain known SH2 domains, such as the calcium ATPases SERCA 1 and 2 [55], and the SV40 large T antigen [56]. Like the insulin receptor, the ability of the IRS proteins to mediate intracellular signaling is also regulated by the action of protein tyrosine phosphatases (PTPases) that dephosphorylate key tyrosine residues in the IRS proteins. Further, some PTPases, such as SHP2, contain SH2 domains and can bind directly to IRS-1 on two p-Tyr residues near the C-terminus [53], which then allows the enzyme special affinity for IRS proteins and ability to dephosphorylate the phosphotyrosines that mediate the binding of PI3K and Grb2.

Regulation of IRS Protein Function

In addition to signal transduction by tyrosine phosphorylation, IRS proteins undergo serine phosphorylation in response to insulin and other stimuli, such as cytokines or free fatty acids [57]. There are over 70 potential serine phosphorylation sites in IRS-1, and in general, serine phosphorylation negatively regulates IRS signaling by inhibiting insulin receptor ability to phosphorylate IRS proteins on tyrosine residues. Many IRS kinases, such as Akt [58], MAPK [59], S6 kinase [60] and c-Jun-N-terminal kinase (JNK) [61], are activated by insulin, suggesting that some serine phosphorylation of the IRS proteins might represent a normal negative feedback mechanism for the insulin signaling pathway (Figs. 2.2 and 2.3).

The exact molecular mechanisms by which serine phosphorylation alters IRS-1 function are multiple. Thus, serine phosphorylation can interfere in a *cis* manner with the functional domains of IRS-1 that are proximal to or surround the phosphoserine (see Fig. 2.3). For instance, the phosphorylation of serine 307 of IRS-1, which is located in the PTB domain, has been correlated with negative regulation of insulin signaling [62]. The in vitro phosphorylation of this residue is sufficient to disrupt the interaction between the IR and IRS-1 in yeast tri-hybrid assay [61, 63]. The phosphorylation of Ser270, also within the PTB domain, has been shown to promote the interaction of IRS-1 with 14-3-3 proteins, which might also interfere with the phosphotyrosine binding function of the PTB domain [64]. In addition, a recent in vivo study has shown that decreased phosphorylation at Ser612 by MAPK is correlated with increased phosphorylation tyrosine 608 [59]. Serine phosphorylation has also been shown to alter intracellular localization [65] and induce degradation of IRS proteins [66].

Although many studies have demonstrated the negative effects of serine phosphorylation, there is evidence that some serine phosphorylation events might positively or bidirectionally regulate insulin signaling. For instance, the phosphorylation of Ser302 of IRS-1 has been shown to have both positive [67] and negative [63] effects on insulin signaling, whereas phosphorylation by Rho kinase on Ser632 of IRS-1 improves insulin action [68]. Other studies have shown that serine phosphorylation of IRS-1 by Akt on serine 612 enhances IRS signaling [69]. The role of serine phosphorylation of IRS-2 and other IRS proteins in regulating insulin action remains to be determined.

Each of the IRS Isoforms May Have Specific Biological Functions

Although the IRS proteins are highly homologous and possess many similar tyrosine phosphorylation motifs, studies in knockout mice and knockout cell lines indicate that the various IRS proteins serve complementary, rather than redundant, roles in insulin/IGF-1 signaling (reviewed in [70]). *Irs-1* knockout mice exhibit defective insulin action primarily in muscle and a generalized defect in body growth due to IGF-1 resistance [71], whereas *Irs-2* knockout mice have greater defects in insulin signaling in the liver and also altered growth, but only in a few tissues, such as certain neurons [72] and pancreatic β-cells [73]. Likewise at the cellular level, IRS-1 knockout pre-adipocytes exhibit defects in differentiation [74], whereas IRS-2 knockout preadipocytes differentiate normally, but fail to respond to insulin-stimulated glucose transport [75]. These knockout studies clearly indicate that the IRS proteins constitute a critical node such that the deletion of each isoform has different biological consequences.

Indeed, these differences in isoform function may influence the relative oncogenic properties of the IRS molecules. IRS-1, in particular, may play a critical role suggesting a closer link to IGF-1 receptor signaling [71]. For example, in human breast cancer high levels of IRS-1 expression correlate with poor differentiation (Grade 3) and positive lymph node status [76, 77]. IRS-1 levels are increased by estrogen and decreased by estrogen antagonists, such as tamoxifen [78]. Thus, it has been postulated that IRS-1 upregulation may play a critical role in ER-positive breast cancer. Indeed, in patients with ER positive breast cancer, higher levels of IRS-1 expression correlates with a poorer outcome [79]. Transgenic mouse models have also demonstrated that mammary-specific overexpression of IRS-1 results in a twofold increase in the incidence of adenocarcinoma of the breast when compared to littermate mice with mammary-specific overexpression of IRS-2 [80].

IRS-1 may also play a role in cancers of the GI tract. In particular, IGF-1/IRS-1 is critical to pancreatic tumorigenesis, and this occurs via the PI3K pathway [81]. In addition, the overexpression of either IRS-1 [82, 83] or IRS-2 [84] have been linked with the development of human hepatocellular carcinoma. Conversely, inhibition of IRS-1 signaling with a dominant negative mutant caused increased apoptosis in a human hepatocellular carcinoma cell line [85].

IRS-1 may also facilitate crosstalk between the IGF-1R and another important oncogenic tyrosine kinase, such as the epidermal growth factor receptor (EGFR) [86]. EGFR mutation or amplification plays a large role in many types of cancer, with the HER2/*neu* (also known as *erbB2*) subtype being prominent in cancers of the breast and lung (reviewed in [87]). Unfortunately, EGFR inhibitors have shown mixed results in human trials due to drug resistance. The mechanism of this resistance may be from increased expression of both IRS-1 and IGF-1 receptor, which maintain signal through the PI3K pathways despite nearly complete inhibition of erbB2 receptors with either the small molecule gefitinib or the monoclonal antibody erbitux [86]. This upregulation of IRS-1 activity can be ablated with inhibitors of IGF-1 receptor activity [88].

While IRS-1 has been the most studied of the IRS proteins, the other IRS isoforms may also have a role in oncogenesis. Forced IRS-2 expression has been linked with increased metastatic potential of human breast carcinoma cells in rodent xenograft models [89] and may also play a role in mediating PTEN-driven cancers [90]. IRS-3 does not play a role in human cancer, since no known IRS-3 homolog exists in humans [91]. IRS-4 has been linked with rare pediatric leukemias [92], but is otherwise thought to play a fairly minor role in IR/IGF-1 signaling, since IRS-4 knockout mice have a very mild phenotype [93].

Biochemical studies have revealed several molecular mechanisms by which the IRS proteins could exert their specific effects. Both tissue specific knockdown and Cre-lox mediated knockout of hepatic IRS-1 and IRS-2 reveal that both IRS-1 and IRS-2 are required to maintain full activation of Akt via PI3K [94]. However, IRS-1 and IRS-2 have different and complementary roles in the regulation of gene expression. For example, acute knockdown of IRS-1 or IRS-2 in the liver by adenoviral short hairpin RNAs demonstrated that decreased hepatic IRS-1 correlates with increased expression of genes involved in gluconeogenesis, whereas downregulation of hepatic IRS-2 results in enhanced expression of genes involved with lipogenesis [94].

These differences in gene expression and cellular function might come about from the different signals generating from binding various SH2-containing partners with greater affinity. For instance, IRS-1 can bind Abl and SHP-2, whereas IRS-2 cannot [95]. In addition, IRS-1 has been shown to bind to several SH2 proteins, such as Grb2, Crk and phospholipase Cγ (PLCγ), with greater affinity than IRS-2 [95]. The IRS proteins also differ in their cellular compartmentalization [96, 97] and activation kinetics [98]. IRS-2 is structurally different from the other IRS proteins in that it can bind to the insulin receptor through a unique kinase regulatory loop binding (KRLB) domain, which might contribute to some of its specific effects [99].

The IRS proteins may also facilitate growth factor signaling and oncogenesis in non-canonical ways. For instance, although IRS-1 has no intrinsic kinase activity, its overexpression can transform mouse embryonic fibroblasts [100]. This effect has been suggested to be due to the fact that IRS-1 binds to SV40 large T antigen. Indeed, IRS-1 has been suggested to be required for SV40-induced transformation [101], although this effect may be cell type dependent, since IRS-1 deficiency does not block the ability of SV40 large T antigen to immortalize brown preadipocytes [102].

Phosphoinositide 3-Kinase

The first SH2 domain protein identified to interact with IRS-1 was the Class IA form of PI3K [41]. This enzyme consists of a regulatory and catalytic subunit, each of which occurs in several isoforms (Fig. 2.4). The activation of the catalytic subunit depends on interaction of the two SH2 domains in the regulatory subunit with specific phosphotyrosine motifs in the IRS proteins of the sequence (pY)MXM and (pY)XXM [103]. Inhibitors of PI3K or transfection with dominant negative

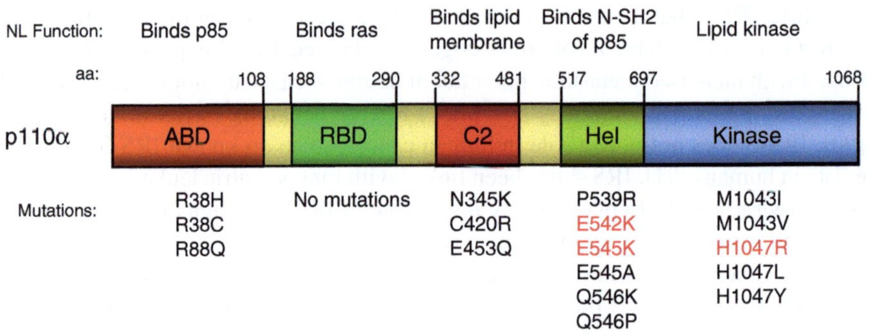

Fig. 2.4 Structure, functions and known oncogenic mutations of p110. Structural features and the Class IA catalytic subunits of PI3K (p110). These come in α-, β- and δ-isoforms, all of which have similar structures, but slightly different tissue distribution (noted in text). The normal functions and oncogenic mutations of each domain are noted above and below the molecule as shown. *ABD* adapter binding domain; *RBD ras* binding domain; *C2* lipid binding domain

constructs of the enzyme block virtually all of insulin's metabolic actions, including stimulation of glucose transport, glycogen synthesis, lipid synthesis, and adipocyte differentiation [104, 105] highlighting the pivotal role of this enzyme in the metabolic actions of insulin and IGF-1 (Figs. 2.1 and 2.5).

PI3K Mediates Growth Factor Signaling by Generating PIP$_3$

PI3K activates critical regulators of insulin signaling by catalyzing the formation of the lipid second messenger phosphatidylinositol (3,4,5) trisphosphate (PI(3,4,5)P$_3$ or PIP$_3$) in the cell (Fig. 2.5). Proteins with PH domains can bind to PIP$_3$ and become localized to the same region, which allows for their activation. Among these proteins with PH domains are the AGC superfamily of serine/threonine protein kinases, guanine nucleotide exchange proteins of the Rho family of GTPases, and the TEC family of tyrosine kinases, including BTK and ITK. Perhaps the most critical of the AGC kinases to insulin action is PIP$_3$-dependent protein kinase-1 (PDK-1) which is, in part, responsible for the activation of Akt/PKB and atypical PKCs. PDK1 phosphorylates the activation loops of Akt/PKB on Thr308 and PKCζ on Thr410 to enable function of these kinases [106, 107]. Akt, however, requires a second phosphorylation on Ser473 for full activation. Because PDK1 is unable to phosphorylate Ser473, the existence of a PDK2 was postulated. The identity of PDK2 was mysterious for quite some time, (see [108] for review), though it is believed that the Rictor mammalian target of rapamycin (mTOR) complex has been proposed to serve as the PDK2 for Akt. This mTOR complex is insensitive to rapamycin and is necessary for Ser473 phosphorylation in *Drosophila* and human cells [109]. The full actions of Akt in oncogenesis will be reviewed in another chapter.

The positive actions of PI3K are negatively regulated at the level of PIP$_3$ by phospholipid phosphatases, such as PTEN and SH2-containing inositol 5′-phosphatase 2 (SHIP2), which dephosphorylate and inactivate PIP$_3$. PTEN dephosphorylates

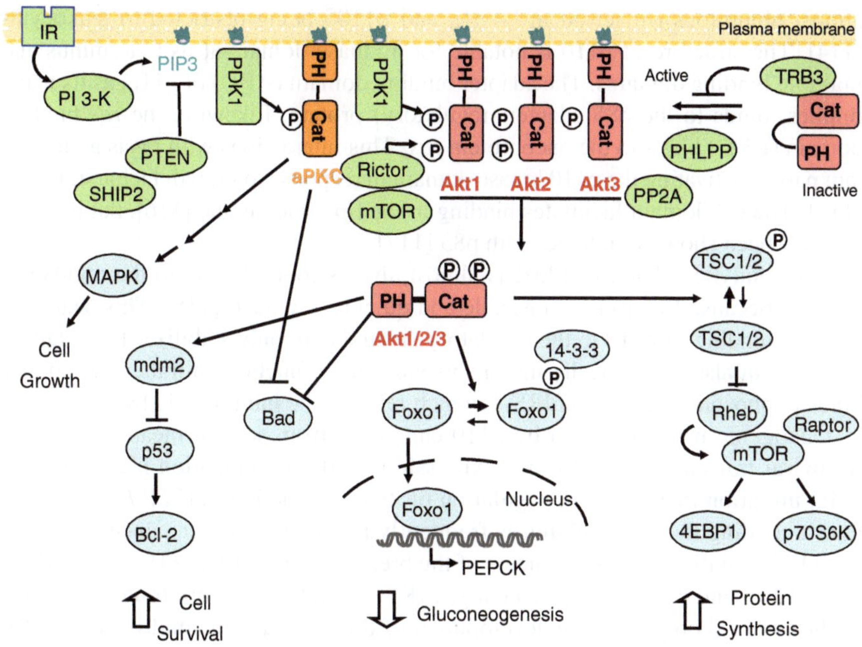

Fig. 2.5 Downstream effectors of PI3-kinase. The three Akt isoforms (in *red*) share the same structural organization: a PH domain required for binding to phospholipids and a catalytic domain, which becomes active upon phosphorylation (P) on two residues (T308 and S473 for Akt1, T309 And S474 for Akt2) or one residue (T305) for Akt3. In *green* are represented the upstream regulators of Akt activity. In *blue* are shown the downstream targets of Akt, which are involved in the control of the metabolic functions regulated by the Akt isoforms

phosphoinositides on the 3′-position, whereas SHIP2 dephosphorylates the 5′-position. PTEN has been shown to downregulate PI3K signaling in various cellular systems and in intact animals [110, 111]. Not surprisingly, inactivating/silencing mutations in the negative regulator PTEN [112] are associated with many human cancers and are linked with poorer treatment outcomes [113]. Such increased activity through PI3K mediators such as Akt and mTOR activity are central to the mechanism of this pathway's oncogenic activity.

The Heterodimeric Components of PI3K Have Unique Roles in Growth Factor Signaling and Oncogenesis: p110 as a Proto-oncogene

PI 3-kinase exists as a heterodimer consisting of a catalytic subunit of 110 kDa and an SH2-containing regulatory subunit, the most common of which are 85 kDa (Fig. 2.4). The three different catalytic subunits, p110α, β, and δ are derived from three different genes and show different tissue distribution, with the α and β forms almost ubiquitous (reviewed in [105]), and p110δ being restricted to leukocytes [114]. The structure of p110 is notable for a kinase domain at its C-terminus and multiple binding domains. The adapter binding domain (ABD) of p110, as its name implies, binds to the p85 adapter (regulatory) protein. Likewise, the *ras* binding domain (RBD) binds to the oncoprotein *ras*. This interactions with ras is an important part of activating the p110 kinase domain in response to growth factor signaling [115]. The C2 domain facilitates binding to the lipid membrane [116], but has also recently been shown to interact with p85 [117].

The catalytic subunit of PI3K is almost always found bound to the regulatory subunit, because free p110 is unstable and quickly degraded [118]. This near irreversible binding of p110 to the regulatory subunits not only stabilizes the catalytic subunit, but also allosterically inhibits its enzymatic function until the heterodimer binds to phosphotyrosines on IRS-1, which relieves the inhibition [118].

Oncogenic transformation by p110 can come from several means, including retroviral transduction [119], overexpression [120], amplification [121], or by a point mutation that alters the regulation of its kinase activity [122]. *PIK3CA*, the gene encoding the p110 subunit is frequently mutated in human cancers and has been linked with the human cancers of the breast [123], ovary [124], cervix [125], liver [126], and colon [127]. Recently, PIK3CA mutations were found to be one of the critical components in development of the glioblastoma multiforme [128].

There are several known oncogenic mutations in p110. The normal functional structure and oncogenic mutations of p110 are detailed in Fig. 2.4. Recent crystallographic evidence from two different groups have shed light on the mechanisms of these mutations [129]. For instance, although the ABD binds p85, the known oncogenic mutations in the ABD (R38H, R38C and R88Q) are not near the interface with p85, but are rather near the interface with the N-terminal portion of the kinase. Thus, mutations in the ABD may enhance the activity of the kinase domain by yet undetermined mechanisms. Likewise, the C2 domain has been shown to be critical for lipid membrane binding. Indeed, while the C420R mutation results in increased affinity for the lipid membrane, other mutations in the C2 region alter the binding of C2 with p85, thus altering the negative regulation of p85 on p110.

The so-called "hot-spot" mutations of p110 occur at E542K and E545K in the helical domain and H1047R in the kinase domain. These mutations are the most frequent oncogenic mutations of p110 [117, 130]. The mutations of the helical domain disrupt the inhibitory binding of the N-terminal SH2 domain of p85–p110. In the basal state, this N-terminal SH2 domain of p85 is bound tightly to the helical domain p110. This inhibition continues until the SH2 domain binds phosphotyrosine moieties, like those on IRS-1 after insulin stimulation. This binding of the SH2 domain releases the inhibition on p110. Thus, mutations of the helical domain prevent the proper inhibition of p110 in the basal state, leading to constitutive activation of PI3K. Conversely, mutations in the C-terminus of p85 can also prevent the basal inhibition; although such mutations are rare, they appear to relatively frequent in PI3K-dependent cancers such as gliobalstoma multiforme [128]. The mechanism of activation of the H1047R hotspot mutation is still not known, but it is posited that it induces conformational changes similar to *ras* in the activation loop, thus mimicking the positive regulatory effect of ras on p110 [131].

Recent evidence suggests that the different isoforms of the p110 catalytic subunit have specific biologic functions. The alpha isoform is the most studied of the p110 subunits and appears to be critical for metabolic homeostasis [132] and in some cases oncogenic transformation [120]. Germline knockouts of either p110α or p110β are early embryonic lethal [133, 134], indicating that each isoform has a unique biological function, since the loss of single isoform could not be adequately compensated by the expression of the other isoforms. Overexpression approaches have identified isoform-specific functions of p110, where p110α might have a more important role in platelet-derived growth factor (PDGF) signaling, while p110β has been suggested to have a more important role in mediating insulin-mediated glucose uptake [135, 136]. However, studies using liver specific knockout approaches have indicated that p110α, rather than p110β has a major role in control glucose metabolism ([137] and Rotter and Kahn, unpublished data). The p110α isoform has also been shown to be critical for glucose homeostasis by both isoform specific small molecule inhibitors [138] or by tissue-specific kinase-dead knock-in mice [132]. A tissue specific knockout of the p110α isoform has also demonstrated its critical role in angiogenesis [139]. The p110β isoform, on the other hand, is central to the development of prostate adenocarcinoma as demonstrated by both knockout [137] and shRNA models [140].

The p85 Subunit as a Proto-oncogene

Although the p110 catalytic subunit of PI3K and the PIP_3 phosphatase PTEN can function as oncogenes when mutated, the role of the p85 regulatory subunit of PI3K in oncogenesis is less clear [141]. As mentioned previously, Class I_A PI3K is an obligate heterodimer with an SH2-containing regulatory subunit and a p110 catalytic subunit [142]. At least eight isoforms of the regulatory subunit of PI3K have been identified, which are derived from three distinct genes [143]. *Pik3r1* encodes 65–75% of the regulatory subunits, mostly in the form of p85α, and is also responsible for producing splice isoforms, p55α, and p50α. Each of the *Pik3r1* gene products can also be expressed with or without a spliced 24 nucleotide insert resulting in 8 additional in-frame amino acids [143]. While p85α is expressed ubiquitously, p55α and p50α are expressed primarily in skeletal muscle and liver, respectively. *Pik3r2* produces p85β and accounts for roughly 20% of the regulatory subunits in most cells [144], though this percentage may actually be higher based on recent studies using mass spectroscopy [145]. *Pik3r3* encodes p55PIK, which is similar in structure to p55α, but is expressed at very low levels in most tissues [146].

The p85, and indeed all Class IA regulatory subunits can bind, stabilize and inhibits the p110 catalytic subunit until RTK activation [118]. This mechanism occurs through the two SH2 domains in the C-terminus of the molecule. Between the two SH2 domains is a rigid alpha-coil structure called the inter-SH2 (iSH2) domain. In addition to normal phosphotyrosine binding, the N-terminal SH2 inhibits p110 in the basal state, as explained earlier (see sections above: p110 as a proto-oncogene). The binding of p85–p110 is facilitated by the interaction between the iSH2 domain of p85 and the ABD, helical and C2 domains of p110 [129].

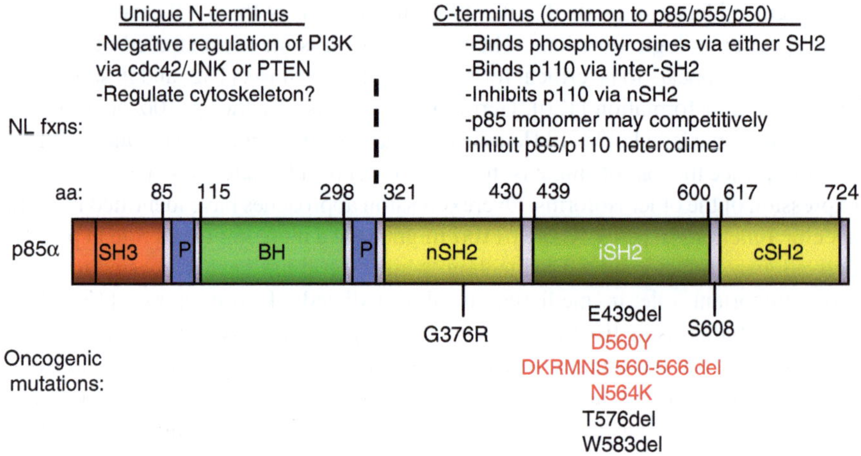

Fig. 2.6 Structure, functions and known oncogenic mutations of p85. Structural features and the Class IA regulatory subunits of PI3K (p85). All regulatory subunits (p85/55/p50) share a common C-terminus, but p85 has a unique N-terminus with an SH3 domain (binds proline-rich domains), two proline-rich domains and a BH (*bcr*-homology). The BH domain is similar in structure to the Rho-GTPase activating protein (GAP) domain of the breakpoint cluster region (bcr) protein and can bind activated cdc42, but has no intrinsic GAP activity because it lacks certain conserved residues in the switch domain. The N-terminal SH2 domain (nSH2) and C-terminal SH2 domains both bind phosphotyrosines, but the nSH2 along with the interSH2 (iSH2) bind p110 and inhibit the intrinsic activity of the kinase. *nSH2* N-terminal SH2 domain; *cSH2* C-terminal SH2 domain; *iSH2* inter-SH2 domain; *BH* bcr homology domain; *P* proline rich domain; *SH3 src* homology domain 3

Oncogenic mutations in p85 occur when p85 is prevented from inhibiting p110, leading to unchecked PI3K activity [147]. The gliobastoma multiforme genome revealed that Pik3r1 was one of the most frequented mutated genes leading to these devastating cancers [128]. The mutations occur chiefly within the iSH2 domain, as depicted in Fig. 2.6. Thus, the general mechanism of these mutations is posited to be the disruption of the inhibitory interaction between p85 and p110 mediated via the N-terminal SH2 domain (nSH2) or the inter-SH2 domain, since these two domains are required for the basal inhibition of p110 by p85. Interestingly, deletion mutations of the iSH2 domain in a murine lymphoma model [148], as well as in human ovarian cancer, colon cancer [149] have demonstrated oncogenicity.

The p85 Subunit as a Negative Regulator of Growth Factor Signaling

Human data indicates that p85 may also act as a tumor suppressor in vivo. For instance, a functional missense mutation in *Pik3r1* that results in hypomorphic p85 expression [150] has been strongly linked to colon cancer [151]. *Pik3r1* is located on human chromosome 5q13, a region that is commonly deleted in cancers that utilize the PI3K pathways for growth, such as breast [152], ovary [153], thyroid [154], stomach [155] and liver [156]. These deletions are often heterozygous, thus, if native p85 does indeed act as a tumor suppressor, then it must result from a loss of heterozygosity mechanism.

Knockout studies have suggested that p85 is a potent negative regulator of growth factor signaling [141] (Fig. 2.6). Mice with heterozygous deletion of *Pik3rl* [157], the gene encoding p85α and its shorter isoforms p55α and p50α as well as mice with a liver-specific knockout of *Pik3r1* (L-Pik3r1KO) display increased hepatic Akt activation and improved insulin sensitivity despite an overall decrease in PI3K activity [158]. In addition, mice that are heterozygous for both *Pik3r1* and *Pten* display increased Akt and S6 activation, and a twofold increase of intestinal neoplasia compared to *Pten* heterozygotes alone [159].

What could account for this seemingly contradictory set of functions of p85? The mechanism of this negative regulation by the p85 monomer in these situations appear to be multiple. We and others have previously shown that in most cells there is a stiochometric imbalance between p85 and p110, with the former being in excess of the latter [160, 161]. This imbalance results in a net inhibition of binding of the p85–p110 heterodimer to receptor phosphotyrosines [160]. The p85 monomer also has significant effects independent of its regulation of the p110, including the sequestration of IRS proteins [162] and positive regulation of PTEN function [158] (for a review, please see [1]).

We are currently investigating the extent to which reduction of *Pik3r1* alone can function to modify tumor growth and development in vivo. In mice with liver specific deletion of *Pik3r1* (L-Pik3r1KO), over 85% develop hepatocellular carcinoma by 14 months of age, often with aggressive characteristics including lung metastases (Taniguchi and Kahn, unpublished data). The formation of these liver tumors correlates with increased levels of PIP_3, increased Akt activation, increased PTEN phosphorylation and decreased PTEN protein expression. Reviewing cancer databases, we also find that p85α expression is reduced in several human cancers, including prostate, lung, breast and hepatocellular carcinoma (Oncomine database, Taniguchi and Kahn, unpublished data). Thus, *Pik3r1* haploinsufficiency may have a role in human oncogenesis, resulting in decreased Pik3r1 mRNA and protein in many types of human cancers.

Conclusion

The insulin/IGF-1 signaling pathway is a powerful, evolutionarily conserved set of signals that controls metabolism, cell differentiation and growth of an organism. Not surprisingly, the dysregulation or mutation of any of the components of this pathway can lead to oncogenesis. In this chapter, we reviewed how the insulin/IGF-1 pathway can be thought of in terms of a "critical node" model, which allows us to better appreciate the different biological effects of the various molecular isoforms and their roles in cancer. These knowledge gained from multiple knockout and knockdown experiments have led us to understand how each of these nodes – the receptors, the insulin substrate receptors, and the two components of PI3K may also be potential chemotherapeutic targets.

Clinical trials of IGF-1 receptor inhibitors have proved promising and may be useful in treatment of cancers of the breast, lung, prostate, liver and pancreas [163]. While no approach has yet been found for clinically targeting IRS-1 or IRS-2, the targeting of PI3K, especially p110 may revolutionize cancer treatment. The p110α subunit appears to a significant role in growth factor signaling, both for metabolism and growth. The trade-off for targeting p110α may be the development of diabetes, as we and others have shown p110α to be critical for metabolic homeostasis. However, the careful dissection of the PI3K pathways revealed that p110β may play a larger role in certain forms of cancer (prostate). Thus, targeting p110β could provide an effective chemotherapeutic without being overtly diabetogenic.

The information gleaned from understanding these signaling nodes also provides a wealth of information for developing novel targets. Currently, many of the kinase targets are ATP-binding domains, which often target multiple kinases of similar ilk [164]. For instance, SF-1226, a PI3K inhibitor currently in clinical trials, inhibits not only Class I PI3K, but mTOR, DNA-PK, PLK-1, CK2, ATM, and PIM-1. A solution to this may be to develop molecules to the helical domain of p110, which could mimic the inhibitory effects of p85 on p110. Such a molecule may be more unique to p110 since it does not target the kinase active site, and might thus provide more specificity. It is clear that we are just beginning capitalize on decades of research on the insulin/IGF-1 signaling pathway to treat human cancer. Hopefully, study in this area will continue to provide insight into the basic science of tumors and to the clinical management of patients with cancer.

References

1. Taniguchi CM, Emanuelli B, Kahn CR (2006) Critical nodes in signalling pathways: insights into insulin action. Nat Rev Mol Cell Biol 7:85–96
2. Avruch J (1998) Insulin signal transduction through protein kinase cascades. Mol Cell Biochem 182:31–48
3. Barone BB, Yeh HC, Snyder CF, Peairs KS, Stein KB et al (2008) Long-term all-cause mortality in cancer patients with preexisting diabetes mellitus: a systematic review and meta-analysis. JAMA 300:2754–2764
4. Whitlock G, Lewington S, Sherliker P, Clarke R, Emberson J et al (2009) Body-mass index and cause-specific mortality in 900,000 adults: collaborative analyses of 57 prospective studies. Lancet 373:1083–1096
5. Renehan AG, Tyson M, Egger M, Heller RF, Zwahlen M (2008) Body-mass index and incidence of cancer: a systematic review and meta-analysis of prospective observational studies. Lancet 371:569–578
6. Vairaktaris E, Spyridonidou S, Goutzanis L, Vylliotis A, Lazaris A et al (2007) Diabetes and oral oncogenesis. Anticancer Res 27:4185–4193
7. Wunderlich FT, Luedde T, Singer S, Schmidt-Supprian M, Baumgartl J et al (2008) Hepatic NF-kappa B essential modulator deficiency prevents obesity-induced insulin resistance but synergizes with high-fat feeding in tumorigenesis. Proc Natl Acad Sci USA 105:1297–1302

8. Zhang B, Roth RA (1992) The insulin receptor-related receptor. Tissue expression, ligand binding specificity, and signaling capabilities. J Biol Chem 267:18320–18328
9. Becker AB, Roth RA (1990) Insulin receptor structure and function in normal and pathological conditions. Annu Rev Med 41:99–115
10. Hedo JA, Kahn CR, Hayashi M, Yamada KM, Kasuga M (1983) Biosynthesis and glycosylation of the insulin receptor. Evidence for a single polypeptide precursor of the two major subunits. J Biol Chem 258:10020–10026
11. Baron V, Kaliman P, Gautier N, Van Obberghen E (1992) The insulin receptor activation process involves localized conformational changes. J Biol Chem 267:23290–23294
12. Ablooglu AJ, Kohanski RA (2001) Activation of the insulin receptor's kinase domain changes the rate-determining step of substrate phosphorylation. Biochemistry 40:504–513
13. Goren HJ, White MF, Kahn CR (1987) Separate domains of the insulin receptor contain sites of autophosphorylation and tyrosine kinase activity. Biochemistry 26:2374–2382
14. Desbois-Mouthon C, Sert-Langeron C, Magre J, Oreal E, Blivet MJ et al (1996) Deletion of Asn281 in the alpha-subunit of the human insulin receptor causes constitutive activation of the receptor and insulin desensitization. J Clin Endocrinol Metab 81:719–727
15. Elchebly M, Payette P, Michaliszyn E, Cromlish W, Collins S et al (1999) Increased insulin sensitivity and obesity resistance in mice lacking the protein tyrosine phosphatase-1B gene. Science 283:1544–1548
16. Klaman LD, Boss O, Peroni OD, Kim JK, Martino JL et al (2000) Increased energy expenditure, decreased adiposity, and tissue-specific insulin sensitivity in protein-tyrosine phosphatase 1B-deficient mice. Mol Cell Biol 20:5479–5489
17. Zinker BA, Rondinone CM, Trevillyan JM, Gum RJ, Clampit JE et al (2002) PTP1B antisense oligonucleotide lowers PTP1B protein, normalizes blood glucose, and improves insulin sensitivity in diabetic mice. Proc Natl Acad Sci USA 99:11357–11362
18. Rondinone CM, Trevillyan JM, Clampit J, Gum RJ, Berg C et al (2002) Protein tyrosine phosphatase 1B reduction regulates adiposity and expression of genes involved in lipogenesis. Diabetes 51:2405–2411
19. Gum RJ, Gaede LL, Koterski SL, Heindel M, Clampit JE et al (2003) Reduction of protein tyrosine phosphatase 1B increases insulin-dependent signaling in ob/ob mice. Diabetes 52:21–28
20. Ueki K, Kondo T, Tseng YH, Kahn CR (2004) Central role of suppressors of cytokine signaling proteins in hepatic steatosis, insulin resistance, and the metabolic syndrome in the mouse. Proc Natl Acad Sci USA 101:10422–10427
21. Ueki K, Kondo T, Kahn CR (2004) Suppressor of cytokine signaling 1 (SOCS-1) and SOCS-3 cause insulin resistance through inhibition of tyrosine phosphorylation of insulin receptor substrate proteins by discrete mechanisms. Mol Cell Biol 24:5434–5446
22. Emanuelli B, Peraldi P, Filloux C, Sawka-Verhelle D, Hilton D et al (2000) SOCS-3 is an insulin-induced negative regulator of insulin signaling. J Biol Chem 275:15958–15991
23. Emanuelli B, Peraldi P, Filloux C, Chavey C, Freidinger K et al (2001) SOCS-3 inhibits insulin signaling and is up-regulated in response to tumor necrosis factor-alpha in the adipose tissue of obese mice. J Biol Chem 276:47944–47949
24. Wick KR, Werner ED, Langlais P, Ramos FJ, Dong LQ et al (2003) Grb10 inhibits insulin-stimulated insulin receptor substrate (IRS)-phosphatidylinositol 3-kinase/Akt signaling pathway by disrupting the association of IRS-1/IRS-2 with the insulin receptor. J Biol Chem 278:8460–8467
25. Dong H, Maddux BA, Altomonte J, Meseck M, Accili D et al (2005) Increased hepatic levels of the insulin receptor inhibitor, PC-1/NPP1, induce insulin resistance and glucose intolerance. Diabetes 54:367–372
26. Sutherland KD, Lindeman GJ, Visvader JE (2007) Knocking off SOCS genes in the mammary gland. Cell Cycle 6:799–803
27. McClain DA (1992) Mechanism and role of insulin receptor endocytosis. Am J Med Sci 304:192–201
28. Friedman JE, Ishizuka T, Liu S, Farrell CJ, Bedol D et al (1997) Reduced insulin receptor signaling in the obese spontaneously hypertensive Koletsky rat. Am J Physiol 273:E1014–E1023

29. Mathieu MC, Clark GM, Allred DC, Goldfine ID, Vigneri R (1997) Insulin receptor expression and clinical outcome in node-negative breast cancer. Proc Assoc Am Physicians 109:565–571
30. Sesti G, Tullio AN, D'Alfonso R, Napolitano ML, Marini MA et al (1994) Tissue-specific expression of two alternatively spliced isoforms of the human insulin receptor protein. Acta Diabetol 31:59–65
31. Pashmforoush M, Yoshimasa Y, Steiner DF (1994) Exon 11 enhances insulin binding affinity and tyrosine kinase activity of the human insulin proreceptor. J Biol Chem 269:32639–32648
32. Vogt B, Carrascosa JM, Ermel B, Ullrich A, Haring HU (1991) The two isotypes of the human insulin receptor (HIR-A and HIR-B) follow different internalization kinetics. Biochem Biophys Res Commun 177:1013–1018
33. Kosaki A, Pillay TS, Xu L, Webster NJ (1995) The B isoform of the insulin receptor signals more efficiently than the A isoform in HepG2 cells. J Biol Chem 270:20816–20823
34. Frasca F, Pandini G, Scalia P, Sciacca L, Mineo R et al (1999) Insulin receptor isoform A, a newly recognized, high-affinity insulin-like growth factor II receptor in fetal and cancer cells. Mol Cell Biol 19:3278–3288
35. Yamaguchi Y, Flier JS, Yokota A, Benecke H, Backer JM et al (1991) Functional properties of two naturally occurring isoforms of the human insulin receptor in Chinese hamster ovary cells. Endocrinology 129:2058–2066
36. Vella V, Pandini G, Sciacca L, Mineo R, Vigneri R et al (2002) A novel autocrine loop involving IGF-II and the insulin receptor isoform-A stimulates growth of thyroid cancer. J Clin Endocrinol Metab 87:245–254
37. Leibiger B, Leibiger IB, Moede T, Kemper S, Kulkarni RN et al (2001) Selective insulin signaling through A and B insulin receptors regulates transcription of insulin and glucokinase genes in pancreatic beta cells. Mol Cell 7:559–570
38. Ohlsson C, Kley N, Werner H, LeRoith D (1998) p53 regulates insulin-like growth factor-I (IGF-I) receptor expression and IGF-I-induced tyrosine phosphorylation in an osteosarcoma cell line: interaction between p53 and Sp1. Endocrinology 139:1101–1107
39. Girnita L, Girnita A, Brodin B, Xie Y, Nilsson G et al (2000) Increased expression of insulin-like growth factor I receptor in malignant cells expressing aberrant p53: functional impact. Cancer Res 60:5278–5283
40. Frasca F, Pandini G, Sciacca L, Pezzino V, Squatrito S et al (2008) The role of insulin receptors and IGF-I receptors in cancer and other diseases. Arch Physiol Biochem 114:23–37
41. Sun XJ, Rothenberg P, Kahn CR, Backer JM, Araki E et al (1991) Structure of the insulin receptor substrate IRS-1 defines a unique signal transduction protein. Nature 352:73–77
42. Sun XJ, Wang LM, Zhang Y, Yenush L, Myers MG Jr et al (1995) Role of IRS-2 in insulin and cytokine signalling. Nature 377:173–177
43. Lavan BE, Lane WS, Lienhard GE (1997) The 60-kDa phosphotyrosine protein in insulin-treated adipocytes is a new member of the insulin receptor substrate family. J Biol Chem 272:11439–11443
44. Fantin VR, Sparling JD, Slot JW, Keller SR, Lienhard GE et al (1998) Characterization of insulin receptor substrate 4 in human embryonic kidney 293 cells. J Biol Chem 273:10726–10732
45. Cai D, Dhe-Paganon S, Melendez PA, Lee J, Shoelson SE (2003) Two new substrates in insulin signaling, IRS5/DOK4 and IRS6/DOK5. J Biol Chem 278:25323–25330
46. Lehr S, Kotzka J, Herkner A, Sikmann A, Meyer HE et al (2000) Identification of major tyrosine phosphorylation sites in the human insulin receptor substrate Gab-1 by insulin receptor kinase in vitro. Biochemistry 39:10898–10907
47. Wick MJ, Dong LQ, Hu D, Langlais P, Liu F (2001) Insulin receptor-mediated p62dok tyrosine phosphorylation at residues 362 and 398 plays distinct roles for binding GTPase-activating protein and Nck and is essential for inhibiting insulin-stimulated activation of Ras and Akt. J Biol Chem 276:42843–42850
48. Baumann CA, Ribon V, Kanzaki M, Thurmond DC, Mora S et al (2000) CAP defines a second signalling pathway required for insulin-stimulated glucose transport. Nature 407:202–207
49. Gustafson TA, He W, Craparo A, Schaub CD, O'Neill TJ (1995) Phosphotyrosine-dependent interaction of SHC and insulin receptor substrate 1 with the NPEY motif of the insulin receptor via a novel non-SH2 domain. Mol Cell Biol 15:2500–2508

50. Björnholm M, He AR, Attersand A, Lake S, Liu SC et al (2002) Absence of functional insulin receptor substrate-3 (IRS-3) gene in humans. Diabetologia 45:1697–702
51. Virkamaki A, Ueki K, Kahn CR (1999) Protein-protein interaction in insulin signaling and the molecular mechanisms of insulin resistance. J Clin Invest 103:931–943
52. Skolnik EY, Lee CH, Batzer A, Vicentini LM, Zhou M et al (1993) The SH2/SH3 domain-containing protein GRB2 interacts with tyrosine-phosphorylated IRS1 and Shc: implications for insulin control of ras signalling. EMBO J 12:1929–1936
53. Myers MG Jr, Mendez R, Shi P, Pierce JH, Rhoads R et al (1998) The COOH-terminal tyrosine phosphorylation sites on IRS-1 bind SHP-2 and negatively regulate insulin signaling. J Biol Chem 273:26908–26914
54. Sun XJ, Pons S, Asano T, Myers MG Jr, Glasheen E et al (1996) The Fyn tyrosine kinase binds Irs-1 and forms a distinct signaling complex during insulin stimulation. J Biol Chem 271:10583–10587
55. Algenstaedt P, Antonetti DA, Yaffe MB, Kahn CR (1997) Insulin receptor substrate proteins create a link between the tyrosine phosphorylation cascade and the Ca^{2+}-ATPases in muscle and heart. J Biol Chem 272:23696–23702
56. Fei ZL, D'Ambrosio C, Li S, Surmacz E, Baserga R (1995) Association of insulin receptor substrate 1 with simian virus 40 large T antigen. Mol Cell Biol 15:4232–4239
57. Zick Y (2005) Ser/Thr phosphorylation of IRS proteins: a molecular basis for insulin resistance. Sci STKE 2005(268):pe4
58. Li J, DeFea K, Roth RA (1999) Modulation of insulin receptor substrate-1 tyrosine phosphorylation by an Akt/phosphatidylinositol 3-kinase pathway. J Biol Chem 274:9351–9356
59. Bard-Chapeau EA, Hevener AL, Long S, Zhang EE, Olefsky JM et al (2005) Deletion of Gab1 in the liver leads to enhanced glucose tolerance and improved hepatic insulin action. Nat Med 11:567–571
60. Harrington LS, Findlay GM, Gray A, Tolkacheva T, Wigfield S et al (2004) The TSC1-2 tumor suppressor controls insulin-PI3K signaling via regulation of IRS proteins. J Cell Biol 166:213–223
61. Aguirre V, Uchida T, Yenush L, Davis R, White MF (2000) The c-Jun NH(2)-terminal kinase promotes insulin resistance during association with insulin receptor substrate-1 and phosphorylation of Ser(307). J Biol Chem 275:9047–9054
62. Hirosumi J, Tuncman G, Chang L, Gorgun CZ, Uysal KT et al (2002) A central role for JNK in obesity and insulin resistance. Nature 420:333–336
63. Werner ED, Lee J, Hansen L, Yuan M, Shoelson SE (2004) Insulin resistance due to phosphorylation of insulin receptor substrate-1 at serine 302. J Biol Chem 279:35298–35305
64. Craparo A, Freund R, Gustafson TA (1997) 14-3-3 (epsilon) interacts with the insulin-like growth factor I receptor and insulin receptor substrate I in a phosphoserine-dependent manner. J Biol Chem 272:11663–11669
65. Tirosh A, Potashnik R, Bashan N, Rudich A (1999) Oxidative stress disrupts insulin-induced cellular redistribution of insulin receptor substrate-1 and phosphatidylinositol 3-kinase in 3T3-L1 adipocytes. A putative cellular mechanism for impaired protein kinase B activation and GLUT4 translocation. J Biol Chem 274:10595–10602
66. Pederson TM, Kramer DL, Rondinone CM (2001) Serine/threonine phosphorylation of IRS-1 triggers its degradation: possible regulation by tyrosine phosphorylation. Diabetes 50:24–31
67. Giraud J, Leshan R, Lee YH, White MF (2004) Nutrient-dependent and insulin-stimulated phosphorylation of insulin receptor substrate-1 on serine 302 correlates with increased insulin signaling. J Biol Chem 279:3447–3454
68. Furukawa N, Ongusaha P, Jahng WJ, Araki K, Choi CS et al (2005) Role of Rho-kinase in regulation of insulin action and glucose homeostasis. Cell Metab 2:119–129
69. Paz K, Liu YF, Shorer H, Hemi R, LeRoith D et al (1999) Phosphorylation of insulin receptor substrate-1 (IRS-1) by protein kinase B positively regulates IRS-1 function. J Biol Chem 274:28816–28822
70. Sesti G, Federici M, Hribal ML, Lauro D, Sbraccia P et al (2001) Defects of the insulin receptor substrate (IRS) system in human metabolic disorders. FASEB J 15:2099–2111

71. Araki E, Lipes MA, Patti M-E, Bruning JC, Haag BL III et al (1994) Alternative pathway of insulin signlaing in targeted disruption of the IRS-1 gene. Nature 372:186–190
72. Kubota N, Terauchi Y, Tobe K, Yano W, Suzuki R et al (2004) Insulin receptor substrate 2 plays a crucial role in beta cells and the hypothalamus. J Clin Invest 114:917–927
73. Withers DJ, Gutierrez JS, Towery H, Burks DJ, Ren JM et al (1998) Disruption of IRS-2 causes type 2 diabetes in mice. Nature 391:900–904
74. Tseng YH, Butte AJ, Kokkotou E, Yechoor VK, Taniguchi CM et al (2005) Prediction of preadipocyte differentiation by gene expression reveals role of insulin receptor substrates and necdin. Nat Cell Biol 7:601–611
75. Miki H, Yamauchi T, Suzuki R, Komeda K, Tsuchida A et al (2001) Essential role of insulin receptor substrate 1 (IRS-1) and IRS-2 in adipocyte differentiation. Mol Cell Biol 21:2521–2532
76. Chang Q, Li Y, White MF, Fletcher JA, Xiao S (2002) Constitutive activation of insulin receptor substrate 1 is a frequent event in human tumors: therapeutic implications. Cancer Res 62:6035–6038
77. Koda M, Sulkowska M, Kanczuga-Koda L, Sulkowski S (2005) Expression of insulin receptor substrate 1 in primary breast cancer and lymph node metastases. J Clin Pathol 58:645–649
78. Jackson JG, White MF, Yee D (1998) Insulin receptor substrate-1 is the predominant signaling molecule activated by insulin-like growth factor-I, insulin, and interleukin-4 in estrogen receptor-positive human breast cancer cells. J Biol Chem 273:9994–10003
79. Rocha RL, Hilsenbeck SG, Jackson JG, VanDenBerg CL, Weng C et al (1997) Insulin-like growth factor binding protein-3 and insulin receptor substrate-1 in breast cancer: correlation with clinical parameters and disease-free survival. Clin Cancer Res 3:103–109
80. Dearth RK, Cui X, Kim HJ, Kuiatse I, Lawrence NA et al (2006) Mammary tumorigenesis and metastasis caused by overexpression of insulin receptor substrate 1 (IRS-1) or IRS-2. Mol Cell Biol 26:9302–9314
81. Asano T, Yao Y, Shin S, McCubrey J, Abbruzzese JL et al (2005) Insulin receptor substrate is a mediator of phosphoinositide 3-kinase activation in quiescent pancreatic cancer cells. Cancer Res 65:9164–9168
82. Longato L, de la Monte S, Kuzushita N, Horimoto M, Rogers AB et al (2009) Overexpression of insulin receptor substrate-1 and hepatitis Bx genes causes premalignant alterations in the liver. Hepatology 49:1935–1943
83. Tanaka S, Wands JR (1996) Insulin receptor substrate 1 overexpression in human hepatocellular carcinoma cells prevents transforming growth factor beta1-induced apoptosis. Cancer Res 56:3391–3394
84. Boissan M, Beurel E, Wendum D, Rey C, Lecluse Y et al (2005) Overexpression of insulin receptor substrate-2 in human and murine hepatocellular carcinoma. Am J Pathol 167:869–877
85. Tanaka S, Wands JR (1996) A carboxy-terminal truncated insulin receptor substrate-1 dominant negative protein reverses the human hepatocellular carcinoma malignant phenotype. J Clin Invest 98:2100–2108
86. Knowlden JM, Jones HE, Barrow D, Gee JM, Nicholson RI et al (2008) Insulin receptor substrate-1 involvement in epidermal growth factor receptor and insulin-like growth factor receptor signalling: implication for Gefitinib ('Iressa') response and resistance. Breast Cancer Res Treat 111:79–91
87. Citri A, Yarden Y (2006) EGF-ERBB signalling: towards the systems level. Nat Rev Mol Cell Biol 7:505–516
88. Guix M, Faber AC, Wang SE, Olivares MG, Song Y et al (2008) Acquired resistance to EGFR tyrosine kinase inhibitors in cancer cells is mediated by loss of IGF-binding proteins. J Clin Invest 118:2609–2619
89. Nagle JA, Ma Z, Byrne MA, White MF, Shaw LM (2004) Involvement of insulin receptor substrate 2 in mammary tumor metastasis. Mol Cell Biol 24:9726–9735
90. Szabolcs M, Keniry M, Simpson L, Reid LJ, Koujak S et al (2009) Irs2 inactivation suppresses tumor progression in Pten+/- mice. Am J Pathol 174:276–286

91. Laustsen PG, Michael MD, Crute BE, Cohen SE, Ueki K et al (2002) Lipoatrophic diabetes in Irs1(–/–)/Irs3(–/–) double knockout mice. Genes Dev 16:3213–3222
92. Karrman K, Kjeldsen E, Lassen C, Isaksson M, Davidsson J et al (2009) The t(X;7)(q22;q34) in paediatric T-cell acute lymphoblastic leukaemia results in overexpression of the insulin receptor substrate 4 gene through illegitimate recombination with the T-cell receptor beta locus. Br J Haematol 144:546–551
93. Fantin VR, Wang Q, Lienhard GE, Keller SR (2000) Mice lacking insulin receptor substrate 4 exhibit mild defects in growth, reproduction, and glucose homeostasis. Am J Physiol Endocrinol Metab 278:E127–E133
94. Taniguchi CM, Ueki K, Kahn R (2005) Complementary roles of IRS-1 and IRS-2 in the hepatic regulation of metabolism. J Clin Invest 115:718–727
95. Sun XJ, Pons S, Wang LM, Zhang Y, Yenush L et al (1997) The IRS-2 gene on murine chromosome 8 encodes a unique signaling adapter for insulin and cytokine action. Mol Endocrinol 11:251–262
96. Inoue G, Cheatham B, Emkey R, Kahn CR (1998) Dynamics of insulin signaling in 3T3-L1 adipocytes. Differential compartmentalization and trafficking of insulin receptor substrate (IRS)-1 and IRS-2. J Biol Chem 273:11548–11555
97. Sun H, Tu X, Prisco M, Wu A, Casiburi I et al (2003) Insulin-like growth factor I receptor signaling and nuclear translocation of insulin receptor substrates 1 and 2. Mol Endocrinol 17:472–486
98. Ogihara T, Shin BC, Anai M, Katagiri H, Inukai K et al (1997) Insulin receptor substrate (IRS)-2 is dephosphorylated more rapidly than IRS-1 via its association with phosphatidylinositol 3-kinase in skeletal muscle cells. J Biol Chem 272:12868–12873
99. Sawka-Verhelle D, Tartare-Deckert S, White MF, Van Obberghen E (1996) Insulin receptor substrate-2 binds to the insulin receptor through its phosphotyrosine-binding domain and through a newly identified domain comprising amino acids 591–786. J Biol Chem 271:5980–5983
100. D'Ambrosio C, Keller SR, Morrione A, Lienhard GE, Baserga R et al (1995) Transforming potential of the insulin receptor substrate 1. Cell Growth Differ 6:557–562
101. DeAngelis T, Chen J, Wu A, Prisco M, Baserga R (2006) Transformation by the simian virus 40 T antigen is regulated by IGF-I receptor and IRS-1 signaling. Oncogene 25:32–42
102. Tseng YH, Kriauciunas KM, Kokkotou E, Kahn CR (2004) Differential roles of insulin receptor substrates in brown adipocyte differentiation. Mol Cell Biol 24:1918–1929
103. Myers MG Jr, Backer JM, Sun XJ, Shoelson S, Hu P et al (1992) IRS-1 activates phosphatidylinositol 3′-kinase by associating with src homology 2 domains of p85. Proc Natl Acad Sci USA 89:10350–10354
104. Cheatham B, Vlahos CJ, Cheatham L, Wang L, Blenis J et al (1994) Phosphatidylinositol 3-kinase activation is required for insulin stimulation of pp 70 S6 kinase, DNA synthesis, and glucose transporter translocation. Mol Cell Biol 14:4902–4911
105. Shepherd PR, Withers DJ, Siddle K (1998) Phosphoinositide 3-kinase: the key switch mechanism in insulin signalling. Biochem J 333(Pt 3):471–490
106. Alessi DR, James SR, Downes CP, Holmes AB, Gaffney PR et al (1997) Characterization of a 3-phosphoinositide-dependent protein kinase which phosphorylates and activates protein kinase Balpha. Curr Biol 7:261–269
107. Le Good JA, Ziegler WH, Parekh DB, Alessi DR, Cohen P et al (1998) Protein kinase C isotypes controlled by phosphoinositide 3-kinase through the protein kinase PDK1. Science 281:2042–2045
108. Woodgett JR (2005) Recent advances in the protein kinase B signaling pathway. Curr Opin Cell Biol 17:150–157
109. Sarbassov DD, Guertin DA, Ali SM, Sabatini DM (2005) Phosphorylation and regulation of Akt/PKB by the rictor-mTOR complex. Science 307:1098–1101
110. Maehama T, Dixon JE (1999) PTEN: a tumour suppressor that functions as a phospholipid phosphatase. Trends Cell Biol 9:125–128
111. Nakashima N, Sharma PM, Imamura T, Bookstein R, Olefsky JM (2000) The tumor suppressor PTEN negatively regulates insulin signaling in 3T3-L1 adipocytes. J Biol Chem 275:12889–12895

112. Yao YJ, Ping XL, Zhang H, Chen FF, Lee PK et al (1999) PTEN/MMAC1 mutations in hepatocellular carcinomas. Oncogene 18:3181–3185
113. Schmitz KJ, Wohlschlaeger J, Lang H, Sotiropoulos GC, Malago M et al (2008) Activation of the ERK and AKT signalling pathway predicts poor prognosis in hepatocellular carcinoma and ERK activation in cancer tissue is associated with hepatitis C virus infection. J Hepatol 48:83–90
114. Vanhaesebroeck B, Welham MJ, Kotani K, Stein R, Warne PH et al (1997) P110delta, a novel phosphoinositide 3-kinase in leukocytes. Proc Natl Acad Sci USA 94:4330–4335
115. Rodriguez-Viciana P, Warne PH, Dhand R, Vanhaesebroeck B, Gout I et al (1994) Phosphatidylinositol-3-OH kinase as a direct target of Ras. Nature 370:527–532
116. Rizo J, Sudhof TC (1998) C2-domains, structure and function of a universal Ca^{2+}-binding domain. J Biol Chem 273:15879–15882
117. Huang CH, Mandelker D, Schmidt-Kittler O, Samuels Y, Velculescu VE et al (2007) The structure of a human p110alpha/p85alpha complex elucidates the effects of oncogenic PI3Kalpha mutations. Science 318:1744–1748
118. Yu J, Zhang Y, McIlroy J, Rordorf-Nikolic T, Orr GA et al (1998) Regulation of the p85/p110 phosphatidylinositol 3'-kinase: stabilization and inhibition of the p110alpha catalytic subunit by the p85 regulatory subunit. Mol Cell Biol 18:1379–1387
119. Chang HW, Aoki M, Fruman D, Auger KR, Bellacosa A et al (1997) Transformation of chicken cells by the gene encoding the catalytic subunit of PI 3-kinase. Science 276:1848–1850
120. Zhao JJ, Liu Z, Wang L, Shin E, Loda MF et al (2005) The oncogenic properties of mutant p110alpha and p110beta phosphatidylinositol 3-kinases in human mammary epithelial cells. Proc Natl Acad Sci USA 102:18443–18448
121. Miyake T, Yoshino K, Enomoto T, Takata T, Ugaki H et al (2008) PIK3CA gene mutations and amplifications in uterine cancers, identified by methods that avoid confounding by PIK3CA pseudogene sequences. Cancer Lett 261:120–126
122. Samuels Y, Wang Z, Bardelli A, Silliman N, Ptak J et al (2004) High frequency of mutations of the PIK3CA gene in human cancers. Science 304:554
123. Wu G, Xing M, Mambo E, Huang X, Liu J et al (2005) Somatic mutation and gain of copy number of PIK3CA in human breast cancer. Breast Cancer Res 7:R609–R616
124. Campbell IG, Russell SE, Choong DY, Montgomery KG, Ciavarella ML et al (2004) Mutation of the PIK3CA gene in ovarian and breast cancer. Cancer Res 64:7678–7681
125. Zhang A, Maner S, Betz R, Angstrom T, Stendahl U et al (2002) Genetic alterations in cervical carcinomas: frequent low-level amplifications of oncogenes are associated with human papillomavirus infection. Int J Cancer 101:427–433
126. Lee JW, Soung YH, Kim SY, Lee HW, Park WS et al (2005) PIK3CA gene is frequently mutated in breast carcinomas and hepatocellular carcinomas. Oncogene 24:1477–1480
127. Guo XN, Rajput A, Rose R, Hauser J, Beko A et al (2007) Mutant PIK3CA-bearing colon cancer cells display increased metastasis in an orthotopic model. Cancer Res 67:5851–5858
128. McLendon R, Friedman A, Bigner D, Van Meir EG, Brat DJ et al (2008) Comprehensive genomic characterization defines human glioblastoma genes and core pathways. Nature 455(7216):1061–1068
129. Miled N, Yan Y, Hon WC, Perisic O, Zvelebil M et al (2007) Mechanism of two classes of cancer mutations in the phosphoinositide 3-kinase catalytic subunit. Science 317:239–242
130. Denley A, Kang S, Karst U, Vogt PK (2008) Oncogenic signaling of class I PI3K isoforms. Oncogene 27:2561–2574
131. Engelman JA, Chen L, Tan X, Crosby K, Guimaraes AR et al (2008) Effective use of PI3K and MEK inhibitors to treat mutant Kras G12D and PIK3CA H1047R murine lung cancers. Nat Med 14:1351–1356
132. Foukas LC, Claret M, Pearce W, Okkenhaug K, Meek S et al (2006) Critical role for the p110alpha phosphoinositide-3-OH kinase in growth and metabolic regulation. Nature 441:366–370
133. Bi L, Okabe I, Bernard DJ, Wynshaw-Boris A, Nussbaum RL (1999) Proliferative defect and embryonic lethality in mice homozygous for a deletion in the p110alpha subunit of phosphoinositide 3-kinase. J Biol Chem 274:10963–10968

134. Bi L, Okabe I, Bernard DJ, Nussbaum RL (2002) Early embryonic lethality in mice deficient in the p110beta catalytic subunit of PI 3-kinase. Mamm Genome 13:169–172
135. Asano T, Kanda A, Katagiri H, Nawano M, Ogihara T et al (2000) p110beta is up-regulated during differentiation of 3T3-L1 cells and contributes to the highly insulin-responsive glucose transport activity. J Biol Chem 275:17671–17676
136. Siddhanta U, McIlroy J, Shah A, Zhang Y, Backer JM (1998) Distinct roles for the p110alpha and hVPS34 phosphatidylinositol 3'-kinases in vesicular trafficking, regulation of the actin cytoskeleton, and mitogenesis. J Cell Biol 143:1647–1659
137. Jia S, Liu Z, Zhang S, Liu P, Zhang L et al (2008) Essential roles of PI(3)K-p110beta in cell growth, metabolism and tumorigenesis. Nature 454:776–779
138. Knight ZA, Gonzalez B, Feldman ME, Zunder ER, Goldenberg DD et al (2006) A pharmacological map of the PI3-K family defines a role for p110alpha in insulin signaling. Cell 125:733–747
139. Graupera M, Guillermet-Guibert J, Foukas LC, Phng LK, Cain RJ et al (2008) Angiogenesis selectively requires the p110alpha isoform of PI3K to control endothelial cell migration. Nature 453:662–666
140. Wee S, Wiederschain D, Maira SM, Loo A, Miller C et al (2008) PTEN-deficient cancers depend on PIK3CB. Proc Natl Acad Sci USA 105:13057–13062
141. Luo J, Cantley LC (2005) The negative regulation of phosphoinositide 3-kinase signaling by p85 and it's implication in cancer. Cell Cycle 4:1309–1312
142. Engelman JA, Luo J, Cantley LC (2006) The evolution of phosphatidylinositol 3-kinases as regulators of growth and metabolism. Nat Rev Genet 7:606–619
143. Antonetti DA, Algenstaedt P, Kahn CR (1996) Insulin receptor substrate 1 binds two novel splice variants of the regulatory subunit of phosphatidylinositol 3-kinase in muscle and brain. Mol Cell Biol 16:2195–2203
144. Ueki K, Yballe CM, Brachmann SM, Vicent D, Watt JM et al (2002) Increased insulin sensitivity in mice lacking p85beta subunit of phosphoinositide 3-kinase. Proc Natl Acad Sci USA 99:419–424
145. Geering B, Cutillas PR, Nock G, Gharbi SI, Vanhaesebroeck B (2007) Class IA phosphoinositide 3-kinases are obligate p85-p110 heterodimers. Proc Natl Acad Sci USA 104:7809–7814
146. Zhang L, Huang J, Yang N, Greshock J, Liang S et al (2007) Integrative genomic analysis of phosphatidylinositol 3'-kinase family identifies PIK3R3 as a potential therapeutic target in epithelial ovarian cancer. Clin Cancer Res 13:5314–5321
147. Shekar SC, Wu H, Fu Z, Yip SC, Nagajyothi F et al (2005) Mechanism of constitutive phosphoinositide 3-kinase activation by oncogenic mutants of the p85 regulatory subunit. J Biol Chem 280:27850–27855
148. Jimenez C, Jones DR, Rodriguez-Viciana P, Gonzalez-Garcia A, Leonardo E et al (1998) Identification and characterization of a new oncogene derived from the regulatory subunit of phosphoinositide 3-kinase. EMBO J 17:743–753
149. Philp AJ, Campbell IG, Leet C, Vincan E, Rockman SP et al (2001) The phosphatidylinositol 3'-kinase p85alpha gene is an oncogene in human ovarian and colon tumors. Cancer Res 61:7426–7429
150. Almind K, Delahaye L, Hansen T, Van Obberghen E, Pedersen O et al (2002) Characterization of the Met326Ile variant of phosphatidylinositol 3-kinase p85alpha. Proc Natl Acad Sci USA 99:2124–2128
151. Li L, Plummer SJ, Thompson CL, Tucker TC, Casey G (2008) Association between phosphatidylinositol 3-kinase regulatory subunit p85alpha Met326Ile genetic polymorphism and colon cancer risk. Clin Cancer Res 14:633–637
152. Richard F, Pacyna-Gengelbach M, Schluns K, Fleige B, Winzer KJ et al (2000) Patterns of chromosomal imbalances in invasive breast cancer. Int J Cancer 89:305–310
153. Tavassoli M, Steingrimsdottir H, Pierce E, Jiang X, Alagoz M et al (1996) Loss of heterozygosity on chromosome 5q in ovarian cancer is frequently accompanied by TP53 mutation and identifies a tumour suppressor gene locus at 5q13.1-21. Br J Cancer 74:115–119

154. Roque L, Rodrigues R, Pinto A, Moura-Nunes V, Soares J (2003) Chromosome imbalances in thyroid follicular neoplasms: a comparison between follicular adenomas and carcinomas. Genes Chromosom Cancer 36:292–302
155. Achille A, Baron A, Zamboni G, Di Pace C, Orlandini S et al (1998) Chromosome 5 allelic losses are early events in tumours of the papilla of Vater and occur at sites similar to those of gastric cancer. Br J Cancer 78:1653–1660
156. Katoh H, Shibata T, Kokubu A, Ojima H, Loukopoulos P et al (2005) Genetic profile of hepatocellular carcinoma revealed by array-based comparative genomic hybridization: identification of genetic indicators to predict patient outcome. J Hepatol 43:863–874
157. Mauvais-Jarvis F, Ueki K, Fruman DA, Hirshman MF, Sakamoto K et al (2002) Reduced expression of the murine p85alpha subunit of phosphoinositide 3-kinase improves insulin signaling and ameliorates diabetes. J Clin Invest 109:141–149
158. Taniguchi CM, Tran TT, Kondo T, Luo J, Ueki K et al (2006) Phosphoinositide 3-kinase regulatory subunit p85alpha suppresses insulin action via positive regulation of PTEN. Proc Natl Acad Sci USA 103:12093–12097
159. Luo J, Sobkiw CL, Logsdon NM, Watt JM, Signoretti S et al (2005) Modulation of epithelial neoplasia and lymphoid hyperplasia in PTEN+/- mice by the p85 regulatory subunits of phosphoinositide 3-kinase. Proc Natl Acad Sci USA 102:10238–10243
160. Ueki K, Fruman DA, Brachmann SM, Tseng YH, Cantley LC et al (2002) Molecular balance between the regulatory and catalytic subunits of phosphoinositide 3-kinase regulates cell signaling and survival. Mol Cell Biol 22:965–977
161. Barbour LA, Mizanoor Rahman S, Gurevich I, Leitner JW, Fischer SJ et al (2005) Increased P85alpha is a potent negative regulator of skeletal muscle insulin signaling and induces in vivo insulin resistance associated with growth hormone excess. J Biol Chem 280:37489–37494
162. Luo J, Field SJ, Lee JY, Engelman JA, Cantley LC (2005) The p85 regulatory subunit of phosphoinositide 3-kinase down-regulates IRS-1 signaling via the formation of a sequestration complex. J Cell Biol 170(3):455–464
163. Pollak M (2008) Insulin and insulin-like growth factor signalling in neoplasia. Nat Rev Cancer 8:915–928
164. Yuan TL, Cantley LC (2008) PI3K pathway alterations in cancer: variations on a theme. Oncogene 27:5497–5510

Chapter 3
The Mechanisms and Impact of Obesity and Insulin Resistance on Breast Cancer Incidence

Deborah J. Clegg

Introduction: Prevalence of Obesity

According to estimates by the International Association for the Study of Obesity provided in April 2007, approximately 40–50% of men and 25–35% of women in the EU were overweight (defined as a BMI between 25.0 and 29.9 kg/m^2), and an additional 15–25% of men and 15–25% of women were obese (BMI = 30.0 kg/m^2) (International Association for the Study of Obesity (2007) Adult overweight and obesity in the European Union). Similarly, in 2004, approximately 34.1% of the US population were overweight and about 32.2% were obese [1]. Obesity is a risk factor for several chronic diseases, most notably hypertension, type II diabetes, dyslipidemia, coronary heart disease (CHD), and accumulating evidence suggests a risk factor for certain types of cancer.

Women in the United States have among the highest breast cancer rates in the world, and breast cancer is the most common cancer among American women [1]. This is not due to increased genetic susceptibility, as less than 10% of breast cancers are attributed to gene mutations such as BRCA1. The rising rate of obesity and interactions between low-penetrance cancer-susceptibility genes and environmental factors including nutrition and lifestyle are thought to be major contributors to the increased risk for breast cancer seen in American women. The frequency of breast cancer in Western societies parallels the prevalence of consumption of diets high in fat, obesity, insulin resistance, and the prevalence of the metabolic syndrome. In spite of considerable effort by the scientific and healthcare professionals to understand and successfully treat obesity, its incidence continues to rise and the obesity-related costs to society are staggering [2, 3].

D.J. Clegg (✉)
Department of Internal Medicine, University of Texas Southwestern Medical Center, 5323 Harry Hines Blvd., Dallas, TX 75390–8854, USA
e-mail: deborah.clegg@utsouthwestern.edu

I.G. Fantus (ed.), *Insulin Resistance and Cancer: Epidemiology, Cellular and Molecular Mechanisms and Clinical Implications*, Energy Balance and Cancer 1, DOI 10.1007/978-1-4419-9911-5_3,

Obesity is associated with increased breast cancer mortality [4–6], and it is estimated that 20% of cancer deaths in women over 50 are related to excess body weight [7]. Breast cancer accounts for 31% of all cancers and 15% of cancer deaths among women in the U.S., with over 200,000 women reportedly newly diagnosed with breast cancer each year [8]. The age of onset of obesity, weight gain over time, and distribution of body fat have also been found to be important in determining the risk of breast cancer [9–11]. There is an expanding literature emphasizing the importance of stromal cells to the pathogenesis of various cancers. Adipocytes constitute the major stromal cell population in the breast microenvironment and many recent studies have implicated adipocytes as critical for both normal mammary gland morphogenesis as well as in the pathogenesis of breast cancer (reviewed [12]). This chapter will examine evidence demonstrating that the incidence of breast cancer and its mortality is linked to body weight, body fat distribution, adipocytokines, inflammation, diet, and insulin sensitivity. We will briefly discuss proposed mechanisms by which these factors combine to increase the risk and prevalence of breast cancer.

Etiology of Breast Cancer

Most of the risk factors linked to breast cancer relate to hormonal stimulation of the breast and include being female, early age of menarche, late age of menopause, nulliparity or late first full-term pregnancy, increased height, and a family history of breast cancer [13]. Circulating estrogens are synthesized in the stromal cells of the adipose tissue by enzymatic aromatization of C19 steroid androstenedione to yield estrone, and this occurs even after menopause, when ovarian production of estrogen has ceased (reviewed by Rose [14]). In fact, adipose tissue can be considered an "extraovarian tissue" where there is a conversion of estrogen to the more potent estradiol (reviewed by Rose [14, 15]), and this conversion is thought to be more prevalent in obese individuals. Obesity-related increases in circulating estrogens have been associated with an elevated breast cancer risk and enhanced progression of estrogen receptor (ER)-positive cancers [16]. Additionally, an increased body mass index (BMI), a measure of obesity, is also correlated with a decrease in the sex hormone binding globulin (SHBG). Decreased SHBG allows increased levels of free estrogen available for receptor activation.

In addition to hormonal status, breast cancer is also stimulated by a number of growth hormones and cytokines, which may increase risk when present in excessive amounts. For example, breast cancer may be promoted by insulin and insulin-like growth factor-1 (IGF-1), both of which are elevated in insulin-resistant states including diabetes and obesity (see below). In support of this, non–insulin-dependent diabetes mellitus has been associated with an increased relative risk of breast cancer of 1.25 [17].

Obesity and Postmenopausal Breast Cancer

With few exceptions in the postmenopausal years, obesity is strongly correlated with breast cancer risk. The American Cancer Society's large prospective Cancer Prevention Study II found that increasing BMI substantially increased breast cancer mortality and contributed to 30–50% of breast cancer deaths in the U.S. [18]. Additionally, both the Framingham Study and The Nurses' Health Study showed a direct correlation between current BMI and postmenopausal breast cancer risk, associated with "early" weight gain, weight gain that began when women were in their early and mid-twenties [19]. An estimated 16 % of postmenopausal breast cancer could be attributed to early weight gain. It is important to question the influence of obesity on breast cancer risk in the postmenopausal cancer. Is obesity (rampant in Western culture) the primary causal factor or is obesity a confounder of other factors in a typical Western lifestyle? Only limited data are available, but they suggest that obesity is an independent risk factor across populations.

Obesity and Premenopausal Breast Cancer

Data from epidemiological studies suggest that premenopausal obesity is protective against breast cancer. There are additional data, however, from studies that found no effect of BMI at diagnosis on premenopausal risk [20–22]. In premenopausal women, a large number of prospective and case-controlled studies from highly disparate populations indicate an inverse correlation between body weight and breast cancer risk. In the New York University Women's Health Study and EPIC Study, premenopausal breast cancer risk was inversely correlated with BMI; however, when waist and hip circumference were taken into consideration, there was an *increased* relative risk for breast cancer [23–25](for a detailed discussion on waist and hip circumference, please see below). A study of 1,000 women with premenopausal breast cancer found that obesity was associated with high-grade estrogen receptor negative (ER-) breast cancer and with a 2.5-fold increase in 5-year mortality [26]. Consistently, BMI in low (Taiwan and Japan) and moderate (Brazil, Greece, and Yugoslavia) risk countries had a positive correlation with premenopausal breast cancer [27]. Finally, in a population case control study in Alberta, they found in nulliparous women, increased BMI increases breast cancer risk. However, in parous women, increased BMI decreases risk [28].

An admittedly tenuous interpretation of these data may be as follows: In populations of low-risk and low-BMI women, obesity increases the incidence of premenopausal breast cancer. In high risk, obese populations, there may be a promotional effect of central adiposity (discussed in the next section). An important exception may be women who have BRCA1 mutations in whom weight loss between ages 18 and 30 was strongly protective of breast cancer risk between ages 30 and 40 [29].

Body Fat Distribution and Breast Cancer

Another important unanswered question is whether the increased risk for breast cancer is associated with overall increased obesity/adiposity or with a specific distribution of body fat. BMI is a general measure of obesity, whereas measuring the wait to hip ratio (WHR) and/or the waist circumference (WC) provides a measure of where the adipose tissue is distributed throughout the body. Adipose tissue is accrued in two distinct patterns, either in the Android or visceral (apple) adipose depots (which is highly correlated with the diseases associated with the metabolic syndrome [30]); or as Gynoid or subcutaneous (pear) adipose depots, which has no association with cancer or metabolic syndrome [31]. Unfortunately, WHR is only weakly correlated with the amount of adipose tissue in the visceral (VAT) or intra-abdominal adipose tissue depot [32, 33]. Waist circumference is superior to the WHR for assessing VAT [33]. Two reports by Okosun et al. indicate that fasting plasma insulin and glucose levels, and other biochemical elements of the insulin resistance syndrome, are associated with the waist circumference rather than the WHR [34, 35]. The Nurses Health Study [36]of breast cancer risk in relation to anthropomorphic features found the following: (1) Increased WC is associated with a reduction in premenopausal breast cancer risk (Q5 vs. Q1 multivariate RR 0.6 [0.37–0.98]); (2) WC, hip circumference, and WHR were all associated with increased risk for postmenopausal breast cancer; (3) the positive relation between WC and risk of breast cancer was monotonic (p trend = 0.007), and the multivariate relative risk was 1.05 for every 2 in. (51-mm) increase in WC.

There are racial and ethnic differences associated with cancer prevalence [37]; African American women have more abdominal obesity [37, 38] and a greater WC than Caucasian women [38–44]. Compared with Caucasian women, African American women are generally more obese, as reflected in higher body weight, BMI, and percentage of body fat. African American have a greater WC and higher subcutaneous adipose tissue (SAT) values, but similar visceral adipose tissue (VAT) levels. It follows that for a given amount of total body fat mass, African American women have less VAT than Caucasian women [40]. In the Carolina Breast Cancer Study [45], increased BMI is associated with a reduced risk for premenopausal Caucasian but not African American women, but increased WHR is associated with increased risk for premenopausal women in both Caucasian and African American women. African American women are more likely to present with advanced disease than Caucasian women.

Body adiposity measurements vary with study population (i.e., lean versus obese, young versus aged), and not all studies include or use similar methodologies to determine body composition, making strong conclusions about body fat distribution and its contribution to breast cancer elusive. One additional caveat is that as women age, they naturally accrue more adipose tissue in the central or VAT depot. Therefore, visceral obesity is common in postmenopausal women [46] and separating obesity per sé from visceral obesity is extremely difficult in this population. Nonetheless, what can be concluded is that insulin resistance, which is associated with visceral obesity, is a risk factor for breast cancer. Therefore, fat accrual in the visceral adipose depot would be expected to be associated with susceptibility for breast cancer.

Obesity and Breast Cancer Prognosis

As previously discussed, there is solid evidence that obesity is associated with increased mortality with respect to breast cancer. In a comprehensive review [47] as well as in a more recent study [48], women with increased body weight and BMI are significantly more prone to disease recurrence and death at 5 or 10 years after diagnosis [48]. Importantly, women who gain weight after diagnosis are also significantly more likely to succumb to the disease [47]. Unlike conflicting data on obesity and menopausal status, obesity and breast cancer prognosis appears to be important in both pre and postmenopausal women, as indicated in a study of premenopausal cancer patients, which indicated that the higher the BMI, the more likely women are to die of their disease [26]. As with almost any other medical condition, obesity is a comorbid factor that may alter treatment strategies and consequences, which for breast cancer patients may include wound healing, lymphedema, congestive heart failure, endometrial cancer, sentinel node biopsy failure, and insufficient chemotherapy [47, 49, 50].

Insulin Resistance and Breast Cancer

In addition to the previously discussed role of adipose tissue in estrogen synthesis and the potential impact this has on carcinogenesis, there are a number of other mechanisms by which obesity may increase breast cancer. Visceral adipose tissue is associated with hyperinsulinemia and the insulin resistance syndromes. There is both experimental and epidemiological support for insulin resistance increasing breast cancer risk [16]; however, the molecular mechanisms by which insulin and insulin resistance affect mammary carcinogenesis are currently not well understood. Although the main function of insulin is linked to glucose metabolism, there is evidence of a mitogenic function [51] and an insulin potentiation of fatty acid metabolism [52, 53], which may affect breast cancer development. Elevated plasma insulin is associated with more aggressive cancer and a worsening outcome regardless of menopausal or ER status [54]. High insulin is correlated with increased postmenopausal breast cancer mortality [55].

African Americans have a higher prevalence of insulin resistance and type II diabetes, but the association between insulin resistance and obesity is weaker [56]. Furthermore, in a meta-analysis of type II diabetes and breast cancer risk [57], breast cancer prevalence is higher (3.7%) in women recently diagnosed with type II diabetes, than women not diagnosed with type II diabetes (3.1%). The mean interval between breast cancer diagnosis and diagnosis of type II diabetes is 7.9 years, suggesting that risk is increased in the pre-diabetic phase [58]. Type II diabetes appears to be most strongly related to ER+ breast cancer (Nurses Health Study [59]).

There are several mechanisms by which insulin may increase breast cancer risk (see Fig. 3.1). One of the primary defects underlying insulin resistance is an impairment in postreceptor pathways of insulin action, resulting in a downregulation of IRS-1 signaling by excess free fatty acids [60].

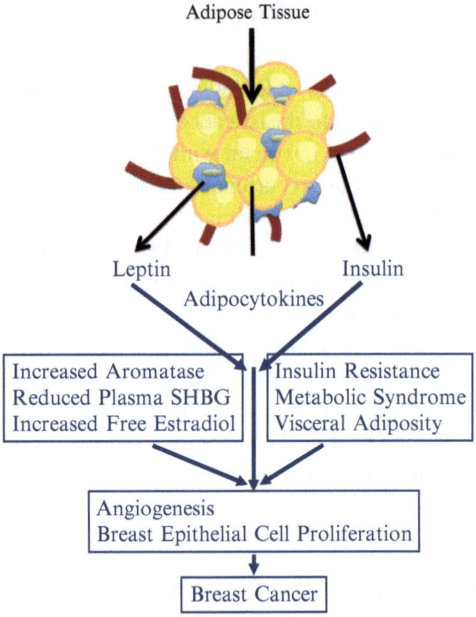

Fig. 3.1 When visceral adiposity is accrued due to excess caloric consumption this is associated with the metabolic syndrome and insulin resistance. Additionally, there is an increase in aromatase and a reduction in SHBG, leading to increased free estradiol levels. All of these factors together or indpendently can influence angiogenesis and breast epithelial cell proliferation leading to mammary gland carcinogenesis. The initiator may be increased dietary fatty acids, obesity, visceral adiposity, and/or leading to insulin resistance

Insulin-Like Growth Factor (IGF)

In recent years, it has become evident that the IGF system plays a role in cancer development and progression [61, 62]. Epidemiological studies have shown that elevated IGF-I plasma concentrations are associated with a higher risk for several cancers, including carcinomas of the breast, colon, prostate, and lung [63–65]. Moreover, the IGF system has been found to be dysregulated in a variety of malignancies by several mechanisms, including IGF-IR overexpression and autocrine/paracrine production of IGF-IR ligands, IGF-I and IGF-II [61]. Finally, studies carried out in transgenic mice have found that abnormal expression of the IGF-IR or its ligands (IGFII and IGF-I) may be linked with cancer initiation in various organs.

Insulin and IGF-1 exert a mitogenic effect on normal and neoplastic breast epithelial cells [16]. Insulin reduces circulating IGF-binding proteins, IGFBP-1 and IGFBP-3, which increases the bioavailable levels of IGF-1 [66]. Furthermore, both insulin and IGF-1 increase ovarian androgen synthesis and inhibit production of SHBG. Increased androgen synthesis provides the substrate for aromatization into estrogen in the adipose tissue [66]. Decreased SHBG allows more free, bioavailable estrogen to circulate. Thus, obesity results in the increase of three stimulators of breast cell proliferation: insulin, IGF-1, and estrogen.

Inflammation and Breast Cancer

The contribution of obesity to breast cancer causation and progression has been hypothesized to be due to increased inflammation in adipose stromal cells, which leads to increased production and release of pro-inflammatory mediators and adipokines by adipose tissues. These cellular effects are mechanistically linked by activation of pro-inflammatory, pro-mitotic, and anti-apoptotic transcription factors that are considered key regulators of the response to inflammation. Women who are immunosuppressed because of HIV infection develop breast cancer at a very low rate prior to the introduction of protease inhibitors, which restores immunocompetence. Furthermore, immunosuppressed transplant recipients also manifest a reduced risk of breast cancer. It is apparent that breast cancer arises and progresses in the pro-inflammatory milieu.

Cancer initiation and progression is associated with chronic inflammation and macrophage activation. Adipose tissue macrophage infiltration increases following consumption of diets high in fat (see discussion below), and macrophages participate in inflammatory pathways that are activated in adipose tissues of obese individuals. Evidence derived from clinical and epidemiological studies implicates macrophages in cancer, where macrophages appear to be directly involved in tumor progression and metastasis. High levels of these tumor-associated macrophages correlate with poor prognosis in over 80% of studies published [67].

Proinflammatory cytokines are secreted from inflamed adipocytes, which signal to initiated and/or otherwise damaged epithelial cells to promote neoplastic cell proliferation and enhance tumorgenesis. These cellular effects are mechanistically linked by activation of NF-κB, a pro-inflammatory, pro-mitotic, and anti-apoptotic transcription factor that is considered a key regulator of the response to inflammation. NF-κB is a transcription factor that promotes expression of many inflammatory cytokines. Its transcriptional activity is inhibited through its sequestration in the cytoplasm by IκB. IκBs bind to NF-κB dimers and sterically block the function of their nuclear localization sequences, thereby causing their cytoplasmic retention. The NF-κB/IκB complex can also shuttle between the cytoplasm and the nucleus in unstimulated cells, but nuclear export of the complex is more efficient and therefore, the NF-κB/IκB complex is mainly cytoplasmic in the basal state. Inflammatory signaling through TNFα, IL-1R, or TLR results in the phosphorylation and degredation of IκB, which frees NF-κB allowing it to translocate to the nucleus and induce inflammatory gene expression. Recent studies indicate that the effects of conventional cancer therapeutics could be enhanced by natural and synthetic NF-κB inhibitors, such as IκB, suggesting that downregulation of NF-κB could sensitize cancer cells to conventional therapeutics Specifically, Patel et al. generated breast cancer cells overexpressing IκB and found that these mutant cells, when compared to parent cells, express fewer anti-apoptotic proteins and are more sensitive to taxol-induced apoptosis [68]. Therefore, focusing on NF-κB inhibitors, such as IkB, provides a novel preventive and therapeutic strategy against human cancers. The NF-κB signaling system, therefore, may represent a critical intracellular pathway linking obesity and breast cancer development.

Adipose Tissue and the Role of Adipokines in Breast Cancer

In the 1980 and early 1990, various studies attempted to define how mammary adipose tissue could influence breast cancer development. Elliott and colleagues [69] have shown that the adipocyte-rich environments could facilitate SP1 (a murine mammary carcinoma cell line) growth after injection into mice. When the SP1 cells were injected subcutaneously or peritoneally outside of a fat pad, no growth or metastases were observed. Addition of adipose cells with the SP1 injections into the peritoneal cavity and subcutaneous regions led to growth and metastasis. There is therefore a strict dependence on adipose-rich environments for tumor propagation in vivo. Further studies revealed that adipocytes promote the estrogen-dependent growth of SP1 cells, with a concomitant induction of hormone and growth factor receptor expression in the breast cancer cells [69]. In vitro work by Johnston et al. [70] demonstrated the possibilities that both pre- and mature adipocytes have the potential to affect growth and differentiation of malignant breast cells.

Adipose tissue secretes a wide range of enzymes, hormones, and growth factors, including a number of adipocyte-derived biologically active polypeptides, which were grouped together by Matsuzawa et al. [71, 72] and termed adipokines. The adipokines constitute a group of polypeptide factors and cytokines that are produced exclusively, or substantially, by mature adipocytes in adipose tissue or by macrophages as a direct result of interactions with adipocytes. There are several adipokines that include leptin, adiponectin, tumor necrosis factor-alpha (TNF-α), interleukin-6 (IL-6), collagen VI, vascular endothelial growth factor (VEGF), and hepatocyte growth factor (HGF) that may have an effect on tumor growth in the mammary gland and thereby mediate the connection between obesity and breast cancer (Figs. 3.1 and 3.2) [72]. Moreover, several studies have raised the possibility that adipose tissue can act as an effector organ that influences both cancer risk and tumor behavior most probably via adipokine secretion. As important adipocyte-derived endocrine and paracrine effectors, the adipokines such as leptin and adiponectin can regulate mammary epithelial cell behavior. However, very little is known about roles of adipokines on fatty acid uptake and metabolism in breast cancer cells.

Leptin

Leptin is produced in adipose tissue and its secretion is directly proportional to the degree of adiposity [73]. Leptin is expressed by the adipose cells as well as to some

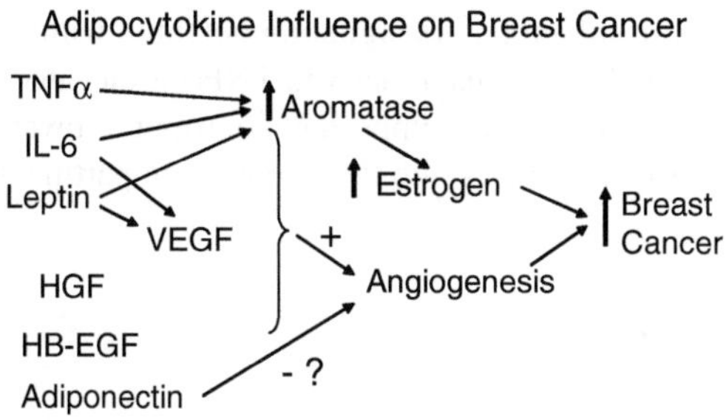

Fig. 3.2 Increased adiposity leads to increased release of adipocytokines. These together or independently cause an increase in aromatase expression which converts androgens to estrogen. Adipocytokines also have an influence on angiogenesis. Both of these pathways, increased estrogen and angiogenesis, lead to increased breast cancer incidence

very low level by other cell types. The levels of this hormone are closely linked to BMI, regardless of a woman's age or reproductive status [74, 75]. Leptin stimulates estrogen biosynthesis by induction of aromatase activity. Leptin can interfere with insulin signaling under some circumstances, and in type II diabetics, plasma leptin levels were frequently found to be correlated with the degree of insulin resistance, a relationship that is independent of BMI and body fat mass [76, 77].

Leptin has been linked to increased breast cancer risk [78–81]. Leptin also alters the rate of cell proliferation and modifies the expression of genes linked to the cell cycle, such as cyclin D1, PPAR, and ERα and ERß in vitro [82]. Leptin has a direct mitogenic effect on human breast cancer cells [83], and leptin's involvement in the insulin resistance syndrome suggests that leptin and insulin may act synergistically to stimulate breast cancer growth and metastasis. Thus, insulin resistance is accompanied by hyperleptinemia, which results in increased signaling activity of these proteins at target sites, which potentially include breast epithelial tissue and vascular endothelial cells. Genetically obese, leptin-deficient mice, or mice lacking a functional leptin receptor fail to develop oncogene-induced mammary tumors [84, 85]. However, this is mostly attributed to the fact that lack of functional leptin signaling causes a complete lack of development of the ductal epithelium in these mice; hence, a direct in vivo effect of leptin remains to be demonstrated. Leptin receptors are, however, expressed by benign and malignant breast cells [81, 86].

Tumor necrosis factor-alpha (TNFα)

Adipose tissue TNFα expression is also positively correlated with visceral adipose tissue and plasma insulin concentrations [87, 88], and TNFα is produced by adipose-associated macrophages [89]. TNFα acts both as an autocrine and as a paracrine factor regulating the production of several cytokines and other adipokines [90].

In light of its potent pro-inflammatory signaling potential within a fat pad, it is very likely that adipocyte- and macrophage-derived TNFα is elevated due to locally dysfunctional adipose tissue which is an important contributor toward enhanced growth potential of tumor lesions invading into the stromal compartment.

Interleukin-6 (IL-6)

Leukocytes and human adipocytes secrete sizeable amounts of IL-6, and plasma IL-6 positively correlates with BMI [91]. As much as 50% of total systemic IL-6 is likely to be derived from adipose tissue. Insulin resistance has also been associated with human adipose tissue-derived IL-6 ([91], and other references therein). Like leptin and TNFα, IL-6 can stimulate estrogen biosynthesis by the induction of aromatase activity [92].

Heparin-Binding Epidermal Growth Factor-Like Growth Factor

Heparin-binding epidermal growth factor-like growth factor (HB-EGF) is secreted by mammary epithelial cells [93] and adipose tissue (in obese mice) [94]. HB-EGF promotes endothelial cell migration and angiogenesis through [95] induction of VEGF [95]. Additionally, HB-EGF acts as an endothelial cell mitogen and inhibitor of apoptosis [96], and regulates expansion and contraction of adipose mass [97].

Hepatocyte Growth Factor (HGF)

HGF disrupts cell–cell adhesion and increases motility and promotes angiogenesis [98, 99]. HGF's receptor, met, is found on both endothelial and epithelial cells [100], and circulating plasma levels correlate with BMI [101], thus providing another link between adipose tissue/obesity/and carcinogenesis.

Adiponectin

Adiponectin is secreted exclusively by adipose tissue and it is present at relatively high levels in the serum [102]. However, its plasma levels are reversely associated with BMI [103]. Reduced adiponectin levels have recently been linked to increased breast cancer risk [104]. Adiponectin has anti-inflammatory properties and promotes insulin sensitivity [105]. Adiponectin may be critical for regulating tissue sensitivity to insulin as a decline in adiponectin precedes insulin resistance [106]. We have recently highlighted a novel and important contribution of adiponectin (APN) in mammary tumor development and angiogenesis, indicating that APN has potent angio-mimetic properties in tumor vascularization [107]. However, in tumors deprived of APN, this anti-angiogenic stress results in an adaptive response that fuels tumor growth via mobilization of circulating endothelial progenitor cells and the development of mechanisms enabling massive cell proliferation despite a chronically hypoxic microenvironment.

Collagen VI

Collagen VI is another factor that is associated with adipose tissue and carcinogenesis. Using purified fragments of collagen VI as well as collagen VI null mice crossed with a widely used breast cancer model (the transgenic MMTV-PyMT mouse), it has been shown that collagen VI enhances tumor growth by providing pro-proliferative and pro-survival signals to the malignant ductal epithelial cells [108]. Curtailing the local production of collagen VI (which is dramatically upregulated during cancer progression) and its cleavage products significantly reduces tumor growth. These studies provide some of the first genetic evidence to suggest that a stromal extracellular matrix protein can modulate tumor behavior and offer a potential link between the epidemiological association of increased adipocyte mass and breast cancer.

Angiogenic Factors

Growth of tumors in the mammary gland is dependent on angiogenesis, or new blood vessel formation, for its development and metastasis [109]. Among the adipokines, leptin, TNFα, VEGF, HGF, HB-EGF, and adiponectin have all been reported to be angiogenic in vitro or in vivo [109]. While not directly angiogenic, Il-6 stimulates VEGF synthesis [109]. The area of adipokine-mediated angiogenesis for developing tumors may be an important therapeutic area in the future.

Nutrients/Fatty Acids and Breast Cancer

At least one-third of all human cancers are associated with diet [110], although the role of specific fatty acids and cancer risk has been under investigated. As previously discussed, obesity (caused predominantly by increased consumption of diets high in fat) has a complex interrelationship with breast cancer risk and metastasis.

The contribution of diet and nutrition status to cancer risk has been a major focus of research as well as public health policy. Studies have been carried out to demonstrate that cancer is largely a preventable disease, and the incidence of cancer can be reduced substantially by means of dietary modification. Additionally, different types of epidemiological designs such as correlation studies, observational studies, cohort, case–control studies, and controlled trials in selected groups have been employed to obtain sufficient proof of causal relationships between dietary modification and cancer. This offers the prospect for initiating primary and secondary nutritional prevention measures for control and prevention of cancers.

The difficulty of most epidemiological studies attempting to determine the role diet, obesity, and breast cancer is discriminating among issues of increased adiposity, distribution of adiposity, adiposity relative to increased calories versus decreased energy expenditure, and adiposity due to increased fat intake. Essentially, all of the epidemiological studies relative to these issues have examined breast cancer incidence or mortality relative to consumption of a variety of fats, in some cases normalized to caloric intake and/or BMI. Among the most compelling data showing a correlation between incidence rates and fat consumption are international comparisons. For example, Prentice suggests that the 5.5-fold difference in incidence between Japan and the USA can be explained by differences in fat consumption [111]. In one prospective study, Knekt et al. followed a cohort of Finnish women (age 20–69 years) for 20 years, and found that energy adjusted for total fat intake was positively associated with breast cancer incidence [112].

Industrial societies, such as the US, have moved to consumption of diets enriched in fat leading to a positive energy balance, making obesity a national crisis. Prior to the rapid onset of obesity, the major dietary fat consumed was butter and/or saturated fat. Based on nutritional recommendations to reduce the amount of saturated fat (for cardiovascular benefits), healthcare professional encouraged consumption of diets high in polyunsaturated fat (PUFA) and monounsaturated fat (olive and cannula oil). High-fat intake is associated with increased premenopausal breast cancer mortality [55]. Therefore, obesity, the change in dietary fatty acid consumption, and increased breast cancer incidence are tightly correlated. Dietary factors are believed to influence the risk and progression of breast cancer, either through effects on hormonal status or via direct tumor-promoting carcinogenic effects.

The "susceptibility" of the target tissue for any particular carcinogen may relate to the presence of a susceptible cell type, proliferation of that cell type, rate of DNA repair, or susceptibility to DNA damage as a function of the nutritional and hormonal state. There is a paucity of data on the cellular mechanisms elicited by dietary fat in breast cancer cells. For some types of breast cancer, dietary intervention (altering the types of fatty acids consumed) may be enough to stave off formation of metastatic tumors. For others, long-term therapy which targets the molecular mechanisms that underlie the metastasis-promoting effects of dietary fats may be beneficial. Dietary fats have profound hormonal sequelae and the effects of the fatty acids may be on initiation, promotion, and/or metastasis.

Types of Fatty Acids

There are only modest links between dietary fat consumption and breast cancer, and this is confounded by the fact that most humans consume diets that are made of mixtures of food types and fatty acid sources. While some animal studies have shown that n-6 PUFAs promote tumorigenesis [113–117], this has not been demonstrated in humans [118]. In a meta-analysis, Fay et al [119] reported on data from 97 animal experiments, involving a total of 12,803 mice or rats, which studied the effects of different dietary fatty acids on the development of breast cancer. This analysis showed that n-6 PUFAs have a strong tumor-enhancing effect, whereas the direct associations with the other types of fatty acids were weak. Saturated fats are associated with increased breast cancer risk in women [120]. Lastly, with respect to n-3 PUFAs, the data are equally conflicting. n-3 PUFAs are protective in some [121, 122], but not all studies [123, 124]. Therefore, there are no consistent data with respect to the influence specific fatty acids have on breast cancer and is an area of research that is still warranted.

Timing of Fatty Acid Exposure

There are conflicting data the age at which different types of fatty acids are consumed, and the potential impact on carcinogenesis. The breast undergoes extensive changes during development and throughout life primarily due to hormonal changes. The mammary gland is especially prone to hormonal influences at dramatic stages of development such as puberty. It has been proposed that most women develop subclinical breast cancer at an early, premenopausal age, and that diet, especially increased amounts of fat and overnutrition, play an important role in the progression from such putative preneoplastic lesions to clinical disease. Therefore, understanding when the mammary gland is most sensitive to different types of fatty acids continues to be an area of needed research.

Potential Mechanism for Fatty Acids to Impact Carcinogenesis

Nonendocrine mechanisms have been proposed to explain how fatty acids may impact mammary tumorigenesis, based primarily upon reports demonstrating increased mitotic activity in normal and neoplastic mammary gland cells after addition of various fatty acids to the culture media [125, 126]. The fatty acid composition of the mammary gland cell membranes reflects, quantitatively and qualitatively, the composition and amount of fatty acids in the diet [127]. In order to exert metabolic effects, fatty acids must be taken up by cells and metabolized effectively to different classes of cellular lipids (triacylglycerols, phospholipids, etc.) for incorporation into different cellular and intracellular compartments. Alterations in the composition of cell membranes by the different fatty acids may change membrane-associated biophysical phenomena, such as membrane fluidity, permeability, transport processes, receptor availability, intracellular communication, and/or enzyme activity, which ultimately may provide a favorable environment for high mitotic activity [128].

Is Weight Loss a Viable Mechanism for Reducing Breast Cancer Risk and Increasing Survival?

Physical Activity

Convincing evidence now supports a probable preventive role for physical activity in postmenopausal breast cancer. The mechanisms by which long-term physical activity affect risk, however, remain unclear. Regular exercise offers protection against all causes of mortality, primarily by protection against atherosclerosis and insulin resistance. Additionally, exercise may exert some of its beneficial health effects by inducing anti-inflammatory actions. A case–control trial conducted in Los Angeles county included 1,883 postmenopausal breast cancer cases and 1,628 controls and found that breast cancer risk is reduced among women who maintained, on average, 17.6 metabolic equivalent of energy expenditure (MET)-hr of activity/week from menarche onward. BMI (adjusted for physical activity) is not a risk factor for those without a family history of breast cancer [129].

Weight Loss

One prediction based on the findings that obesity may enhance carcionogenesis, might be that weight loss would decrease the relative risk. Loss of weight, regardless of when it was initially gained during adulthood, was associated with lower risk of postmenopausal breast cancer compared with weight maintenance [130–132]. Although the biochemical and epidemiological data would suggest that weight loss in adulthood may decrease the risk of breast cancer, particularly in postmenopausal women, there are very few prospective studies to verify this hypothesis. However, there are data from the Iowa Women's Health Study that suggest that weight loss may actually be protective [133]. Postmenopausal women who had an intentional weight loss of 20 lb or more were found to have a significantly decreased risk of breast cancer. Furthermore, women who had weight loss and were not currently overweight had risks similar to non-overweight women who had never lost weight [133]. This verifies a previous study that showed weight loss of greater than 20 lb significantly decreased cancer-related mortalities [134]. Long-term intervention trials to decrease incidence or to alter prognosis are not yet available. However, small-scale trials indicate that weight reduction in the breast cancer patient population is achievable [135, 136]. Therefore, based on these studies, one could conclude that modest weight loss is also associated with improvement in metabolic profiles.

Dietary Restriction

Dietary/energy restriction (DER) is arguably the most potent physiological approach to the prevention of experimentally induced breast cancer that has been identified to date [137–139]. However, DER does not have to be sufficiently severe to elicit weight loss in order to confer protection against breast cancer; rather the key feature of DER in this regard is to provide limited access to nutrients (reviewed in [138]). Furthermore, the literature suggests that the protective effects of DER are NOT due (entirely or even in part) to decreased calorie consumption per sé, because there is still a chemo-protective effect in animals that receive the same number of calories as long as these calories are provided with limited access. It has been suggested that DER exerts its effect by altering one or more aspects of cell cycle regulation, due to the findings that energy restriction inhibits cell proliferation and increases cell death due to apoptosis [137]. Note that in a large meta-analysis of spontaneous mammary tumors in mice, energy restriction uniformly reduces tumor incidence. However, the beneficial effect is reduced with prolonged periods of DER treatment. This suggests that dietary restriction may delay but not prevent tumor formation. Importantly, the only study included in that meta-analysis that did not find any protective effect used the lowest level of energy restriction (23%) and the longest duration (2.5 years) [140].

Conclusion

Breast cancer is the most common cancer among American women. Obesity is associated with increased breast cancer mortality, and it is estimated that 20% of cancer deaths in women over 50 are related to excess body weight. Consumption of high-fat, calorically dense food is implicated as one of the most important environmental factors leading to obesity. Preliminary data suggest that consumption of high-fat diets induces adipose-associated inflammation, and increased production of mitogenic adipocytokines, all contributing to a pro-inflammatory microenvironment that is favorable for breast cancer development and progression. Adipose tissue constitutes the major stromal cell population in the breast microenvironment and many recent studies have implicated adipocytes as critical for both normal mammary gland morphogenesis as well as in the pathogenesis of breast cancer. This review focused on the underlying molecular mechanisms that link obesity with increased cancer incidence and metastasis. We discussed the role of adipose tissue, body fat distribution, inflammation, insulin resistance, and diet/nutrients and their impact on altering the susceptibility to carcinogenesis by exploring the mechanisms by which these factors modify cancer incidence, and prognosis. For many types of cancer, including breast cancer, metastatic "seeding" appears to be an early event that has already occurred by the time the primary tumor is detected. Sometimes, it can take years before these seeded cells develop into full-blown metastatic tumors. It is not known whether exposure to high-fat diets, obesity, and increased inflammation associated with both the consumption of the high-fat diet and obesity, enhances breast cancer incidence and causes the switch from a dormant (or very slow-proliferating) seed cell into a rapidly proliferating tumor cell. There are conflicting data with respect to the optimal amount of body fat, and a recent study even suggests that small amounts of body fat may be protective for women against breast cancer premenopausally; however, in the postmenopausal years, increased body fat enhances the risk of carcinogenesis. Thus, there is a need to understand the associations between dietary fatty acid consumption, body fat/obesity, and disease risk at the epidemiological, cellular, and molecular levels.

Acknowledgments Dedication: I would like to dedicate this chapter in loving memory of Carol Benoit.

References

1. Ogden CL, Carroll MD, Curtin LR, McDowell MA, Tabak CJ, Flegal KM (2006) Prevalence of overweight and obesity in the United States, 1999–2004. JAMA 295:1549–1555
2. Flegal KM, Carroll MD, Ogden CL, Johnson CL (2002) Prevalence and trends in obesity among US adults, 1999–2000. JAMA 288:1723–1727
3. Ogden CL, Carroll MD, Flegal KM (2003) Epidemiologic trends in overweight and obesity. Endocrinol Metab Clin North Am 32:741–760
4. Goodwin PJ, Boyd NF (1990) Body size and breast cancer prognosis: a critical review of the evidence. Breast Cancer Res Treat 16:205–214
5. Borugian MJ, Sheps SB, Kim-Sing C, Olivotto IA, Van Patten C, Dunn BP, Coldman AJ, Potter JD, Gallagher RP, Hislop TG (2003) Waist-to-hip ratio and breast cancer mortality. Am J Epidemiol 158:963–968
6. Cleveland RJ, Eng SM, Abrahamson PE, Britton JA, Teitelbaum SL, Neugut AI, Gammon MD (2007) Weight gain prior to diagnosis and survival from breast cancer. Cancer Epidemiol Biomarkers Prev 16:1803–1811
7. Calle EE, Rodriguez C, Walker-Thurmond K, Thun MJ (2003) Overweight, obesity, and mortality from cancer in a prospectively studied cohort of U.S. adults. N Engl J Med 348:1625–1638
8. Jemal A, Murray T, Samuels A, Ghafoor A, Ward E, Thun MJ (2003) Cancer statistics, 2003. CA Cancer J Clin 53:5–26
9. Hunter D, Willett W (1993) Re: Dietary fat and breast cancer. J Natl Cancer Inst 85:1776–1777
10. Hunter DJ, Willett WC (1993) Diet, body size, and breast cancer. Epidemiol Rev 15:110–132
11. Morabia A, Wynder EL (1990) Epidemiology and natural history of breast cancer. Implications for the body weight-breast cancer controversy. Surg Clin North Am 70:739–752
12. Rose DP, Komninou D, Stephenson GD (2004) Obesity, adipocytokines, and insulin resistance in breast cancer. Obes Rev 5:153–165
13. Medina D (2005) Mammary developmental fate and breast cancer risk. Endocr Relat Cancer 12:483–495

14. Rose DP (1993) Diet, hormones, and cancer. Annu Rev Public Health 14:1–17
15. Bulun SE, Simpson ER (1994) Regulation of aromatase expression in human tissues. Breast Cancer Res Treat 30:19–29
16. Stephenson GD, Rose DP (2003) Breast cancer and obesity: an update. Nutr Cancer 45:1–16
17. Wolf I, Sadetzki S, Catane R, Karasik A, Kaufman B (2005) Diabetes mellitus and breast cancer. Lancet Oncol 6:103–111
18. Petrelli JM, Calle EE, Rodriguez C, Thun MJ (2002) Body mass index, height, and postmenopausal breast cancer mortality in a prospective cohort of US women. Cancer Causes Control 13:325–332
19. Huang Z, Hankinson SE, Colditz GA, Stampfer MJ, Hunter DJ, Manson JE, Hennekens CH, Rosner B, Speizer FE, Willett WC (1997) Dual effects of weight and weight gain on breast cancer risk. JAMA 278:1407–1411
20. Chow LW, Lui KL, Chan JC, Chan TC, Ho PK, Lee WY, Leung LH, Sy WM, Yeung CC, Yung AK (2005) Association between body mass index and risk of formation of breast cancer in Chinese women. Asian J Surg 28:179–184
21. Adebamowo CA, Ogundiran TO, Adenipekun AA, Oyesegun RA, Campbell OB, Akang EU, Rotimi CN, Olopade OI (2003) Obesity and height in urban Nigerian women with breast cancer. Ann Epidemiol 13:455–461
22. Shu XO, Jin F, Dai Q, Shi JR, Potter JD, Brinton LA, Hebert JR, Ruan Z, Gao YT, Zheng W (2001) Association of body size and fat distribution with risk of breast cancer among Chinese women. Int J Cancer 94:449–455
23. Lahmann PH, Lissner L, Berglund G (2004) Breast cancer risk in overweight postmenopausal women. Cancer Epidemiol Biomarkers Prev 13:1414
24. Lahmann PH, Hoffmann K, Allen N, van Gils CH, Khaw KT, Tehard B, Berrino F, Tjonneland A, Bigaard J, Olsen A, Overvad K, Clavel-Chapelon F, Nagel G, Boeing H, Trichopoulos D, Economou G, Bellos G, Palli D, Tumino R, Panico S, Sacerdote C, Krogh V, Peeters PH, Bueno-de-Mesquita HB, Lund E, Ardanaz E, Amiano P, Pera G, Quiros JR, Martinez C, Tormo MJ, Wirfalt E, Berglund G, Hallmans G, Key TJ, Reeves G, Bingham S, Norat T, Biessy C, Kaaks R, Riboli E (2004) Body size and breast cancer risk: findings from the European Prospective Investigation into Cancer And Nutrition (EPIC). Int J Cancer 111:762–771
25. Tehard B, Lahmann PH, Riboli E, Clavel-Chapelon F (2004) Anthropometry, breast cancer and menopausal status: use of repeated measurements over 10 years of follow-up-results of the French E3N women's cohort study. Int J Cancer 111:264–269
26. Daling JR, Malone KE, Doody DR, Johnson LG, Gralow JR, Porter PL (2001) Relation of body mass index to tumor markers and survival among young women with invasive ductal breast carcinoma. Cancer 92:720–729
27. Pathak DR, Whittemore AS (1992) Combined effects of body size, parity, and menstrual events on breast cancer incidence in seven countries. Am J Epidemiol 135:153–168
28. Friedenreich CM, Courneya KS, Bryant HE (2002) Case-control study of anthropometric measures and breast cancer risk. Int J Cancer 99:445–452
29. Kotsopoulos J, Olopado OI, Ghadirian P, Lubinski J, Lynch HT, Isaacs C, Weber B, Kim-Sing C, Ainsworth P, Foulkes WD, Eisen A, Sun P, Narod SA (2005) Changes in body weight and the risk of breast cancer in BRCA1 and BRCA2 mutation carriers. Breast Cancer Res 7:R833–843
30. Wajchenberg BL (2000) Subcutaneous and visceral adipose tissue: their relation to the metabolic syndrome. Endocr Rev 21:697–738
31. McCarty MF (2003) A paradox resolved: the postprandial model of insulin resistance explains why gynoid adiposity appears to be protective. Med Hypotheses 61:173–176
32. Bonora E, Micciolo R, Ghiatas AA, Lancaster JL, Alyassin A, Muggeo M, DeFronzo RA (1995) Is it possible to derive a reliable estimate of human visceral and subcutaneous abdominal adipose tissue from simple anthropometric measurements? Metabolism 44:1617–1625
33. Raikkonen K, Matthews KA, Kuller LH (1999) Anthropometric and psychosocial determinants of visceral obesity in healthy postmenopausal women. Int J Obes Relat Metab Disord 23:775–782

34. Okosun IS, Cooper RS, Prewitt TE, Rotimi CN (1999) The relation of central adiposity to components of the insulin resistance syndrome in a biracial US population sample. Ethn Dis 9:218–229
35. Okosun IS, Liao Y, Rotimi CN, Prewitt TE, Cooper RS (2000) Abdominal adiposity and clustering of multiple metabolic syndrome in White, Black and Hispanic Americans. Ann Epidemiol 10:263–270
36. Huang Z, Willett WC, Colditz GA, Hunter DJ, Manson JE, Rosner B, Speizer FE, Hankinson SE (1999) Waist circumference, waist:hip ratio, and risk of breast cancer in the Nurses' Health Study. Am J Epidemiol 150:1316–1324
37. Zillikens MC, Conway JM (1990) Anthropometry in blacks: applicability of generalized skinfold equations and differences in fat patterning between blacks and whites. Am J Clin Nutr 52:45–51
38. Berman DM, Rodrigues LM, Nicklas BJ, Ryan AS, Dennis KE, Goldberg AP (2001) Racial disparities in metabolism, central obesity, and sex hormone-binding globulin in postmenopausal women. J Clin Endocrinol Metab 86:97–103
39. Hill JO, Sidney S, Lewis CE, Tolan K, Scherzinger AL, Stamm ER (1999) Racial differences in amounts of visceral adipose tissue in young adults: the CARDIA (Coronary Artery Risk Development in Young Adults) study. Am J Clin Nutr 69:381–387
40. Despres JP, Couillard C, Gagnon J, Bergeron J, Leon AS, Rao DC, Skinner JS, Wilmore JH, Bouchard C (2000) Race, visceral adipose tissue, plasma lipids, and lipoprotein lipase activity in men and women: the Health, Risk Factors, Exercise Training, and Genetics (HERITAGE) family study. Arterioscler Thromb Vasc Biol 20:1932–1938
41. Ryan AS, Nicklas BJ, Berman DM (2002) Racial differences in insulin resistance and mid-thigh fat deposition in postmenopausal women. Obes Res 10:336–344
42. Torrens JI, Skurnick J, Davidow AL, Korenman SG, Santoro N, Soto-Greene M, Lasser N, Weiss G (2004) Ethnic differences in insulin sensitivity and beta-cell function in premenopausal or early perimenopausal women without diabetes: the Study of Women's Health Across the Nation (SWAN). Diabetes Care 27:354–361
43. Hoffman DJ, Wang Z, Gallagher D, Heymsfield SB (2005) Comparison of visceral adipose tissue mass in adult African Americans and whites. Obes Res 13:66–74
44. Araneta MR, Barrett-Connor E (2005) Ethnic differences in visceral adipose tissue and type 2 diabetes: Filipino, African-American, and white women. Obes Res 13:1458–1465
45. Hall IJ, Newman B, Millikan RC, Moorman PG (2000) Body size and breast cancer risk in black women and white women: the Carolina Breast Cancer Study. Am J Epidemiol 151:754–764
46. Piche ME, Weisnagel SJ, Corneau L, Nadeau A, Bergeron J, Lemieux S (2005) Contribution of abdominal visceral obesity and insulin resistance to the cardiovascular risk profile of postmenopausal women. Diabetes 54:770–777
47. Chlebowski RT (2002) Breast cancer risk reduction: strategies for women at increased risk. Annu Rev Med 53:519–540
48. Loi S, Milne RL, Friedlander ML, McCredie MR, Giles GG, Hopper JL, Phillips KA (2005) Obesity and outcomes in premenopausal and postmenopausal breast cancer. Cancer Epidemiol Biomarkers Prev 14:1686–1691
49. Colleoni M, Rotmensz N, Robertson C, Orlando L, Viale G, Renne G, Luini A, Veronesi P, Intra M, Orecchia R, Catalano G, Galimberti V, Nole F, Martinelli G, Goldhirsch A (2002) Very young women (<35 years) with operable breast cancer: features of disease at presentation. Ann Oncol 13:273–279
50. Derossis AM, Fey JV, Cody HS III, Borgen PI (2003) Obesity influences outcome of sentinel lymph node biopsy in early-stage breast cancer. J Am Coll Surg 197:896–901
51. Papa V, Belfiore A (1996) Insulin receptors in breast cancer: biological and clinical role. J Endocrinol Invest 19:324–333
52. Miyaoka K, Kuwasako T, Hirano K, Nozaki S, Yamashita S, Matsuzawa Y (2001) CD36 deficiency associated with insulin resistance. Lancet 357:686–687
53. Hajri T, Han XX, Bonen A, Abumrad NA (2002) Defective fatty acid uptake modulates insulin responsiveness and metabolic responses to diet in CD36-null mice. J Clin Invest 109:1381–1389

54. Goodwin PJ, Ennis M, Pritchard KI, Trudeau ME, Koo J, Madarnas Y, Hartwick W, Hoffman B, Hood N (2002) Fasting insulin and outcome in early-stage breast cancer: results of a prospective cohort study. J Clin Oncol 20:42–51
55. Borugian MJ, Sheps SB, Kim-Sing C, Van Patten C, Potter JD, Dunn B, Gallagher RP, Hislop TG (2004) Insulin, macronutrient intake, and physical activity: are potential indicators of insulin resistance associated with mortality from breast cancer? Cancer Epidemiol Biomarkers Prev 13:1163–1172
56. Okosun IS (2001) Racial differences in rates of type 2 diabetes in American women: how much is due to differences in overall adiposity? Ethn Health 6:27–34
57. Larsson SC, Mantzoros CS, Wolk A (2007) Diabetes mellitus and risk of breast cancer: a meta-analysis. Int J Cancer 121:856–862
58. Lipscombe LL, Goodwin PJ, Zinman B, McLaughlin JR, Hux JE (2006) Increased prevalence of prior breast cancer in women with newly diagnosed diabetes. Breast Cancer Res Treat 98:303–309
59. Michels KB, Solomon CG, Hu FB, Rosner BA, Hankinson SE, Colditz GA, Manson JE (2003) Type 2 diabetes and subsequent incidence of breast cancer in the Nurses' Health Study. Diabetes Care 26:1752–1758
60. Agarwal N, Sharma BC (2005) Insulin resistance and clinical aspects of non-alcoholic steatohepatitis (NASH). Hepatol Res 33:92–96
61. Pollak MN, Schernhammer ES, Hankinson SE (2004) Insulin-like growth factors and neoplasia. Nat Rev Cancer 4:505–518
62. LeRoith D, Roberts CT Jr (2003) The insulin-like growth factor system and cancer. Cancer Lett 195:127–137
63. Hankinson SE, Willett WC, Colditz GA, Hunter DJ, Michaud DS, Deroo B, Rosner B, Speizer FE, Pollak M (1998) Circulating concentrations of insulin-like growth factor-I and risk of breast cancer. Lancet 351:1393–1396
64. Ma J, Pollak MN, Giovannucci E, Chan JM, Tao Y, Hennekens CH, Stampfer MJ (1999) Prospective study of colorectal cancer risk in men and plasma levels of insulin-like growth factor (IGF)-I and IGF-binding protein-3. J Natl Cancer Inst 91:620–625
65. Chan JM, Stampfer MJ, Giovannucci E, Gann PH, Ma J, Wilkinson P, Hennekens CH, Pollak M (1998) Plasma insulin-like growth factor-I and prostate cancer risk: a prospective study. Science 279:563–566
66. Guastamacchia E, Resta F, Triggiani V, Liso A, Licchelli B, Ghiyasaldin S, Sabba C, Tafaro E (2004) Evidence for a putative relationship between type 2 diabetes and neoplasia with particular reference to breast cancer: role of hormones, growth factors and specific receptors. Curr Drug Targets Immune Endocr Metabol Disord 4:59–66
67. Bingle L, Brown NJ, Lewis CE (2002) The role of tumour-associated macrophages in tumour progression: implications for new anticancer therapies. J Pathol 196:254–265
68. Patel NM, Nozaki S, Shortle NH, Bhat-Nakshatri P, Newton TR, Rice S, Gelfanov V, Boswell SH, Goulet RJ Jr, Sledge GW Jr, Nakshatri H Jr (2000) Paclitaxel sensitivity of breast cancer cells with constitutively active NF-kappaB is enhanced by IkappaBalpha super-repressor and parthenolide. Oncogene 19:4159–4169
69. Elliott BE, Tam SP, Dexter D, Chen ZQ (1992) Capacity of adipose tissue to promote growth and metastasis of a murine mammary carcinoma: effect of estrogen and progesterone. Int J Cancer 51:416–424
70. Johnston PG, Rondinone CM, Voeller D, Allegra CJ (1992) Identification of a protein factor secreted by 3T3-L1 preadipocytes inhibitory for the human MCF-7 breast cancer cell line. Cancer Res 52:6860–6865
71. Funahashi T, Nakamura T, Shimomura I, Maeda K, Kuriyama H, Takahashi M, Arita Y, Kihara S, Matsuzawa Y (1999) Role of adipocytokines on the pathogenesis of atherosclerosis in visceral obesity. Intern Med 38:202–206
72. Rajala MW, Scherer PE (2003) Minireview: The adipocyte–at the crossroads of energy homeostasis, inflammation, and atherosclerosis. Endocrinology 144:3765–3773
73. Zhang Y, Proenca R, Maffei M, Barone M, Leopold L, Friedman JM (1994) Positional cloning of the mouse obese gene and its human homologue. Nature 372:425–432

74. Kolaczynski JW, Ohannesian JP, Considine RV, Marco CC, Caro JF (1996) Response of leptin to short-term and prolonged overfeeding in humans. J Clin Endocrinol Metab 81:4162–4165
75. Thomas T, Burguera B, Melton LJ 3rd, Atkinson EJ, O'Fallon WM, Riggs BL, Khosla S (2000) Relationship of serum leptin levels with body composition and sex steroid and insulin levels in men and women. Metabolism 49:1278–1284
76. Fischer S, Hanefeld M, Haffner SM, Fusch C, Schwanebeck U, Kohler C, Fucker K, Julius U (2002) Insulin-resistant patients with type 2 diabetes mellitus have higher serum leptin levels independently of body fat mass. Acta Diabetol 39:105–110
77. Wauters M, Considine RV, Yudkin JS, Peiffer F, De Leeuw I, Van Gaal LF (2003) Leptin levels in type 2 diabetes: associations with measures of insulin resistance and insulin secretion. Horm Metab Res 35:92–96
78. Marttunen MB, Andersson S, Hietanen P, Karonen SL, Koistinen HA, Koivisto VA, Tiitinen A, Ylikorkala O (2000) Antiestrogenic tamoxifen and toremifene increase serum leptin levels in postmenopausal breast cancer patients. Maturitas 35:175–179
79. Tessitore L, Vizio B, Jenkins O, De Stefano I, Ritossa C, Argiles JM, Benedetto C, Mussa A (2000) Leptin expression in colorectal and breast cancer patients. Int J Mol Med 5:421–426
80. Ozet A, Arpaci F, Yilmaz MI, Ayta H, Ozturk B, Komurcu S, Yavuz AA, Tezcan Y, Acikel C (2001) Effects of tamoxifen on the serum leptin level in patients with breast cancer. Jpn J Clin Oncol 31:424–427
81. Hu X, Juneja SC, Maihle NJ, Cleary MP (2002) Leptin–a growth factor in normal and malignant breast cells and for normal mammary gland development. J Natl Cancer Inst 94:1704–1711
82. Okumura M, Yamamoto M, Sakuma H, Kojima T, Maruyama T, Jamali M, Cooper DR, Yasuda K (2002) Leptin and high glucose stimulate cell proliferation in MCF-7 human breast cancer cells: reciprocal involvement of PKC-alpha and PPAR expression. Biochim Biophys Acta 1592:107–116
83. Rose DP, Gilhooly EM, Nixon DW (2002) Adverse effects of obesity on breast cancer prognosis, and the biological actions of leptin (review). Int J Oncol 21:1285–1292
84. Cleary MP, Juneja SC, Phillips FC, Hu X, Grande JP, Maihle NJ (2004) Leptin receptor-deficient MMTV-TGF-alpha/Lepr(db)Lepr(db) female mice do not develop oncogene-induced mammary tumors. Exp Biol Med (Maywood) 229:182–193
85. Cleary MP, Phillips FC, Getzin SC, Jacobson TL, Jacobson MK, Christensen TA, Juneja SC, Grande JP, Maihle NJ (2003) Genetically obese MMTV-TGF-alpha/Lep(ob)Lep(ob) female mice do not develop mammary tumors. Breast Cancer Res Treat 77:205–215
86. Laud K, Gourdou I, Pessemesse L, Peyrat JP, Djiane J (2002) Identification of leptin receptors in human breast cancer: functional activity in the T47-D breast cancer cell line. Mol Cell Endocrinol 188:219–226
87. Hotamisligil GS, Arner P, Caro JF, Atkinson RL, Spiegelman BM (1995) Increased adipose tissue expression of tumor necrosis factor-alpha in human obesity and insulin resistance. J Clin Invest 95:2409–2415
88. Miyazaki Y, Pipek R, Mandarino LJ, DeFronzo RA (2003) Tumor necrosis factor alpha and insulin resistance in obese type 2 diabetic patients. Int J Obes Relat Metab Disord 27:88–94
89. Weisberg SP, McCann D, Desai M, Rosenbaum M, Leibel RL, Ferrante AW Jr (2003) Obesity is associated with macrophage accumulation in adipose tissue. J Clin Invest 112:1796–1808
90. Coppack SW (2001) Pro-inflammatory cytokines and adipose tissue. Proc Nutr Soc 60:349–356
91. Kern PA, Ranganathan S, Li C, Wood L, Ranganathan G (2001) Adipose tissue tumor necrosis factor and interleukin-6 expression in human obesity and insulin resistance. Am J Physiol Endocrinol Metab 280:E745–751
92. Purohit A, Newman SP, Reed MJ (2002) The role of cytokines in regulating estrogen synthesis: implications for the etiology of breast cancer. Breast Cancer Res 4:65–69
93. Martinez-Lacaci I, De Santis M, Kannan S, Bianco C, Kim N, Wallace-Jones B, Wechselberger C, Ebert AD, Salomon DS (2001) Regulation of heparin-binding EGF-like growth factor expression in Ha-ras transformed human mammary epithelial cells. J Cell Physiol 186:233–242

94. Matsumoto S, Kishida K, Shimomura I, Maeda N, Nagaretani H, Matsuda M, Nishizawa H, Kihara S, Funahashi T, Matsuzawa Y, Yamada A, Yamashita S, Tamura S, Kawata S (2002) Increased plasma HB-EGF associated with obesity and coronary artery disease. Biochem Biophys Res Commun 292:781–786
95. Abramovitch R, Neeman M, Reich R, Stein I, Keshet E, Abraham J, Solomon A, Marikovsky M (1998) Intercellular communication between vascular smooth muscle and endothelial cells mediated by heparin-binding epidermal growth factor-like growth factor and vascular endothelial growth factor. FEBS Lett 425:441–447
96. Tran J, Rak J, Sheehan C, Saibil SD, LaCasse E, Korneluk RG, Kerbel RS (1999) Marked induction of the IAP family antiapoptotic proteins survivin and XIAP by VEGF in vascular endothelial cells. Biochem Biophys Res Commun 264:781–788
97. Hausman GJ, Richardson RL (2004) Adipose tissue angiogenesis. J Anim Sci 82:925–934
98. Rosen EM, Grant DS, Kleinman HK, Goldberg ID, Bhargava MM, Nickoloff BJ, Kinsella JL, Polverini P (1993) Scatter factor (hepatocyte growth factor) is a potent angiogenesis factor in vivo. Symp Soc Exp Biol 47:227–234
99. Lamorte L, Royal I, Naujokas M, Park M (2002) Crk adapter proteins promote an epithelial-mesenchymal-like transition and are required for HGF-mediated cell spreading and breakdown of epithelial adherens junctions. Mol Biol Cell 13:1449–1461
100. Tuck AB, Park M, Sterns EE, Boag A, Elliott BE (1996) Coexpression of hepatocyte growth factor and receptor (Met) in human breast carcinoma. Am J Pathol 148:225–232
101. Rehman J, Considine RV, Bovenkerk JE, Li J, Slavens CA, Jones RM, March KL (2003) Obesity is associated with increased levels of circulating hepatocyte growth factor. J Am Coll Cardiol 41:1408–1413
102. Scherer PE, Williams S, Fogliano M, Baldini G, Lodish HF (1995) A novel serum protein similar to C1q, produced exclusively in adipocytes. J Biol Chem 270:26746–26749
103. Stefan N, Stumvoll M (2002) Adiponectin – its role in metabolism and beyond. Horm Metab Res 34:469–474
104. Miyoshi Y, Funahashi T, Kihara S, Taguchi T, Tamaki Y, Matsuzawa Y, Noguchi S (2003) Association of serum adiponectin levels with breast cancer risk. Clin Cancer Res 9:5699–5704
105. Kubota N, Terauchi Y, Yamauchi T, Kubota T, Moroi M, Matsui J, Eto K, Yamashita T, Kamon J, Satoh H, Yano W, Froguel P, Nagai R, Kimura S, Kadowaki T, Noda T (2002) Disruption of adiponectin causes insulin resistance and neointimal formation. J Biol Chem 277:25863–25866
106. Stefan N, Vozarova B, Funahashi T, Matsuzawa Y, Weyer C, Lindsay RS, Youngren JF, Havel PJ, Pratley RE, Bogardus C, Tataranni PA (2002) Plasma adiponectin concentration is associated with skeletal muscle insulin receptor tyrosine phosphorylation, and low plasma concentration precedes a decrease in whole-body insulin sensitivity in humans. Diabetes 51:1884–1888
107. *Landskroner-Eiger* S, *Qian, B., Muise, E.S, Nawrocki, A.R., Berger, J.P., Fine, E.J., Koba, W., Deng, Y., Pollard, J.W. and P.E. Scherer: Proanglogenic contribution of adiponectin towards mammary tumor growth in vivo. Clin Canc Res in press, 2009*
108. Iyengar P, Espina V, Williams TW, Lin Y, Berry D, Jelicks LA, Lee H, Temple K, Graves R, Pollard J, Chopra N, Russell RG, Sasisekharan R, Trock BJ, Lippman M, Calvert VS, Petricoin EF 3rd, Liotta L, Dadachova E, Pestell RG, Lisanti MP, Bonaldo P, Scherer PE (2005) Adipocyte-derived collagen VI affects early mammary tumor progression in vivo, demonstrating a critical interaction in the tumor/stroma microenvironment. J Clin Invest 115:1163–1176
109. Schneider BP, Miller KD (2005) Angiogenesis of breast cancer. J Clin Oncol 23:1782–1790
110. Doll R, Peto R (1981) The causes of cancer: quantitative estimates of avoidable risks of cancer in the United States today. J Natl Cancer Inst 66:1191–1308
111. Prentice RL, Kakar F, Hursting S, Sheppard L, Klein R, Kushi LH (1988) Aspects of the rationale for the Women's Health Trial. J Natl Cancer Inst 80:802–814
112. Knekt P, Albanes D, Seppanen R, Aromaa A, Jarvinen R, Hyvonen L, Teppo L, Pukkala E (1990) Dietary fat and risk of breast cancer. Am J Clin Nutr 52:903–908

113. Carroll KK (1991) Dietary fat and cancer. CMAJ 144:572
114. Hopkins GJ, Carroll KK (1979) Relationship between amount and type of dietary fat in promotion of mammary carcinogenesis induced by 7,12-dimethylbenz[a]anthracene. J Natl Cancer Inst 62:1009–1012
115. Carroll KK, Hopkins GJ (1979) Dietary polyunsaturated fat versus saturated fat in relation to mammary carcinogenesis. Lipids 14:155–158
116. Welsch CW (1992) Relationship between dietary fat and experimental mammary tumorigenesis: a review and critique. Cancer Res 52:2040s–2048s
117. Welsch CW (1992) Dietary fat, calories, and mammary gland tumorigenesis. Adv Exp Med Biol 322:203–222
118. Hunter DJ, Spiegelman D, Adami HO, Beeson L, van den Brandt PA, Folsom AR, Fraser GE, Goldbohm RA, Graham S, Howe GR et al (1996) Cohort studies of fat intake and the risk of breast cancer – a pooled analysis. N Engl J Med 334:356–361
119. Fay MP, Freedman LS, Clifford CK, Midthune DN (1997) Effect of different types and amounts of fat on the development of mammary tumors in rodents: a review. Cancer Res 57:3979–3988
120. Willett WC (1997) Dietary fat intake and cancer risk: a controversial and instructive story. Semin Cancer Biol 8:245–253
121. Eid A, Berry EM (1988) The relationship between dietary fat, adipose tissue composition, and neoplasms of the breast. Nutr Cancer 11:173–177
122. Caygill CP, Charlett A, Hill MJ (1996) Fat, fish, fish oil and cancer. Br J Cancer 74:159–164
123. Holmes MD, Colditz GA, Hunter DJ, Hankinson SE, Rosner B, Speizer FE, Willett WC (2003) Meat, fish and egg intake and risk of breast cancer. Int J Cancer 104:221–227
124. Stripp C, Overvad K, Christensen J, Thomsen BL, Olsen A, Moller S, Tjonneland A (2003) Fish intake is positively associated with breast cancer incidence rate. J Nutr 133:3664–3669
125. Kidwell WR, Monaco ME, Wicha MS, Smith GS (1978) Unsaturated fatty acid requirements for growth and survival of a rat mammary tumor cell line. Cancer Res 38:4091–4100
126. Wicha MS, Liotta LA, Kidwell WR (1979) Effects of free fatty acids on the growth of normal and neoplastic rat mammary epithelial cells. Cancer Res 39:426–435
127. Hillyard L, Rao GA, Abraham S (1980) Effect of dietary fat on fatty acid composition of mouse and rat mammary adenocarcinomas. Proc Soc Exp Biol Med 163:376–383
128. Aylsworth CF, Jone C, Trosko JE, Meites J, Welsch CW (1984) Promotion of 7,12-dimethylbenz[a]anthracene-induced mammary tumorigenesis by high dietary fat in the rat: possible role of intercellular communication. J Natl Cancer Inst 72:637–645
129. Carpenter CL, Ross RK, Paganini-Hill A, Bernstein L (2003) Effect of family history, obesity and exercise on breast cancer risk among postmenopausal women. Int J Cancer 106:96–102
130. Eliassen AH, Colditz GA, Rosner B, Willett WC, Hankinson SE (2006) Adult weight change and risk of postmenopausal breast cancer. JAMA 296:193–201
131. Harvie M, Howell A, Vierkant RA, Kumar N, Cerhan JR, Kelemen LE, Folsom AR, Sellers TA (2005) Association of gain and loss of weight before and after menopause with risk of postmenopausal breast cancer in the Iowa women's health study. Cancer Epidemiol Biomarkers Prev 14:656–661
132. Eng SM, Gammon MD, Terry MB, Kushi LH, Teitelbaum SL, Britton JA, Neugut AI (2005) Body size changes in relation to postmenopausal breast cancer among women on Long Island, New York. Am J Epidemiol 162:229–237
133. Parker ED, Folsom AR (2003) Intentional weight loss and incidence of obesity-related cancers: the Iowa Women's Health Study. Int J Obes Relat Metab Disord 27:1447–1452
134. Williamson DF, Pamuk E, Thun M, Flanders D, Byers T, Heath C (1995) Prospective study of intentional weight loss and mortality in never-smoking overweight US white women aged 40–64 years. Am J Epidemiol 141:1128–1141
135. Djuric Z, DiLaura NM, Jenkins I, Darga L, Jen CK, Mood D, Bradley E, Hryniuk WM (2002) Combining weight-loss counseling with the weight watchers plan for obese breast cancer survivors. Obes Res 10:657–665

136. Goodwin P, Esplen MJ, Butler K, Winocur J, Pritchard K, Brazel S, Gao J, Miller A (1998) Multidisciplinary weight management in locoregional breast cancer: results of a phase II study. Breast Cancer Res Treat 48:53–64
137. Thompson HJ, Jiang W, Zhu Z (1999) Mechanisms by which energy restriction inhibits carcinogenesis. Adv Exp Med Biol 470:77–84
138. Thompson HJ, Zhu Z, Jiang W (2002) Protection against cancer by energy restriction: all experimental approaches are not equal. J Nutr 132:1047–1049
139. Zhu Z, Jiang W, Thompson HJ (2002) An experimental paradigm for studying the cellular and molecular mechanisms of cancer inhibition by energy restriction. Mol Carcinog 35:51–56
140. Dirx MJ, Zeegers MP, Dagnelie PC, van den Bogaard T, van den Brandt PA (2003) Energy restriction and the risk of spontaneous mammary tumors in mice: a meta-analysis. Int J Cancer 106:766–770

Chapter 4
Obesity and Cancer: Epidemiology

Melinda L. Irwin

Introduction

The increase in overweight and obesity in the past few decades is well documented [1]. Observational epidemiologic studies have consistently shown associations between obesity and increased risk of cancer [2, 3]. Studies have also consistently shown associations between obesity at or before the time of cancer diagnosis and increased risk of cancer mortality [4]. Less known is whether weight gain or weight loss affects cancer prognosis [5, 6].

The purpose of this paper is to review the evidence of (1) obesity and cancer risk and mortality, with specific emphasis on the most recent studies of obesity at diagnosis and breast cancer prognosis; (2) weight gain and breast cancer prognosis; and (3) physical activity, diet, and breast cancer prognosis. We will then present a rationale for conducting a large-scale weight loss trial on disease-free survival in women diagnosed with breast cancer. Since a majority of men and women and cancer survivors are overweight, and not participating in recommended levels of physical activity or eating a prudent diet [7], improving these behaviors has the potential to benefit a large number of adults and cancer survivors.

M.L. Irwin (✉)
Department of Epidemiology and Public Health, Yale School of Public Health, 60 College Street, New Haven, CT 06520-8034, USA
e-mail: elinda.irwin@yale.edu

I.G. Fantus (ed.), *Insulin Resistance and Cancer: Epidemiology, Cellular and Molecular Mechanisms and Clinical Implications*, Energy Balance and Cancer 1, DOI 10.1007/978-1-4419-9911-5_4,

Obesity and Cancer Risk and Mortality

Obesity and Cancer Risk

Substantial observational evidence suggests that obesity is associated with increasing risk of many cancers including breast (in postmenopausal women), colon (particularly in men), endometrium, kidney (renal-cell carcinoma), gallbladder (in women), and esophagus (adenocarcinoma) [2, 3]. An association of obesity with cancers of the pancreas, prostate, liver, cervix, ovary, advanced prostate, and on hemotopoietic cancers are inconsistent primarily due to limited number of studies; however, the most recent studies suggest an association [2, 3]. Most of these studies have reported between a 20% and twofold increased risk of cancer with a BMI > 30 kg/m^2 compared with a BMI < 25 kg/m^2, yet most studies show a linear association between BMI and cancer risk [2].

Most recently, Reeves and colleagues examined the association between BMI and incidence of cancer from cancer in more than a million women aged 50–64 years [3]. Higher BMI was associated with significantly increased incidence of postmenopausal breast cancer, endometrial cancer, kidney cancer, and adenocarcinoma of the esophagus. These findings are generally in agreement with accumulated evidence to date, as well as an International Agency for Research on Cancer (IARC) expert panel review in 2002, which examined the epidemiological, clinical, and experimental data of weight and cancer [2].

Interestingly, Reeves and colleagues found no association between BMI and colorectal cancer in postmenopausal women; however, an association between BMI and colorectal cancer was found in men. One hypothesis for the effect modification observed by gender may be that central adiposity, which occurs more often in men, is a stronger predictor of colon cancer risk than total adiposity.

Obesity and Cancer Mortality

Many observational studies have looked at the relationship between weight prior to or at diagnosis and cancer outcomes, and the vast majority of these have demonstrated an increased risk of cancer recurrence and death in men and women who are overweight or obese prior to or at the time of cancer diagnosis [4, 8–10].

In a landmark prospective epidemiological study conducted by the American Cancer Society in over 900,000 U.S. men and women, obesity in adult men and women was associated with increased mortality from cancers of the colon, breast, endometrium, kidney (renal cell), esophagus (adenocarcinoma), gastric cardia, pancreas, prostate, gallbladder, and liver [4]. Estimates from this study suggest 14% of all cancer deaths in men and 20% of all cancer deaths in women from a range of cancer types are attributable to overweight and obesity. Furthermore, there was a

52 and 88% increase in the risk of all cancer death for men and women, respectively, who were severely obese (BMI ≥ 40 kg/m^2) compared with men and women who were normal body weight (BMI < 25 kg/m^2). From these results, it is estimated that 90,000 deaths due to cancer could be prevented each year in the United States if men and women could maintain normal weight.

Recently, two studies observed associations between obesity and increased risk for recurrence and death from colon and prostate cancer. Dignam and colleagues investigated the association between BMI at diagnosis and risk of recurrence, second primary cancer and mortality in 4,288 colon cancer patients [11]. A BMI greater than 35.0 kg/m^2 at diagnosis was associated with a 38 and 49% increased risk of recurrence or death, respectively, as compared to a BMI less than 25 kg/m^2. Wright and colleagues examined BMI in relation to prostate cancer mortality in 287,760 men in the NIH-AARP Diet and Health Study [12]. A significant twofold elevation in prostate cancer mortality was observed in men with BMI levels greater than 35 kg/m^2 as compared with men with BMI levels less than 25 kg/m^2.

Given breast cancer is the most frequently diagnosed invasive cancer among women and given rates of obesity are increasing among women and breast cancer survivors, there has been significant research directed toward the relationship between obesity and breast cancer prognosis. A meta-analysis of these observational studies demonstrated a hazard ratio for breast cancer recurrence at 5 years of 1.78 (95% CI 1.5–2.11) and for breast cancer death at 10 years of 1.36 (95% CI 1.19–1.55) for women in higher BMI categories compared with women at lower BMI categories [13]. The findings that obesity is associated with cancer mortality are apparent even after adjustment for stage at diagnosis and adequacy of treatment.

Association between obesity and breast cancer prognosis in younger women appears to be even stronger; Daling and colleagues [9] reported that women younger than 45 years of age who had invasive breast cancer and a BMI > 25 kg/m^2 were 2.5 times as likely to die of their disease within 5 years of diagnosis compared with women with breast cancer and a BMI < 21 kg/m^2.

Post-Diagnosis Weight Gain and Cancer Mortality

Some epidemiological studies have also shown that weight gain after a cancer diagnosis is associated with an increased risk for recurrence and death compared with maintaining weight after diagnosis [5]. This is especially worrisome given the fact that especially among women treated for breast cancer, a majority of them gain a significant amount of weight in the year following breast cancer diagnosis, and return to prediagnosis weight is rare [14]. Analyses from the Nurses' Health Study showed that median weight gains of 6 and 17 lb from approximately the year before diagnosis to 2 years after diagnosis was related to 35 and 64% higher rates of breast cancer recurrence and death, respectively [5]. The findings were especially apparent in women who never smoked, among women with earlier stage disease, or those who were normal weight before diagnosis.

While these findings are intriguing, not all studies have observed an association between weight gain and poor survival. Caan and colleagues did not observe an association between post-diagnosis weight gain and breast cancer recurrence risk in 1,692 breast cancer survivors enrolled in a prospective cohort study entitled Life After Cancer Epidemiology (LACE) [6]. While being obese 1 year before diagnosis was associated with a 60% increased risk of death from any cause, weight gain up to 4 years after diagnosis was not associated with increased risk of recurrence or death. Furthermore, among the subset of women who lost weight, an increased risk of recurrence and death was observed compared with being weight stable. Thus, they conclude that body weight prior to diagnosis appears to be the strongest predictor of a poor breast cancer prognosis.

Meyerhardt and colleagues, using data from the Cancer and Leukemia Group B (CALGB) 89803 study of 1,053 patients who had stage III colon cancer, demonstrated no association between weight change and survival in colon cancer patients [15]. It is unknown if chemotherapy dose specifications may account for the differences between these studies and the studies showing an increased risk of death with higher BMI and weight gain. Thus, obesity is associated with either poor prognosis or receiving inadequate chemotherapy doses.

Recently, Buist and colleagues examined the association between BMI and receipt of appropriate primary tumor therapy and adjuvant therapy in 897 women diagnosed with breast cancer. They found that receipt of appropriate primary therapy and adjuvant therapy was not associated with BMI in women treated for breast cancer, implying that the majority of studies that have shown an association between obesity and poor prognosis may in fact be true [16].

One concern recently raised by Daniell and colleagues is that being obese, compared with being normal weight, prior to and at cancer diagnosis is associated with earlier tumor metastasis, or more rapid growth of node metastases before diagnosis, as well as differences in hormone receptor status [17]. Thus, these genetic differences in tumors among obese patients may have already influenced the growth of metastic tissue before their initial diagnosis. Therefore, weight gain or loss after diagnosis may not influence prognosis because of the already established genetic alterations.

However, without a methodologically strong weight loss trial conducted in overweight and obese cancer survivors, we are unable to definitively know whether weight loss improves survival or not. Regardless, obesity and weight gain still have adverse effects on risk of other new cancers and overall survival. Specifically, there is evidence that cancer survivors die of noncancer causes at a higher rate than persons in the general population (deaths being primarily from cardiovascular disease and diabetes) [18]. Therefore, surviving cancer requires not only treating the primary cancer but also avoiding second cancers for which patients are at increased risk. To improve overall survival, it is critically important for cancer survivors to prevent obesity. One of the primary methods for preventing or treating obesity and weight gain is by eating a healthy diet and increasing physical activity levels. Physical activity in particular has also been presented as a therapeutic strategy to address both the psychological and physical concerns faced by cancer survivors.

Physical Activity and Cancer Prognosis

There is now consistent evidence that regular exercise is associated with a lower risk of many cancers [19]. Lower risk of both pre- and postmenopausal breast cancer with increased physical activity has been observed in many epidemiological studies, with a 30–40% lower risk of breast cancer in individuals who perform 3–4 h/week of moderate to vigorous activity [20].

Numerous observational studies have also recently been published demonstrating that participation in moderate-intensity recreational physical activity, such as brisk walking, after diagnosis is associated with improved survival in women who develop breast cancer [21–24]. These studies have demonstrated an approximate 50% reduction in the risk of total deaths and risk of breast cancer deaths. These studies also showed that the decreased risk of death associated with physical activity was observed in pre- and postmenopausal women, overweight and normal weight women, and women with stage I–III disease. While any amount of recreational physical activity performed after diagnosis has been associated with a decreased risk of death, the maximal benefit occurred in women who performed the equivalent of brisk walking 3 h per week.

Given that women who are more physically active after diagnosis may have been similarly active before diagnosis, these studies cannot exclude the possibility that physically active individuals who develop breast cancer acquire tumors that are biologically less aggressive. Therefore, being physically active prior to diagnosis may have been associated with an earlier disease stage. Two studies, assessing physical activity in the year prior to diagnosis, observed nonsignificant reduced risks of breast cancer death with higher levels of prediagnosis physical activity [22, 23]. These finding emphasizes the importance of maintaining or increasing physical activity levels after a diagnosis of breast cancer to gain the maximum benefits of physical activity on survival.

Two large observational studies have also demonstrated that participation in 3 h/week of moderate-intensity recreational physical activity after a diagnosis of colon cancer is associated with a 50–63% reduction in the risk of total death and 39–59% reduction in the risk of colon cancer death [25, 26]. The inverse relations between post-diagnosis physical activity and colon cancer mortality remained largely unchanged across strata of sex, BMI, age, disease stage, or year since diagnosis.

In summary, these observational findings of post-diagnosis physical activity and improved survival suggest that exercise may confer additional improvements in breast and colon cancer survival beyond surgery, radiation, and chemotherapy. However, despite this growing body of observational evidence suggesting a strong link between physical activity and cancer survival, there is still the potential for confounding by unknown or poorly characterized variables. For example, physical activity may be a marker of overall health behaviors including adherence to adjuvant treatments. Thus, randomized controlled trials testing the effects of physical activity on cancer survival are necessary and would provide critical information for cancer survivors about whether and how much lifestyle change can affect their prognosis. While a trial of physical activity on cancer survival has yet to be done, a small number of randomized trials of exercise on surrogate/biological markers of survival have been published. The potential adverse effect of low levels of physical activity and obesity on cancer risk and prognosis may be mediated through changes in metabolic (insulin) and sex hormones (androgens and estrogens), growth factors (insulin-like growth factor (IGF)-I and IGFBP-3), adipokines (leptin, adiponectin), and/or inflammation (C-reactive protein) [27]. A growing number of randomized trials have observed clinically meaningful effects of exercise on reducing insulin, IGFs, and sex hormones [28–31].

Diet and Breast Cancer Prognosis

At present, there are hundreds of studies that have investigated nutritional factors in the etiology of various cancers, with some, but not all, suggesting an association between higher fruits and vegetables and lower dietary fat intake with a reduced breast cancer risk [32, 33]. Fewer studies have evaluated nutrition in relation to survival. Several new cohort studies of cancer survivors that include post-diagnosis dietary assessments are now underway as reviewed by Kushi and colleagues [34]. A recent publication by Kwan and colleagues from the Life After Cancer Epidemiology Study examined dietary patterns and breast cancer survival. They observed a prudent dietary pattern (i.e., high intake of fruits, vegetables, whole grains, and poultry) was associated with a 43% reduced risk of overall death ($p=0.02$). In contrast, a Western diet (high intakes of red and processed meats and refined grains) was related to a 53% increased risk of overall death ($p=0.05$) [35].

Two important large-scale multi-site studies evaluated dietary interventions in breast cancer survivors. The Women's Intervention Nutrition Study (WINS) was a randomized trial of a dietary intervention designed to reduce fat intake in 2,437 women with resected, early-stage breast cancer [36]. The low-fat diet group consumed an estimated 33 g total fat/day in comparison with 51 g total fat/day in the usual care group. An interim analysis based on 5 years of follow-up reported that the intervention group had a lower risk of relapse events (HR=0.76, 95% CI 0.60–0.98). Of particular interest, when the results were stratified by the estrogen receptor (ER) status (positive vs. negative) of the women's first breast cancer, a more substantial benefit was observed in women who had ER-negative breast cancer (RR: 0.58, 95% CI: 0.37, 0.91). Women with ER-positive breast cancer who were randomized to the low-fat diet also had fewer second breast cancers, but the result was not statistically significant (RR: 0.85, 95% CI: 0.63, 1.14). However, the updated results from the WINS study (presented at the San Antonio Breast Conference in December 2006, www.sabcs.org) demonstrated a nonsignificant improvement in disease-free survival in the intervention group compared with usual care.

The Women's Healthy Eating and Living (WHEL) study was a randomized clinical trial of high fruit and vegetable and low-fat diet versus usual diet in breast cancer survivors. This trial demonstrated that women randomized to a high fruit and vegetable diet increased consumption of fruits and vegetables, as supported by marked increases in plasma carotenoids, which are biomarkers of fruit and vegetable intake [37]. Despite this apparent adherence, and a 7.3-year follow-up period, rates of second breast cancer were similar in the two dietary arms of this trial (HR = 0.96, 95% CI 0.80–1.14) and mortality was lower, but not significantly so (HR = 0.91, 95% CI 0.72–1.15). The women in the nonintervention arm of this study were consuming 3.8 servings of vegetables and 3.4 servings of fruit at baseline; therefore, this trial was evaluating incremental benefits in cancer survival for consuming very high intakes versus high intakes. The observational evidence commonly suggests that the incremental benefits are largest when intervening in populations with low intakes, so the results of this trial should be interpreted in their proper context (no additional benefit to consuming beyond 5-a-day).

These two trials are by far the largest trials of nutritional interventions in cancer survivors, and while the impact of diet on cancer prognosis is still unclear, it is well known that cancer survivors are often at heightened risk for noncancer chronic diseases such as coronary heart disease. Thus, it is obviously prudent to emphasize dietary patterns associated with lowered all-cause mortality. Also, examining the contribution of both diet and physical activity on all-cause and cancer-specific mortality is important. A recent observational analysis of the nonintervention arm of the WHEL study suggested that the combination of fruit and vegetable intake with physical activity was in deed beneficial [24]. Specifically, breast cancer survivors who consumed 5+ daily servings of fruits and vegetables and who exercised an amount equivalent to walking 30 min 6 days per week had a significant survival advantage. This was not seen in women who engaged in only one behavior (diet or physical activity); rather, the combined influence of diet and physical activity was associated with risk reduction. Notably, only a minority of breast cancer survivors engaged in both health-promoting behaviors, suggesting obvious opportunities for post-diagnosis interventions.

Rationale for Conducting a Large-Scale Weight Loss Trial on Disease-Free Survival in Women with Breast Cancer

Some scientists have posited that weight gain or loss after diagnosis may not influence prognosis because of the already established genetic alterations that occur at initial diagnosis [17]. While two large-scale diet trials on breast cancer prognosis have been conducted [36, 37], neither trial focused on or showed significant weight loss during the intervention. Furthermore, no trial has examined the effect of increasing physical activity after a cancer diagnosis on survival. Thus, the impact of dietary-induced weight loss and physical activity on survival after a cancer diagnosis is unknown. Without a methodologically strong weight loss and physical activity trial conducted in cancer survivors, we are unable to definitively know whether weight loss and physical activity impact survival or not. Given the strong observational evidence suggesting that being overweight or obese and physically inactive is associated with poor prognosis in breast cancer, there is a need to develop clinical trials testing the effect of weight loss and exercise upon breast cancer recurrence and mortality.

Even if a benefit of weight loss and physical activity on disease-free survival is not observed, there are additional benefits including reduced therapy-related complications, improved quality of life, and reduced risk of death from other causes. Oncologists are, therefore, encouraged to counsel patients on maintaining a healthy weight via increased physical activity and eating a prudent diet high in fruits and vegetables, whole grains, and poultry.

Conclusions

Numerous epidemiological studies have observed associations between obesity and cancer risk and mortality. The influence of weight gain or loss on cancer mortality has not been fully characterized in observational studies or clinical trials. There are, clearly, many questions to be answered concerning if weight loss impacts cancer prognosis, who would benefit from lifestyle change, when these lifestyle changes would be most beneficial, and what type of diet and exercise program would be most beneficial. Future research must be done both to establish the efficacy and effectiveness of weight control, nutrition and physical activity to lower cancer recurrence and death, and to understand the biologic mechanisms through which these methods impact cancer development and malignant potential. However, until these studies are conducted, it may well be a benefit for men and women with or without cancer to maintain a healthy weight, eat a prudent diet of fruits and vegetables, whole grains, and poultry, and to exercise 30 min per day [8, 32]. Since a majority of adults and cancer survivors are not currently participating in recommended levels of physical activity or eating a healthy diet, these lifestyle behaviors have the potential to benefit a large number of adults and cancer survivors. Thus, oncologists and primary care physicians should be encouraged to counsel their patients proactively about nutrition, exercise, and weight control.

In conclusion, improved understanding in obesity and lifestyle research will pave the way for weight loss, physical activity, and dietary programs to become a routine component of cancer treatment and recovery, and will hopefully provide the necessary evidence to convince policy makers for the inclusion of weight loss, exercise, and nutrition counseling in cancer management, and second party payers in reimbursing cancer survivors for receipt of their counseling.

References

1. Flegal K, Graubard B, Williamson D et al (2005) Excess deaths associated with underweight, overweight, and obesity. JAMA 293:1861–1867
2. International Agency for Research on Cancer (2002) IARC handbooks of cancer prevention: weight control and physical activity. International Agency for Research on Cancer, Lyon
3. Reeves GK, Pirie K, Beral V et al (2007) Cancer incidence and mortality in relation to body mass index in the Million Women Study: cohort study. BMJ 335(7630):1134

4. Calle EE, Rodriguez C, Walker-Thurmond K, Thun MJ (2003) Overweight, obesity, and mortality from Cancer in a Prospectively Studied Cohort of U.S. Adults. N Engl J Med 348(17):1625–1638
5. Kroenke CH, Chen WY, Rosner B, Holmes MD (2005) Weight, weight gain, and survival after breast cancer diagnosis. J Clin Oncol 23(7):1370–1378
6. Caan BJ, Emond JA, Natarajan L et al (2006) Post-diagnosis weight gain and breast cancer recurrence in women with early stage breast cancer. Breast Cancer Res Treat 99(1):47–57
7. Blanchard CM, Courneya KS, Stein K (2008) Cancer survivors' adherence to lifestyle behavior recommendations and associations with health-related quality of life: results from the American Cancer Society's SCS-II. J Clin Oncol 26(13):2198–2204
8. Doyle C, Kushi LH, Byers T et al (2006) Nutrition and physical activity during and after cancer treatment: an American Cancer Society guide for informed choices. CA Cancer J Clin 56(6):323–353
9. Daling JR, Malone KE, Doody DR, Johnson LG, Gralow JR, Porter PL (2001) Relation of body mass index to tumor markers and survival among young women with invasive ductal breast carcinoma. Cancer 92(4):720–729
10. Chlebowski RT, Aiello E, McTiernan A (2002) Weight loss in breast cancer patient management. J Clin Oncol 20(4):1128–1143
11. Dignam JJ, Polite BN, Yothers G et al (2006) Body mass index and outcomes in patients who receive adjuvant chemotherapy for colon cancer. J Natl Cancer Inst 98(22):1647–1654
12. Wright ME, Chang SC, Schatzkin A et al (2007) Prospective study of adiposity and weight change in relation to prostate cancer incidence and mortality. Cancer 109(4):675–684
13. Goodwin P (1995) In: Bitzer J, Stauber M (eds) Psychosomatic obstetrics and gynecology. Bologna: Monduzzi Editore, International Proceedings Division. Obesity and Cancer Outcomes. pp. 491–496
14. Irwin ML, McTiernan A, Baumgartner RN et al (2005) Changes in body fat and weight after a breast cancer diagnosis: influence of demographic, prognostic, and lifestyle factors. J Clin Oncol 23(4):774–782
15. Meyerhardt JA, Niedzwiecki D, Hollis D et al (2008) Impact of body mass index and weight change after treatment on cancer recurrence and survival in patients with stage III colon cancer: findings from CALGB 89803. J Clin Oncol 26:4109–4115
16. Buist D, Ichikawa L, Prout M et al (2007) Receipt of appropriate primary breast cancer therapy and adjuvant therapy are not associated with obesity in older women with access to health care. J Clin Oncol 25:3428–3436
17. Daniell HW (2009) Weight loss after breast cancer diagnosis may not improve prognosis. J Clin Oncol 27:829–830
18. Carver JR, Shapiro CL, Ng A et al (2007) American Society of Clinical Oncology clinical evidence review on the ongoing care of adult cancer survivors: cardiac and pulmonary late effects. J Clin Oncol 25(25):3991–4008
19. Thune I, Ferberg A (2001) Physical activity and cancer risk: dose-response and cancer, all sites and site specific. Med Sci Sports Exerc 33(6):S530–S550
20. Friedenreich CM, Cust AE (2008) Physical activity and breast cancer risk: impact of timing, type, and dose of activity and population subgroup effects. Br J Sports Med 42(8):636–647
21. Holmes MD, Chen WY, Feskanich D, Kroenke CH, Colditz GA (2005) Physical activity and survival after breast cancer diagnosis. JAMA 293(20):2479–2486
22. Irwin ML (2008) Influence of pre- and post-diagnosis physical activity on survival in breast cancer survivors: the health, eating, activity, and lifestyle (HEAL) study. J Clin Oncol 26(24):1–7
23. Holick CN, Newcomb PA, Trentham-Dietz A et al (2008) Physical activity and survival after diagnosis of invasive breast cancer. Cancer Epidemiol Biomarkers Prev 17(2):379–386
24. Pierce JP, Stefanick ML, Flatt SW et al (2007) Greater survival after breast cancer in physically active women with high vegetable-fruit intake regardless of obesity. J Clin Oncol 25(17):2345–2351

25. Meyerhardt JA, Giovannucci EL, Holmes MD et al (2006) Physical activity and survival after colorectal cancer diagnosis. J Clin Oncol 24(22):3527–3534
26. Meyerhardt JA, Heseltine D, Niedzwiecki D et al (2006) Impact of physical activity on cancer recurrence and survival in patients with stage III colon cancer: findings from CALGB 89803. J Clin Oncol 24(22):3535–3541
27. Hursting SD, Lashinger LM, Colbert LH et al (2007) Energy balance and carcinogenesis: underlying pathways and targets for intervention. Curr Cancer Drug Targets 7(5):484–491
28. Ligibel JA, Campbell N, Partridge A et al (2008) Impact of a mixed strength and endurance exercise intervention on insulin levels in breast cancer survivors. J Clin Oncol 26(6):907–912
29. Irwin ML, Varma K, Alvarez-Reeves M et al (2009) Randomized controlled exercise trial on insulin and IGFs in breast cancer survivors: the Yale Exercise and Survivorship Study. Cancer Epidemiol Biomarkers Prev 18(1):306–313
30. Schmitz KH, Ahmed RL, Hannan PJ, Yee D (2005) Safety and efficacy of weight training in recent breast cancer survivors to alter body composition, insulin, and IGFs. Cancer Epidemiol Biomarkers Prev 14(7):1672–1680
31. McTiernan A, Tworoger SS, Ulrich CM et al (2004) Effect of exercise on serum estrogens in postmenopausal women: a 12-month randomized clinical trial. Cancer Res 64(8):2923–2928
32. Kushi L, Byers T, Doyle C et al (2006) American Cancer Society Guidelines on nutrition and physical activity for cancer prevention. CA Cancer J Clin 56:254–281
33. Prentice R, Caan B, Chlebowski R et al (2006) Low fat dietary pattern and risk of invasive breast cancer: the Women's Health Initiative Randomized Controlled Dietary Modification Trial. JAMA 295(6):629–642
34. Kushi LH, Kwan ML, Lee MM, Ambrosone CB (2007) Lifestyle factors and survival in women with breast cancer. J Nutr 137(1 Suppl):236S–242S
35. Kwan ML, Weltzien E, Kushi LH et al (2008) Dietary patterns and breast cancer recurrence and survival among women with early-stage breast cancer. J Clin Oncol 27:1–8
36. Chlebowski RT, Blackburn GL, Thomson CA et al (2006) Dietary fat reduction and breast cancer outcome: interim efficacy results from the Women's Intervention Nutrition Study. J Natl Cancer Inst 98(24):1767–1776
37. Pierce JP, Natarajan L, Caan BJ et al (2007) Influence of a diet very high in vegetables, fruit, and fiber and low in fat on prognosis following treatment for breast cancer: the Women's Healthy Eating and Living (WHEL) randomized trial [see comment]. JAMA 298(3):289–298

Chapter 5
Insulin, Insulin Resistance, and Cancer Associations

Lorraine Lipscombe

There have been long-standing attempts to elucidate the causes of cancer through observational research. While causation can never be definitively established based on this type of evidence, the impossibility of conducting experimental studies forces us to rely on epidemiologic studies to generate hypotheses regarding key risk factors for cancers. Initially, potential risk factors are considered based on biological hypotheses, preliminary in vitro or animal studies, ecologic observations, or anecdotal evidence. Associations between risk factors and cancer outcomes are then sought through more rigorous observational studies. We must then determine whether such associations represent causative relationships, based on well-established criteria such as biologic plausibility, the strength, specificity and consistency of the association, temporality, and demonstration of a biologic gradient [1]. Recently, epidemiologic associations have emerged between obesity, diabetes, and certain forms of cancer such as those of the breast, colon, and pancreas. Since these conditions are associated with insulin resistance and compensatory hyperinsulinemia, it has been hypothesized that insulin may be a common mediator in these relationships due to its cancer-promoting properties. This chapter will review the growing body of evidence linking obesity and diabetes to the risk of certain cancers and the potential role of hyperinsulinemia in these associations, with a particular focus on cancer of the breast, colon, pancreas, and prostate. As a framework, this review consider these cancers separately, and will discuss the epidemiological evidence linking cancer risk first to obesity, then to insulin resistance and diabetes, followed by a discussion of direct and indirect evidence of the role of hyperinsulinemia in these associations.

L. Lipscombe (✉)
Department of Medicine, University of Toronto, Toronto, ON, Canada
e-mail: lorraine.lipscombe@wchospital.ca

I.G. Fantus (ed.), *Insulin Resistance and Cancer: Epidemiology, Cellular and Molecular Mechanisms and Clinical Implications*, Energy Balance and Cancer 1,
DOI 10.1007/978-1-4419-9911-5_5,

Breast Cancer

Obesity

There is a well-accepted relationship between body mass index (BMI) and risk of breast cancer [2- 4]. Interestingly, the association between BMI and breast cancer risk differs between pre- and postmenopausal women. While there is a strong positive relationship between BMI and postmenopausal breast cancer, BMI has been inversely correlated with premenopausal breast cancer [5, 6]. In 2000, van den Brandt et al. performed a pooled analysis of seven prospective cohort studies of BMI and breast cancer risk involving a total of over 300,000 women [5]. After controlling for dietary, reproductive, and other risk factors, premenopausal women with a BMI>31 kg/m^2 had a relative risk (RR) of 0.54 (95% CI: 0.34–0.85) for breast cancer compared to women with a BMI<21 kg/m^2. In postmenopausal women, a BMI of>28 kg/m^2 was associated with an overall RR of 1.26 (95% CI: 1.09–1.46) [5]. A more recent meta-analysis of obesity and cancer incidence published in 2008 confirmed a significant association between obesity and postmenopausal breast cancer [4]. The protective effect of excess weight in premenopausal women may reflect longer anovular cycles resulting in less estrogen and progesterone exposure [7]. In contrast, the positive association between weight and breast cancer among postmenopausal women has been traditionally attributed to increased peripheral production of estrogens derived from aromatization of androstenedione within the larger adipose stores of obese women [8, 9]. However, more recent evidence suggests that the association between obesity and postmenopausal breast cancer may be mediated via the insulin resistance and hyperinsulinemia associated with obesity.

Insulin Resistance

The hypothesized relationship between insulin resistance and breast cancer may be due to either direct effects of insulin on breast tissue, or indirectly through higher circulating levels of insulin like growth factor-1 (IGF-1) [10, 11] or increased sex steroid availability due to a reduction of sex-hormone-binding globulin [12]. No studies have directly examined the role of biologically-documented insulin resistance on breast cancer risk in humans. However, many studies have explored the link between clinical markers of insulin resistance and breast cancer. For example, insulin resistance is more specifically associated with accumulation of fat in visceral rather than subcutaneous areas. Anthropometric measures such as waist-to-hip ratio (WHR) or waist circumference (WC) have been well-validated as markers of central visceral adiposity and correlate well with insulin resistance [13]. These measures have been used in several studies to assess the specific role of insulin resistance in the link between obesity and breast cancer. Some have found that higher WHR or WC is associated with a higher risk of postmenopausal breast cancer independent of

BMI [14–16], while other studies have failed to demonstrate a relationship [17–20]. A systematic review by Harvie et al. in 2003 examined studies of the relationship between central obesity and pre- and postmenopausal breast cancer [21]. Pooled data from five cohort and three case-control studies found that the lowest WC was associated with a 39% decrease and the lowest WHR with a 24% decrease in post-menopausal breast cancer risk compared to the highest WC or WHR. The relationship was however abolished after adjustment for BMI, which may simply reflect the difficulty separating the independent contribution of these highly correlated measures when both factors have similar effects on cancer risk. In contrast, an association between central obesity and premenopausal breast cancer was only seen *after* adjusting for BMI. These findings suggest that general and central obesity may both have effects on the risk of breast cancer. In premenopausal women, generalized obesity may be unrelated or possibly protective whereas central obesity appears to increase the risk of breast cancer. Conversely, in postmenopausal women both central and generalized obesity are harmful, but an independent effect of central obesity based on anthropometric measures is more difficult to disentangle in this population.

The metabolic syndrome, which is characterized by central obesity, hypertension, dyslipidemia, and hyperglycemia, is a clinical syndrome tightly linked to insulin resistance [13]. In addition to central obesity, some studies have explored the association between other features of metabolic syndrome and risk of breast cancer. For example, hypertension has been associated with a higher risk of breast cancer in some studies [22–24], but not in others [25–27]. Dyslipidemia has also been linked to risk of breast cancer in some studies. Case-control studies have shown an association between high total cholesterol [28–33], high LDL cholesterol [30, 31], and decreased HDL cholesterol [29, 31, 34] and breast cancer. Results from prospective studies are more conflicting with both positive [35] and negative [22, 36] associations, but the majority have failed to support a relationship between dyslipidemia and risk of breast cancer [37–44]. Interestingly, no observational study has considered the association between breast cancer and the metabolic syndrome itself. One small case-control study from Italy did report a higher prevalence of diabetes, hypertension, and dyslipidemia among breast cancer cases compared to controls [45]. However, further studies involving women specifically with the metabolic syndrome, as well as studies using direct assessments of visceral fat, are needed to more adequately address the role of insulin resistance on the risk of breast cancer.

Diabetes Mellitus

Since type 2 diabetes is an important consequence of insulin resistance, several epidemiologic studies have explored the association between diabetes and risk of breast cancer. Case-control and cohort studies have been conducted in Canada [46], the United States [47–54], the United Kingdom [10, 55], Italy [56–58], Japan [59–61], Sweden [62, 63], Denmark [64, 65], Germany [66], Netherlands [67], and Korea [68]. The majority of case-control studies have suggested that breast cancer patients were more likely to have a history of diabetes with odds ratios between 1.10 and 2.15 [47, 50, 53, 57, 58, 62, 66], and in three studies the odds ratios were statistically significant [57, 58, 66]. Ten cohort studies have also documented a higher incidence of breast cancer among women with diabetes [46, 48, 49, 51, 59, 61, 63, 65, 67, 68], and the increase was statistically significant in six studies [46, 48, 59, 63, 65, 68]. A meta-analysis from 2007 of five case-control and 15 cohort studies confirmed a significant 20% increased risk of breast cancer among women with versus without diabetes (relative risk, RR 1.20, 95% confidence interval, CI 1.12–1.28) [69]. A second meta-analysis in the same year included nine case-control and 11 cohort studies, and also documented an overall 15% increased risk of breast cancer associated with diabetes (RR 1.15, 95% CI 1.12, 1.19) [70]. In both reviews similar results were obtained for case-control and cohort studies. Larsson et al. also found no difference in findings when studies were stratified by factors such as definition of diabetes, geographic region, publication year, and adjustment for BMI, physical activity, alcohol intake, and post-menopausal hormone use [69]. Several studies stratified findings by menopausal status [48, 56, 57] or limited their populations to predominantly postmenopausal women [46, 47, 52, 65, 67]. When meta-analysis results were separated by menopausal status, the significant association between diabetes and breast cancer appeared to be limited to postmenopausal women in both reviews [69, 70]. Thus, evidence supports a significant 15–20% increased risk of breast cancer associated with diabetes, which is primarily seen in postmenopausal cases.

Hyperinsulinemia

Despite the mounting body of epidemiologic evidence suggesting an association between obesity, insulin resistance, and diabetes and a higher risk of postmenopausal breast cancer, the mechanism of this association is unclear. Many hypothesize that it is exposure to long-standing hyperinsulinemia that occurs in response to insulin resistance which mediates this association. This hypothesis is supported by evidence that insulin has mitogenic effects on breast tissue [71, 72], and insulin receptors are frequently overexpressed in breast cancer cells [73, 74]. However, indirect effects of insulin resistance, such as higher circulating levels of IGF-1 [10, 11] or increased sex steroid availability due to a reduction of sex-hormone-binding globulin [12], may also contribute to a higher risk of breast cancer. Finally, given the consistent association between diabetes and breast cancer, it is possible that hyperglycemia may increase the risk of breast cancer [75].

There are several lines of evidence that may help to elucidate the role of hyperinsulinemia versus other factors underlying the association between insulin resistance, diabetes, and the risk of breast cancer. First, although diabetes has been associated with a small but significant increased risk of incident breast cancer, insulin concentrations are actually highest before type 2 diabetes develops in insulin-resistant individuals. This state of compensatory hyperinsulinemia may predate diabetes by 10–20 years, until pancreatic beta-cell failure ensues and insulin secretion declines heralding the onset of diabetes [76, 77]. Thus, if insulin is an important mediator underlying the association between diabetes and breast cancer, then the risk of cancer may be greater with earlier diabetes or before diabetes develops when insulin levels are higher. Only one study explored the influence of diabetes duration on the incidence of breast cancer. Using data from the Nurses' Health Study that followed over 100,000 women, Michels et al. documented a statistically significant association between diabetes and subsequent risk of breast cancer, but they did not find a consistent difference in risk based on years since diabetes diagnosis [48]. To examine whether breast cancer risk is higher in the prediabetic phase, another large retrospective study from Canada assessed whether women with newly diagnosed diabetes were more likely to have a history of breast cancer prior to their diagnosis [78]. In this population-based study involving over 500,000 women, women with diabetes were 22% more likely to have previous breast cancer compared to women without diabetes. These data support the observation that breast cancer risk is increased even in the prediabetic phase, supporting an independent role of insulin resistance on the risk of cancer. Other studies have looked at the risk of breast cancer among women with conditions that carry a high risk of future diabetes, such as gestational diabetes [79] and polycystic ovarian syndrome [47, 80, 81]. These syndromes are generally characterized by insulin resistance and hyperinsulinemia but have not progressed to hyperglycemia. Despite small sample sizes in these studies, increased risk of breast cancer has been observed with both of these conditions and the association with gestational diabetes was statistically significant [79].

The insulin hypothesis can also be explored by examining whether treatment with insulin or insulin secretagogues increases the risk of cancer. One Canadian study found that among patients with diabetes, treatment with insulin or a sulfonylurea (an insulin secretagogue) was associated with a significant increase in cancer-related mortality compared to metformin treatment (an insulin sensitizer) [82]. More recently there has been concern regarding higher cancel risk with long-acting insulins, and in particular insulin glargine [83–87], which has higher insulin receptor binding affinity compared to other insulins [88]. There is also some evidence that metformin may be protective against breast cancer, possibly due to its insulin-lowering properties. A case-control study from Scotland found that metformin treatment was associated with a RR of 0.79 (95% CI 0.67–0.93) for overall cancer incidence, and the risk increased with increasing duration of treatment [89]. A more recent systematic review confirmed that metformin is associated with a significant reduction in cancer incidence [90], and one study found that metformin treatment among women with type 2 diabetes and breast cancer was associated with a significant improvement in complete pathologic response following adjuvant chemotherapy [91]. Although there have been no epidemiological studies to date assessing the effect of diabetes treatments on breast cancer specifically, there is some in vitro evidence that metformin directly inhibits the growth of breast cancer cells [92].

Several epidemiologic studies have also examined whether there is a direct link between increased serum levels of insulin or C-peptide (a marker of insulin secretion) and risk of breast cancer. Results from these studies have been mixed. Four case-control studies have demonstrated an association between serum insulin levels and breast cancer [10, 93–95], however two case-control and three cohort studies did not [49, 96–99]. Similarly, C-peptide levels were associated with breast cancer in four case-control studies [100–103], however another five studies found no association [94, 97, 104–106]. A recent meta-analysis summarized the studies of insulin and C-peptide and breast cancer, and upper levels of insulin or C-peptide were associated with a RR 1.26 (95% CI 1.06–1.48) overall for breast cancer risk [107]. However, there was a significant heterogeneity between studies, whereby the RR was only significant for findings from case-control studies (RR 1.81, 95% CI 1.36–2.40) – the association was not significant for cohort studies. Overall, the results of these studies provide suggestive but inconsistent evidence of a link between excess serum insulin and breast cancer risk. This may be partly due to how fasting insulin was measured and how high insulin levels were defined. Despite the American Heart Association's definition of hyperinsulinemia as a fasting insulin concentration of >139 pmol/L [108], this definition was not used in any of the studies. Overall insulin concentrations were lower than this threshold in these study populations; therefore studies may not have been able to detect an effect of high serum insulin on breast cancer risk.

Hyperglycemia

Given the association between diabetes and breast cancer, it is possible that hyperglycemia also plays a role in promoting cancer incidence. Malignant cells use glucose for proliferation [109], and there is an increased metabolism of glucose towards the pentose phosphate pathway [75]. Therefore, higher glucose concentrations may promote carcinogenesis by providing an environment for malignant cell growth. Both type 1 and type 2 diabetes are associated with hyperglycemia, whereas only type 2 diabetes is associated with insulin resistance and relative hyperinsulinemia. If hyperglycemia is the central mediator of breast cancer risk in the setting of diabetes, then one would expect that both type 1 and type 2 diabetes confer a higher risk of breast cancer. While most epidemiologic studies of diabetes and breast cancer have not differentiated between type 1 and type 2 diabetes, three studies have looked specifically at the risk in women with type 1 diabetes [55, 64, 110]. None of these studies found a significant association between type 1 diabetes and risk of breast cancer. Since the vast majority of diabetes cases are due to type 2 diabetes, particularly among postmenopausal women, the lack of association among women with type 1 diabetes may be partly due to inadequate power to detect an effect in this population. Five studies have analyzed the association between fasting glucose concentration and risk of breast cancer [25, 49, 68, 99, 111], and a statistically significant association was found in two studies [99, 111]. However, one of these studies suggested that the risk was increased with fasting glucose concentrations above 7 mmol/L [111], which is the threshold for a diagnosis of diabetes. Thus, while the mechanism underlying the association between diabetes and breast cancer is still unclear, the balance of epidemiologic evidence supports a greater role of insulin resistance and hyperinsulinemia over hyperglycemia.

Breast Cancer Prognosis

There is also some evidence that diabetes and hyperinsulinemia may worsen the prognosis following breast cancer. Studies have found that insulin receptors are frequently overexpressed in breast cancer cells [73, 74, 112], and insulin receptors are associated with higher mortality [112]. In addition, some breast cancers have been reported to express the more sensitive IR-A receptor isoform [113]. This may lead to enhanced sensitivity to the mitogenic effects of insulin, leading to a worse prognosis for breast cancer patients in the setting of hyperinsulinemia. One study by Goodwin et al. reported a direct association between fasting insulin concentrations and risk of recurrence and death in a population of women with breast cancer [114].

Five large studies have examined the association between diabetes and breast cancer mortality [55, 68, 115–117]. Statistically significant associations between diabetes and increased breast cancer mortality were documented in three studies [68, 115, 116]. The meta-analysis by Larsson et al. calculated a summary relative risk of breast cancer mortality associated with diabetes of 1.24 (95% CI 0.95–1.62) [69]. However, because these studies were not limited to patients with breast cancer, this association may be partly driven by an increase in the incidence of breast cancer among women with diabetes. Five studies have specifically examined the influence of preexisting diabetes on all-cause mortality among breast cancer patients, and all studies have documented a worse survival following breast cancer among patients with diabetes [69, 118–122]. A recent meta-analysis confirmed this association, with a pooled hazard ratio of 1.60 (95% CI 1.46–1.78) for diabetes and all-cause mortality following breast cancer [123]. In addition to a potential role of insulin resistance and hyperinsulinemia, diabetes may also worsen all-cause mortality due to less aggressive treatment [121, 122, 124], later stage at diagnosis due to lower screening rates [125], or because of diabetes-related comorbidity. Further studies are needed to differentiate the effect of diabetes on breast cancer prognosis from its effect on all-cause mortality in women with breast cancer.

Colorect.al Cancer

As with breast cancer, there is a growing body of evidence of an association between insulin resistance, diabetes, and colorectal cancer. These associations have also been attributed to the carcinogenic effects of hyperinsulinemia.

Obesity

The relationship between obesity and risk of colorectal cancer has been well-documented, with many studies reporting a significant association between higher BMI and risk of colon cancer [126]. The association appears to be more consistent in men, whereby obesity is associated with a relative of 1.5–2.0 for colorectal cancer when compared to normal BMI [126]. The large European Prospective Investigation into Cancer and Nutrition (EPIC) study reported a significant 55% increase in colon cancer risk for the highest versus lowest BMI quintile in men, but no significant association in women [127]. A recent meta-analysis from 2008 of studies of obesity and cancer incidence confirmed a significant 25% increase in colorectal cancer risk for every 5 kg/m^2 increase in BMI in men, and a weaker, nonsignificant association in women [4].

Insulin Resistance

To determine whether the association between obesity and colon cancer can be explained by insulin resistance, many studies have explored the contribution of anthropometric measures of insulin resistance, such as waist circumference (WC) and WHR to this relationship. Most studies have found a direct association between WC and WHR and colon cancer risk that is independent of BMI [128–132], and higher WC or WHR are more clearly associated with colon cancer than is BMI in women [127, 130–133]. For example, in the aforementioned EPIC study, whereas in women there was no significant association between BMI and risk of colon cancer, a significant 50% increase in risk was seen in women with a higher WHR [127].

Studies have also explored whether other clinical features of insulin resistance increase the risk of colorectal cancer. Unlike with breast cancer, at least four studies have examined whether individuals with the metabolic syndrome have a higher risk of colon cancer, and all have documented significant associations between features of the metabolic syndrome and risk of colorectal cancer [134–137]. Hypertriglyceridemia is a typical component of the metabolic syndrome, and several studies have also assessed the association between serum triglycerides and colon cancer. One Japanese case-control study found that hypertriglyceridemia was associated with a threefold increase in the risk of colorectal carcinoma in situ [138]; however other studies have been inconsistent and only suggestive of an association [128, 136, 139–141]. An association between hypertriglyceridemia and colorectal adenoma risk has also been reported in some studies [142–145]. While no studies have explored the role of direct measures of insulin resistance on colon cancer risk, findings from studies of clinical markers provide indirect evidence that insulin resistance may play a role in the development of colon cancer.

Diabetes Mellitus

Since type 2 diabetes is a major consequence of insulin resistance, several studies have also found an association between diabetes and the risk of colorectal cancer. At least six case-control [50, 146–150] and 12 cohort studies [51, 65, 68, 151–159] have examined the association between diabetes and colon or colorectal cancer incidence. Statistically significant associations have been reported in three case-control [146, 148, 149] and eight cohort studies [65, 68, 151, 152, 156–159], with relative risks (RR) ranging from 1.02 to 2.78. A meta-analysis in 2005 by Larsson et al. reported summary RR of 1.30 (95% CI 1.20–1.40) for the association between diabetes and colorectal cancer risk and results were comparable for colon cancer (RR 1.43, 95% CI 1.28–1.60) and rectal cancer (RR 1.33, 95% CI 1.14–1.54) [69]. No heterogeneity among studies was found and results were similar for case-control and cohort studies and for studies conducted in the United States and Europe. Similar risks were also seen for both men (RR 1.29, 95% CI 1.15–1.44) and for women (RR 1.33, 95% CI 1.23–1.44). Several studies adjusted for other risk factors such as physical activity and BMI [148, 149, 151, 153–155, 159], and results were similar when Larsson et al. restricted their meta-analysis to those studies (RR 1.34, 95% CI 1.20–1.49) [69]. Thus, these findings provide consistent evidence of a 30–40% increased risk of colorectal cancer associated with diabetes.

Hyperinsulinemia

The role of hyperinsulinemia underlying the associations between obesity, diabetes, and colorectal cancer has been explored in several ways. First, studies have examined the relationship between serum insulin or C-peptide and colon cancer. One cohort study found that serum insulin after a 2-h post-glucose load was associated with a significant increase in colon cancer risk (RR 2.0), but the association for fasting insulin was not significant [128]. A Swedish study did not find an association when both fasting and non-fasting insulin samples were considered, but found a nonsignificant trend toward a higher risk of colon cancer with high fasting insulin alone (RR 1.68) [160]. A third study that also used a mixture of fasting and non-fasting samples did not find an association between insulin concentration and colorectal cancer risk [139]. Three studies have assessed the relationship between C-peptide concentrations and colorectal cancer, and all have reported significant associations [161–164]. The Physician's Health Study found that men with a C-peptide concentration in the top quintile had an RR of 2.7 for colorectal cancer compared to those with C-peptide levels in the lowest quintile [163]. Interestingly, in that study the RR increased to 3.4 after controlling for features of the metabolic syndrome, suggesting an independent, stronger effect of hyperinsulinemia on the risk of colorectal cancer. In the Nurses' Health Study, the risk of colon cancer was increased by 76% for women with C-peptide concentrations in the top versus bottom quartile [164]. Another prospective study of women found a threefold higher risk of colorectal cancer for the top quartile of serum C-peptide [161], and a fourfold higher risk for colon cancer alone [162]. A recent meta-analysis summarized studies of the association between insulin or C-peptide and colon cancer, and confirmed a significant overall 35% increase in risk of colon cancer with high serum insulin or C-peptide (95% CI 1.13–1.161) [107].

To further isolate the potential role of hyperinsulinemia versus hyperglycemia underlying the association between diabetes and colorectal cancer, the natural history of type 2 diabetes can be exploited. Since hyperinsulinemia predominates in the initial stages of insulin resistance, whereas insulin levels decline as glucose intolerance worsens [76, 77], one would expect a greater risk of cancer earlier in this course if insulin were the central mediator of this risk. Conversely, a stronger risk might be seen in persons with more long-standing diabetes if hyperglycemia was more important. Supporting the insulin hypothesis, one study found that colon cancer mortality was significantly increased only for patients with impaired glucose tolerance, whereas a nonsignificant trend was observed for patients with diabetes [141]. Only the Nurses' Health Study has examined the impact of diabetes duration on the association between diabetes and risk of colon cancer. Unlike for breast cancer, the risk of colon cancer was greatest in women who were recently diagnosed with diabetes and the effect became attenuated in those with greater than 15 years diabetes duration [151]. Finally, further support for the insulin hypothesis is provided by evidence that insulin or insulin secretagogue treatment is associated with an increased cancer-related mortality [82], and metformin (an insulin sensitizer) is associated with a decrease in cancer incidence [89]. In addition, one study observed that insulin therapy in patients with type 2 diabetes was associated with a 21% increase in colorectal cancer risk with each incremental year of insulin treatment [165]. Taken together, these findings support the hypothesis that hyperinsulinemia is the central underlying mechanism for higher risk of colon cancer among persons with obesity, insulin resistance, and diabetes.

Hyperglycemia

Although hyperinsulinemia appears to be an important risk factor for colon cancer, hyperglycemia may also play a role. At least eight studies have assessed the association between serum glucose concentrations and risk of colon cancer [68, 128, 134, 135, 139, 141, 155, 166], and five have documented significant associations [128, 134, 135, 139, 141, 155]. A meta-analysis of prospective studies comparing colorectal cancer risk between the highest and lowest serum glucose levels found a summary RR of 1.18 (95% CI 1.07–1.31) [107].

A comparable increased risk among persons with type 1 and type 2 diabetes would support a greater role of hyperglycemia versus hyperinsulinemia, which is mainly seen in the setting of type 2 diabetes. However, no studies have examined the risk of colorectal cancer specifically among patients with type 1 diabetes, and most epidemiological studies have not differentiated between types although the majority of cases tend to be type 2. One study from Italy found that the association between diabetes and risk of colon cancer was only significant among persons diagnosed after the age of 40 years, who were more likely to have type 2 diabetes [149]. In summary, while there also appears to be a relationship between glucose concentrations and risk of colorectal cancer, most of the evidence favors a greater role of hyperinsulinemia in the association between colon cancer and diabetes.

Colorectal Cancer Prognosis

The association between diabetes and colorectal cancer mortality in overall populations has been examined in five studies [68, 115, 151, 157, 167], and three studies found significant associations between diabetes and the risk of colorectal cancer deaths [68, 115, 151]. However, because these studies were not limited to patients with colon cancer, these associations may be partly driven by an increased risk of cancer incidence rather than a specific effect of diabetes on cancer prognosis. A meta-analysis of the impact of diabetes on mortality among cancer populations was recently conducted [123], and six studies in colorectal cancer patients were included [121, 168–172]. The summary RR for colorectal mortality was 1.32 (95% CI 1.24–1.41), suggesting that diabetes not only increases the incidence of colorectal cancer but also worsens survival as well.

Pancreatic Cancer

Insulin resistance and hyperinsulinemia have also been implicated in the etiology of pancreatic cancer, and there is a growing body of evidence to support this association. It should be noted that the majority of pancreatic cancers arise from the exocrine pancreas as adenocarcinomas, whereas tumors of the endocrine pancreas are far less common [173]. Thus, most epidemiological studies of pancreatic cancers are predominantly based on exocrine malignancies because endocrine cancers are either excluded or represent only a small fraction of total cases.

Obesity

Several case-control studies in the 1990 examined whether obesity increased the risk of pancreatic cancer, and no relationship was found [174–176]. However, numerous cohort studies since then have documented positive associations between BMI and pancreatic cancer. At least ten prospective cohort studies [177–186] and four more recent case-control studies [187–190] have documented elevated risks of pancreatic cancer for persons with a BMI over 30 compared to a BMI <25, with RR between 1.2 and 3.0. Four prospective studies have failed to document an association [191–194]. A meta-analysis from 2003 of 14 studies on obesity and pancreatic cancer confirmed a summary RR of 1.19 (95% CI 1.10–1.29) for the risk of pancreatic cancer between persons with a BMI >30 versus <22 [195].

Diabetes

There is a large body of evidence suggesting that type 2 diabetes may increase the risk of pancreatic cancer. However, because pancreatic cancer has a long asymptomatic phase, and diabetes is also a consequence of advanced pancreatic cancer, controversy has existed over the direction of this association. Despite numerous epi-demiological studies of positive associations between diabetes and pancreatic cancer risk, reverse causality could not be excluded as a reason for these findings. Many studies have explored the effect of duration of diabetes prior to cancer, to help tease out to what extent diabetes is a risk factor versus a consequence of pancreatic cancer. A meta-analysis from 1995 reviewed 20 studies, and found that diabetes of 5 years or more duration increased the risk of pancreatic cancer twofold (RR 2.0, 95% CI 1.2–3.2) [196]. A more recent meta-analysis from 2005, based on 50 studies, confirmed a slightly weaker but nonetheless significant association between pancreatic cancer and preexisting diabetes of 5 years or more (RR 1.5, 95% CI 1.3–1.8 for 5–9 years, and RR 1.5, 95% CI 1.2.–2.0 for >10 years) [197]. Results were similar for both case-control and cohort studies, lending further strength to a temporal relationship between preexisting diabetes and risk of developing colon cancer.

Hyperinsulinemia

In contrast to the mechanism underlying the risk of breast and colon cancer, the role of insulin versus glucose or some other diabetes-related factor in the risk of pancreatic cancer is less clear. First, animal studies have not supported a direct role of insulin in pancreatic carcinogenesis. Insulin has been shown to promote growth of pancreatic cell lines in vitro [198, 199], however exogenous administration of insulin in the hamster pancreatic cancer model inhibits tumor induction [200]. Two studies have directly examined the association between serum insulin concentration and pancreatic cancer risk in humans [201, 202]. In one study, a twofold increase in risk of cancer was observed for the highest versus lowest quartile of insulin (RR 2.01, 95% CI 1.03–3.93) [201]. In the second study, serum insulin was associated with a higher risk of pancreatic cancer but this was not statistically significant [202]. A recent meta-analysis of these two studies confirmed that the highest versus lowest insulin level was associated with a significant 70% increased risk of pancreatic cancer [107].

There is some animal evidence of an association between indirect measures of insulin resistance and pancreatic cancer. For example, animal studies have found that islet cell turnover, which is associated with insulin resistance, may promote pancreatic carcinogenesis. In hamsters, stimulation of islet cell proliferation increases carcinogenesis [203], and streptozotocin-induced islet cell destruction or treatment with metformin (an insulin sensitizer) inhibits cancer induction [204, 205]. These studies argue for a role of increased islet cell turnover in the setting of insulin resistance, rather than hyperinsulinemia per se, in the relationship between obesity, diabetes, and risk of pancreatic cancer.

Hyperglycemia

Unlike with colon and breast cancer, there is a direct relationship between longer diabetes duration and pancreatic cancer risk [196, 197]. This observation favors a greater role of hyperglycemia or some other factor related to advanced diabetes, rather than hyperinsulinemia, in the etiology of pancreatic cancer. For example, hyperglycemia in susceptible cells results in the overproduction of superoxide by the mitochondrial electron-transport chain, leading to oxidative stress [199]. Animal studies have suggested that oxidative stress may be an important mediator in pancreatic cancer [206–208].

At least four studies have documented a direct association between serum glucose and risk of pancreatic cancer. Two studies examined the relationship between glucose following a 50 gm oral glucose load and pancreatic cancer, and both found that a post-load glucose value of >11.1 mmol/L (the definition of diabetes) was associated with a two to fourfold elevation in risk of pancreatic cancer death [184, 209]. In two other studies, fasting glucose was used and a concentration of 7.0 mmol/L or greater (threshold for diabetes) was associated with an approximate twofold higher risk of pancreatic cancer in both cases [201]. Significant dose–response relationships between glucose levels and pancreatic cancer were also observed in all four studies. A recent meta-analysis of prospective studies of pancreatic cancer and glycemia level found an overall summary RR of 1.98 (95% CI 1.67–2.35) of pancreatic cancer risk for the highest versus lowest glucose level [68, 107]. In addition to the large body of evidence for diabetes and pancreatic cancer, these findings support a role for diabetes and hyperglycemia in pancreatic cancer etiology. There is insufficient data to exclude hyperinsulinemia as an etiology in this association; however the balance of evidence favors greater importance of hyperglycemia or some other diabetes-related cause.

Prostate Cancer

Obesity

Some prospective studies have documented a positive association between BMI and prostate cancer risk [185, 210–216], but many have not supported an association [217–225]. In a recent meta-analysis of BMI and prostate cancer from 2006, a modest association was found when findings were summarized (RR. 1.05, for every 5 kg/m^2 in BMI) [210–215, 216]. Interestingly, for studies that reported results by disease stage, a stronger association was observed for more advanced prostate cancer [226]. A recent Australian cohort study reported a positive association between BMI and aggressive prostate cancer (high-grade), but not with low-grade cancer [227]. Another study found that higher BMI was associated with a higher risk of high-grade prostate cancer but a lower risk of low-grade prostate cancer [228]. It is interesting to note that studies conducted in regions where widespread prostate-specific antigen (PSA) screening is performed have suggested an inverse association between BMI and prostate cancer risk [229–232]. Since PSA screening tends to identify cancer cases at early stages, those studies may have had a greater majority of low-grade prostate cancer cases picked up through screening. Age may also be a modifying factor in the association between obesity and prostate cancer. There is increasing evidence of a clear positive association between obesity and prostate cancer risk in older men, while in younger men there is a less clear and maybe even opposite effect in younger men [230–233].

Obesity is associated with a reduction in the production of testosterone and increased aromatization of testosterone to estradiol in adipose tissue [234]. One study found that inhibiting testosterone decreased the risk of prostate cancer, but the effect was primarily on well-differentiated cancers, whereas the risk of high-grade cancers was unchanged or even increased [235]. Three studies have found that low testosterone is associated with a higher risk of poorly differentiated prostate cancer [236–238]. While the mechanism of these differing effects of testosterone is unclear, these findings are consistent with the evidence for opposing effects of obesity depending on the cancer grade.

Diabetes

Contrary to positive associations observed between diabetes and the risk of other cancers such as those of the breast and colon, a number of studies have noted that prostate cancer risk is lower in patients with diabetes [149, 216, 239–241]. Not all studies have shown statistically significant associations, however a meta-analysis from 2006 of 19 studies confirmed that diabetes was associated with a significantly lower risk of prostate cancer (RR 0.84, 95% CI 0.76–0.93) [242]. In that same year an inverse association was also documented in the large Prostate Cancer Prevention Trial [228]. Diabetes is associated with a reduction in androgen levels [243], possibly due to effects of hyperglycemia on testosterone production. This may explain this protective effect on the risk of pancreatic cancer.

Hyperinsulinemia

Interestingly, despite the inverse relationship between diabetes and prostate cancer, there is some evidence that insulin may play a direct role in the risk of prostate cancer. For instance, like with colon cancer risk, studies have suggested a trend toward decreasing risk of prostate cancer from time of diagnosis of diabetes [239, 240, 244, 245]. Two studies have also documented an association between the metabolic syndrome and increased risk of prostate cancer [246, 247]. In addition, a case-control study from China found a 2.6-fold higher risk of prostate cancer for persons with fasting plasma insulin levels in the top compared to the bottom tertile [248]. Two studies have also found that high plasma insulin was associated with a poorer prognosis or recurrence following prostate cancer [249, 250]. However, one prospective Swedish study did not observe an association between insulin levels and prostate cancer [251], and another study from the United States found a lower risk of prostate cancer associated with the metabolic syndrome [252]. Although not entirely consistent, evidence suggests that hyperinsulinemia may play a role in risk and progression of prostate cancer. The conflicting data on obesity and the protective effects of diabetes on prostate cancer risk may reflect varying contributions of the beneficial effects of low androgen levels and the adverse effects of hyperinsulinemia on cancer promotion.

Other Cancers

Bladder Cancer

There is some evidence of an association between diabetes and risk of bladder cancer. A recent meta-analysis from 2006 of 16 studies indicated that diabetes was associated with a 24% increase in risk of bladder cancer (95% CI 1.08–1.42), but noted that there was significant heterogeneity based on study design whereby a significant relationship was predominantly seen in case-control studies [253]. The mechanism of this possible association is unclear, but the insulin hypothesis has been proposed. For instance, there is evidence that higher plasma IGF-1 concentration is associated with a higher risk of bladder cancer [254, 255]. Obesity has also been linked to risk of bladder cancer in some studies [181, 185, 256] but not others [180, 183]. However, diabetes is also associated with a higher risk of urinary tract infection [257], which may also explain a higher risk of bladder cancer in this population [258]. Further studies are needed to determine the mechanism of this association and the potential role of insulin in the incidence of bladder cancer.

Endometrial Cancer

There is a well-documented association between obesity and risk of endometrial cancer. A recent meta-analysis observed a significant 60% increase in the risk of endometrial cancer in women for every 5 kg/m^2 increase in BMI [4]. Diabetes has also been associated with increased risk of endometrial cancer in several studies, which was confirmed by a meta-analysis by Friberg et al. in 2007 [259]. Based on findings from three cohort and 13 case-control studies, diabetes was associated with a summary RR of 2.10 (95% CI 1.75–2.53) [259]. Findings were weaker but still significant for cohort studies compared to case-control studies, and for studies that included multivariate adjustment compared to those that only adjusted for age. There are several potential mechanisms that have been proposed for this association. First, long-standing insulin resistance may lead to anovulation and increased exposure to unopposed estrogen, which has been shown to increase the risk of endometrial cancer [260, 261]. Second, hyperinsulinemia may also play a role. Insulin has been shown to promote growth of endometrial cells, and high serum insulin and C-peptide levels have been associated with a trend toward higher risk of endometrial

Table 5.1 Summary findings from meta-analyses of associations between obesity, diabetes, hyperinsulinemia, and the risk of certain cancers

	Obesity	Diabetes	Hyperinsulinemia	Other factors
Breast cancer				
Premenopausal	46% ↓* [5]	No significant association [69, 70]	–	Genetic risk factors more common
Postmenopausal	26% ↑ ** [5]	15–20% ↑ [69, 70]	26% ↑ [107]	Excess estrogen: insulin resistance is associated with higher peripheral estrogen production and availability
Colon cancer	25%↑*** [4]	30–40% ↑ [159]	35% ↑ [107]	Hyperglycemia: 18% ↑ risk [107]
Pancreatic cancer	19% ↑ **** [195]	50% ↑ [199]	70% ↑ [107]	Hyperglycemia: 98% ↑ risk [107]
Prostate cancer	5%↑*** [226]	16% ↓ [242]	Conflicting findings [248, 251, 252]	Hypoandrogenemia: lower androgens associated with obesity and diabetes may have protective effects
Bladder cancer	Conflicting findings [180, 181, 183, 185, 256]	24% ↑ [253]	No studies	Higher risk of bladder infection associated with diabetes may increase risk of bladder cancer
Endometrial cancer	60% ↑ *** [4]	210% ↑ [259]	Nonsignificant ↑ [107]	Unopposed estrogen: insulin resistance associated with a higher risk of anovulation

*BMI >31 versus <21; **BMI >28 versus <21; ***for each 5 kg/m^2 BMI increase; ****BMI >30 versus <22

cancer [107, 262]. However, in contrast to studies of other cancers, three studies conducted in women with type 1 diabetes observed strongly positive associations with risk of endometrial cancer (summary RR 3.15, 95% CI 1.07–9.29) [259]. Given that patients with type 1 diabetes are not hyperinsulinemic, these findings argue against the insulin hypothesis and suggest that hyperglycemia or some other diabetes-related factor may influence the risk of endometrial cancer in women with diabetes (Table 5.1).

In summary, there is a growing body of epidemiological evidence of an association between obesity and diabetes, and risk of several epithelial cancers such as cancers of the breast, colon, pancreas, prostate, bladder, and endometrium. Since hyperinsulinemia is strongly associated with these conditions and insulin has well-known growth-promoting effects, insulin has been proposed as a central mediator in these associations. Hyperinsulinemia appears to play a primary role in the risk and prognosis of postmenopausal breast cancer and colorectal cancer, whereas its contribution in other cancers is less clear. Other factors, such as sex steroid hormones, hyperglycemia, and diabetes-related comorbidity may also influence cancer risk and may interact directly or inversely with insulin. Further studies are needed to better explore the role of insulin in these malignancies, and the potential role of insulin-modifying therapies in the treatment and prevention of cancer.

References

1. Bradford-Hill A (1966) The environment and disease: association or causation? Proc Roy Soc Med 58:295
2. Cleary MP, Maihle NJ (1997) The role of body mass index in the relative risk of developing premenopausal versus postmenopausal breast cancer. Proc Soc Exp Biol Med 216:28–43
3. Stephenson GD, Rose DP (2003) Breast cancer and obesity: an update. Nutr Cancer 45:1–16
4. Renehan AG, Tyson M, Egger M, Heller RF, Zwahlen M (2008) Body-mass index and incidence of cancer: a systematic review and meta-analysis of prospective observational studies. Lancet 371:569–578
5. van den Brandt PA, Spiegelman D, Yaun SS, Adami HO, Beeson L, Folsom AR, Fraser G, Goldbohm RA, Graham S, Kushi L, Marshall JR, Miller AB, Rohan T, Smith-Warner SA, Speizer FE, Willett WC, Wolk A, Hunter DJ (2000) Pooled analysis of prospective cohort studies on height, weight, and breast cancer risk. Am J Epidemiol 152:514–527
6. Ursin G, Longnecker MP, Haile RW, Greenland S (1995) A meta-analysis of body mass index and risk of premenopausal breast cancer. Epidemiology 6:137–141
7. Lake JK, Power C, Cole TJ (1997) Women's reproductive health: the role of body mass index in early and adult life. Int J Obes Relat Metab Disord 21:432–438
8. Bray GA (2002) The underlying basis for obesity: relationship to cancer. J Nutr 132:3451S–3455S
9. Bulun SE, Mahendroo MS, Simpson ER (1994) Aromatase gene expression in adipose tissue: relationship to breast cancer. J Steroid Biochem Mol Biol 49:319–326
10. Lawlor DA, Smith GD, Ebrahim S (2004) Hyperinsulinaemia and increased risk of breast cancer: findings from the British Women's Heart and Health Study. Cancer Causes Control 15:267–275
11. Renehan AG, Zwahlen M, Minder C, O'Dwyer ST, Shalet SM, Egger M (2004) Insulin-like growth factor (IGF)-I, IGF binding protein-3, and cancer risk: systematic review and meta-regression analysis. The Lancet 363(9418):1346–1353

12. Nyholm H, Djursing H, Hagen C, Agner T, Bennett P, Svenstrup B (1989) Androgens and estrogens in postmenopausal insulin-treated diabetic women. J Clin Endocrinol Metab 69:946–949
13. Alexander CM, Landsman PB, Teutsch SM, Haffner SM, Third National H, Nutrition Examination S, National Cholesterol Education P (2003) NCEP-defined metabolic syndrome, diabetes, and prevalence of coronary heart disease among NHANES III participants age 50 years and older. Diabetes 52:1210–1214
14. Folsom AR, Kaye SA, Prineas RJ, Potter JD, Gapstur SM, Wallace RB (1990) Increased incidence of carcinoma of the breast associated with abdominal adiposity in postmenopausal women. Am J Epidemiol 131:794–803
15. Huang Z, Willett WC, Colditz GA, Hunter DJ, Manson JE, Rosner B, Speizer FE, Hankinson SE (1999) Waist circumference, waist:hip ratio, and risk of breast cancer in the Nurses' Health Study. Am J Epidemiol 150:1316–1324
16. Kaaks R, van Noord PA, Den Tonkelaar I, Peeters PH, Riboli E, Grobbee DE (1998) Breast-cancer incidence in relation to height, weight and body-fat distribution in the Dutch "DOM" cohort. Int J Cancer 76:647–651
17. den Tonkelaar I, Seidell JC, Collette HJ (1995) Body fat distribution in relation to breast cancer in women participating in the DOM-project. Breast Cancer Res Treat 34:55–61
18. Lahmann PH, Hoffmann K, Allen N, Van Gils CH, Khaw KT, Tehard B, Berrino F, Tjonneland A, Bigaard J, Olsen A, Overvad K, Clavel-Chapelon F, Nagel G, Boeing H, Trichopoulos D, Economou G, Bellos G, Palli D, Tumino R, Panico S, Sacerdote C, Krogh V, Peeters PH, Bueno-de-Mesquita HB, Lund E, Ardanaz E, Amiano P, Pera G, Quiros JR, Martinez C, Tormo MJ, Wirfalt E, Berglund G, Hallmans G, Key TJ, Reeves G, Bingham S, Norat T, Biessy C, Kaaks R, Riboli E (2004) Body size and breast cancer risk: findings from the European Prospective Investigation into Cancer And Nutrition (EPIC). Int J Cancer 111:762–771
19. Morimoto LM, White E, Chen Z, Chlebowski RT, Hays J, Kuller L, Lopez AM, Manson J, Margolis KL, Muti PC, Stefanick ML, McTiernan A (2002) Obesity, body size, and risk of postmenopausal breast cancer: the Women's Health Initiative (United States). Cancer Causes Control 13:741–751
20. Sonnenschein E, Toniolo P, Terry MB, Bruning PF, Kato I, Koenig KL, Shore RE (1999) Body fat distribution and obesity in pre- and postmenopausal breast cancer. Int J Epidemiol 28:1026–1031
21. Harvie M, Hooper L, Howell AH (2003) Central obesity and breast cancer risk: a systematic review. Obes Rev 4:157–173
22. Tornberg SA, Holm LE, Carstensen JM (1988) Breast cancer risk in relation to serum cholesterol, serum beta-lipoprotein, height, weight, and blood pressure. Acta Oncol 27:31–37
23. Soler M, Chatenoud L, Negri E, Parazzini F, Franceschi S, La VC (1999) Hypertension and hormone-related neoplasms in women. Hypertension 34:320–325
24. Largent JA, McEligot AJ, Ziogas A, Reid C, Hess J, Leighton N, Peel D, Anton-Culver H (2006) Hypertension, diuretics and breast cancer risk. J Hum Hypertens 20:727–732
25. Manjer J, Kaaks R, Riboli E, Berglund G (2001) Risk of breast cancer in relation to anthropometry, blood pressure, blood lipids and glucose metabolism: a prospective study within the Malmo Preventive Project. Eur J Cancer Prev 10:33–42
26. Peeters PH, van Noord PA, Hoes AW, Fracheboud J, Gimbrere CH, Grobbee DE (2000) Hypertension and breast cancer risk in a 19-year follow-up study (the DOM cohort). Diagnostic investigation into mammarian cancer. J Hypertens 18:249–254
27. Lindgren AM, Nissinen AM, Tuomilehto JO, Pukkala E (2005) Cancer pattern among hypertensive patients in North Karelia, Finland. Hum Hypertens 19:373–379
28. Basu TK, Williams DC (1975) Plasma and body lipids in patients with carcinoma of the breast. Oncology 31:172–176
29. Bani IA, Williams CM, Boulter PS, Dickerson JW (1986) Plasma lipids and prolactin in patients with breast cancer. Br J Cancer 54:439–446
30. Alexopoulos CG, Blatsios B, Avgerinos A (1987) Serum lipids and lipoprotein disorders in cancer patients. Cancer 60:3065–3070

31. Kumar K, Sachdanandam P, Arivazhagan R (1991) Studies on the changes in plasma lipids and lipoproteins in patients with benign and malignant breast cancer. Biochem Int 23:581–589
32. Kaye JA, Meier CR, Walker AM, Jick H (2002) Statin use, hyperlipidaemia, and the risk of breast cancer. Br J Cancer 86:1436–1439
33. Gerber M, Cavallo F, Marubini E, Richardson S, Barbieri A, Capitelli E, Costa A, de Crastes PA, de Crastes PP, Decarli A (1988) Liposoluble vitamins and lipid parameters in breast cancer. A joint study in northern Italy and southern France. Int J Cancer 42:489–494
34. Kokoglu E, Karaarslan I, Karaarslan HM, Baloglu H (1994) Alterations of serum lipids and lipoproteins in breast cancer. Cancer Lett 82:175–178
35. Dyer AR, Stamler J, Paul O, Shekelle RB, Schoenberger JA, Berkson DM, Lepper M, Collette P, Shekelle S, Lindberg HA (1981) Serum cholesterol and risk of death from cancer and other causes in three Chicago epidemiological studies. J Chron Dis 34:249–260
36. Vatten LJ, Foss OP (1990) Total serum cholesterol and triglycerides and risk of breast cancer: a prospective study of 24,329 Norwegian women. Cancer Res 50:2341–2346
37. Williams RR, Sorlie PD, Feinleib M, McNamara PM, Kannel WB, Dawber TR (1981) Cancer incidence by levels of cholesterol. JAMA 245:247–252
38. Hiatt RA, Friedman GD, Bawol RD, Ury HK (1982) Breast cancer and serum cholesterol. J Natl Cancer Inst 68:885–889
39. Morris DL, Borhani NO, Fitzsimons E, Hardy RJ, Hawkins CM, Kraus JF, Labarthe DR, Mastbaum L, Payne GH (1983) Serum cholesterol and cancer in the Hypertension Detection and Follow-up Program. Cancer 52:1754–1759
40. Schatzkin A, Hoover RN, Taylor PR, Ziegler RG, Carter CL, Albanes D, Larson DB, Licitra LM (1988) Site-specific analysis of total serum cholesterol and incident cancer in the National Health and Nutrition Examination Survey I Epidemiologic Follow-up Study. Cancer Res 48:452–458
41. Gaard M, Tretli S, Urdal P (1994) Risk of breast cancer in relation to blood lipids: a prospective study of 31,209 Norwegian women. Cancer Causes Control 5:501–509
42. Elkhadrawy TM, Ahsan H, Neugut AI (1998) Serum cholesterol and the risk of ductal carcinoma in situ: a case-control study. Eur J Cancer Prev 7:393–396
43. Eliassen AH, Colditz GA, Rosner B, Willett WC, Hankinson SE (2005) Serum lipids, lipid-lowering drugs, and the risk of breast cancer. Arch Intern Med 165:2264–2271
44. Hoyer AP, Engholm G (1992) Serum lipids and breast cancer risk: a cohort study of 5,207 Danish women. Cancer Causes Control 3:403–408
45. Sinagra D, Amato C, Scarpilta AM, Brigandi M, Amato M, Saura G, Latteri MA, Caimi G (2002) Metabolic syndrome and breast cancer risk. Eur Rev Med Pharmacol Sci 6:55–59
46. Lipscombe LL, Goodwin PJ, Zinman B, McLaughlin JR, Hux JE (2006) Diabetes mellitus and breast cancer: a retrospective population-based cohort study. Breast Cancer Res Treat 98:349–356
47. Baron JA, Weiderpass E, Newcomb PA, Stampfer M, Titus-Ernstoff L, Egan KM, Greenberg ER (2001) Metabolic disorders and breast cancer risk (United States). Cancer Causes Control 12:875–880
48. Michels KB, Solomon CG, Hu FB, Rosner BA, Hankinson SE, Colditz GA, Manson JE (2003) Type 2 diabetes and subsequent incidence of breast cancer in the Nurses' Health Study. Diabetes Care 26:1752–1758
49. Mink PJ, Shahar E, Rosamond WD, Alberg AJ, Folsom AR (2002) Serum insulin and glucose levels and breast cancer incidence: the atherosclerosis risk in communities study. Am J Epidemiol 156:349–352
50. O'Mara BA, Byers T, Schoenfeld E (1985) Diabetes mellitus and cancer risk: a multisite case-control study. J Chron Dis 38:435–441
51. Ragozzino M, Melton LJ III, Chu CP, Palumbo PJ (1982) Subsequent cancer risk in the incidence cohort of Rochester, Minnesota, residents with diabetes mellitus. J Chron Dis 35:13–19
52. Sellers TA, Sprafka JM, Gapstur SM, Rich SS, Potter JD, Ross JA, McGovern PG, Nelson CL, Folsom AR (1994) Does body fat distribution promote familial aggregation of adult onset diabetes mellitus and postmenopausal breast cancer? Epidemiology 5:102–108

53. Weiss HA, Brinton LA, Potischman NA, Brogan D, Coates RJ, Gammon MD, Malone KE, Schoenberg JB (1999) Breast cancer risk in young women and history of selected medical conditions. Int J Epidemiol 28:816–823
54. Moseson M, Koenig KL, Shore RE, Pasternack BS (1993) The influence of medical conditions associated with hormones on the risk of breast cancer. Int J Epidemiol 22:1000–1009
55. Swerdlow AJ, Laing SP, Qiao Z, Slater SD, Burden AC, Botha JL, Waugh NR, Morris AD, Gatling W, Gale EA, Patterson CC, Keen H (2005) Cancer incidence and mortality in patients with insulin-treated diabetes: a UK cohort study. Br J Cancer 92:2070–2075
56. Franceschi S, La Vecchia C, Negri E, Parazzini F, Boyle P (1990) Breast cancer risk and history of selected medical conditions linked with female hormones. Eur J Cancer 26:781–785
57. Talamini R, Franceschi S, Favero A, Negri E, Parazzini F, La Vecchia C (1997) Selected medical conditions and risk of breast cancer. Br J Cancer 75:1699–1703
58. Resta F, Triggiani V, Sabba C, Licchelli B, Ghiyasaldin S, Liso A, Schittulli F, Quaranta M, Paradiso A, Tafaro E, Guastamacchia E (2004) The impact of body mass index and type 2 diabetes on breast cancer: current therapeutic measures of prevention. Curr Drug Targets Immune Endocr Metabol Disord 4:327–333
59. Goodman MT, Cologne JB, Moriwaki H, Vaeth M, Mabuchi K (1997) Risk factors for primary breast cancer in Japan: 8-year follow-up of atomic bomb survivors. Prev Med 26:144–153
60. Inoue M, Iwasaki M, Otani T, Sasazuki S, Noda M, Tsugane S (2006) Diabetes mellitus and the risk of cancer: results from a large-scale population-based cohort study in Japan. Arch Intern Med 166:1871–1877
61. Khan M, Mori M, Fujino Y, Shibata A, Sakauchi F, Washio M, Tamakoshi A (2006) Site-specific cancer risk due to diabetes mellitus history: evidence from the Japan Collaborative Cohort (JACC) Study. Asian Pac J Cancer Prev 7:253–259
62. Adami HO, Rimsten A (1978) Prevalence of hypertension and diabetes in breast cancer: a case-control study in 179 patients and age-matched, non-hospitalized controls. Clin Oncol 4:243–249
63. Weiderpass E, Gridley G, Persson I, Nyren O, Ekbom A, Adami HO (1997) Risk of endometrial and breast cancer in patients with diabetes mellitus. Int J Cancer 71:360–363
64. Hjalgrim H, Frisch M, Ekbom A, Kyvik KO, Melbye M, Green A (1997) Cancer and diabetes – a follow-up study of two population-based cohorts of diabetic patients. J Intern Med 241:471–475
65. Wideroff L, Gridley G, Mellemkjaer L, Chow WH, Linet M, Keehn S, Borch-Johnsen K, Olsen JH (1997) Cancer incidence in a population-based cohort of patients hospitalized with diabetes mellitus in Denmark. J Natl Cancer Inst 89:1360–1365
66. Muck BR, Trotnow S, Hommel G (1975) Cancer of the breast, diabetes and pathological glucose tolerance. Arch Gynäkol 220:73–81
67. de Waard F, Baanders-van Halewijn EA (1974) A prospective study in general practice on breast-cancer risk in postmenopausal women. Int J Cancer 14:153–160
68. Jee SH, Ohrr H, Sull JW, Yun JE, Ji M, Samet JM (2005) Fasting serum glucose level and cancer risk in Korean men and women. JAMA 293:194–202
69. Larsson SC, Mantzoros CS, Wolk A (2007) Diabetes mellitus and risk of breast cancer: a meta-analysis. Int J Cancer 121:856–862
70. Xue F, Michels KB (2007) Diabetes, metabolic syndrome, and breast cancer: a review of the current evidence. Am J Clin Nutr 86:s823–s835
71. van der Burg B, Rutteman GR, Blankenstein MA, de Laat SW, van Zoelen EJ (1988) Mitogenic stimulation of human breast cancer cells in a growth factor-defined medium: synergistic action of insulin and estrogen. J Cell Physiol 134:101–108
72. Chappell J, Leitner JW, Solomon S, Golovchenko I, Goalstone ML, Draznin B (2001) Effect of insulin on cell cycle progression in MCF-7 breast cancer cells. Direct and potentiating influence. J Biol Chem 276:38023–38028
73. Belfiore A, Frittitta L, Costantino A, Frasca F, Pandini G, Sciacca L, Goldfine ID, Vigneri R (1996) Insulin receptors in breast cancer. Ann NY Acad Sci 784:173–188

74. Papa V, Belfiore A (1996) Insulin receptors in breast cancer: biological and clinical role. J Endocrinol Invest 19:324–333
75. Dang CV, Semenza GL (1999) Oncogenic alterations of metabolism. Trends Biochem Sci 24:68–72
76. Buchanan TA (2003) Pancreatic beta-cell loss and preservation in type 2 diabetes. Clin Ther 25(Suppl B):32–46
77. Steppel JH, Horton ES (2004) Beta-cell failure in the pathogenesis of type 2 diabetes mellitus. Curr Diab Rep 4:169–175
78. Lipscombe LL, Goodwin PJ, Zinman B, McLaughlin JR, Hux JE (2006) Increased prevalence of prior breast cancer in women with newly diagnosed diabetes. Breast Cancer Res Treat 98:303–309
79. Dawson SI (2004) Long-term risk of malignant neoplasm associated with gestational glucose intolerance. Cancer 100:149–155
80. Balen A (2001) Polycystic ovary syndrome and cancer. Hum Reprod Update 7:522–525
81. Chittenden BG, Fullerton G, Maheshwari A, Bhattacharya S (2009) Polycystic ovary syndrome and the risk of gynaecological cancer: a systematic review. Reprod Biomed Online 19(3):398–405
82. Bowker SL, Majumdar SR, Veugelers P, Johnson JA (2006) Increased cancer-related mortality for patients with type 2 diabetes who use sulfonylureas or insulin. Diabetes Care 29:254–258
83. Colhoun HM (2009) Use of insulin glargine and cancer incidence in Scotland: a study from the Scottish Diabetes Research Network Epidemiology Group. Diabetologia 52(9):1755–1765
84. Currie CJ, Poole CD, Gale EA (2009) The influence of glucose-lowering therapies on cancer risk in type 2 diabetes. Diabetologia 52(9):1766–1777
85. Hemkens LG, Grouven U, Bender R, Gunster C, Gutschmidt S, Selke GW et al (2009) Risk of malignancies in patients with diabetes treated with human insulin or insulin analogues: a cohort study. Diabetologia 52(9):1732–1744
86. Jonasson JM, Ljung R, Talback M, Haglund B, Gudbjornsdottir S, Steineck G (2009) Insulin glargine use and short-term incidence of malignancies-a population-based follow-up study in Sweden. Diabetologia 52(9):1745–1754
87. Suissa S, Azoulay L, Dell'aniello S, Evans M, Vora J, Pollak M (2011) Long-term effects of insulin glargine on the risk of breast cancer. Diabetologia; On-line first May 26th
88. McFarland MS, Cripps R (2010) Diabetes mellitus and increased risk of cancer: focus on metformin and the insulin analogs. Pharmacotherapy 30(11):1159–1178
89. Evans JM, Donnelly LA, Emslie-Smith AM, Alessi DR, Morris AD (2005) Metformin and reduced risk of cancer in diabetic patients. BMJ 330:1304–1305
90. Decensi A, Puntoni M, Goodwin P, Cazzaniga M, Gennari A, Bonanni B et al (2010) Metformin and cancer risk in diabetic patients: a systematic review and meta-analysis. Cancer Prev Res (Phila) 3(11):1451–1461
91. Jiralerspong S, Palla SL, Giordano SH, Meric-Bernstam F, Liedtke C, Barnett CM et al (2009) Metformin and pathologic complete responses to neoadjuvant chemotherapy in diabetic patients with breast cancer. J Clin Oncol 27(20):3297–3302
92. Zakikhani M, Dowling R, Fantus IG, Sonenberg N, Pollak M (2006) Metformin is an AMP kinase-dependent growth inhibitor for breast cancer cells. Cancer Res 66:10269–10273
93. Del Giudice ME, Fantus IG, Ezzat S, McKeown-Eyssen G, Page D, Goodwin PJ (1998) Insulin and related factors in premenopausal breast cancer risk. Breast Cancer Res Treat 47:111–120
94. Hirose K, Toyama T, Iwata H, Takezaki T, Hamajima N, Tajima K (2003) Insulin, insulin-like growth factor-I and breast cancer risk in Japanese women. Asian Pac J Cancer Prev 4:239–246
95. Yam D, Fink A, Mashiah A, Ben-Hur E (1996) Hyperinsulinemia in colon, stomach and breast cancer patients. Cancer Lett 104:129–132
96. Gamayunova VB (1997) Comparative study of blood insulin levels in breast and endometrial cancer patients. Neoplasma 44:123–126
97. Jernstrom H, Barrett-Connor E (1999) Obesity, weight change, fasting insulin, proinsulin, C-peptide, and insulin-like growth factor-1 levels in women with and without breast cancer: the Rancho Bernardo Study. J Womens Health Gend Based Med 8:1265–1272

98. Kaaks R, Lundin E, Rinaldi S, Manjer J, Biessy C, Soderberg S, Lenner P, Janzon L, Riboli E, Berglund G, Hallmans G (2002) Prospective study of IGF-I, IGF-binding proteins, and breast cancer risk, in northern and southern Sweden. Cancer Causes Control 13:307–316
99. Muti P, Quattrin T, Grant BJ, Krogh V, Micheli A, Schunemann HJ, Ram M, Freudenheim JL, Sieri S, Trevisan M, Berrino F (2002) Fasting glucose is a risk factor for breast cancer: a prospective study. Cancer Epidemiol Biomarkers Prev 11:1361–1368
100. Bruning PF, Bonfrer JM, van Noord PA, Hart AA, de Jong-Bakker M, Nooijen WJ (1992) Insulin resistance and breast-cancer risk. Int J Cancer 52:511–516
101. Verheus M, Peeters PH, Rinaldi S, Dossus L, Biessy C, Olsen A, Tjonneland A, Overvad K, Jeppesen M, Clavel-Chapelon F, Tehard B, Nagel G, Linseisen J, Boeing H, Lahmann PH, Arvaniti A, Psaltopoulou T, Trichopoulou A, Palli D, Tumino R, Panico S, Sacerdote C, Sieri S, Van Gils CH, Bueno-de-Mesquita BH, Gonzalez CA, Ardanaz E, Larranaga N, Garcia CM, Navarro C, Quiros JR, Key T, Allen N, Bingham S, Khaw KT, Slimani N, Riboli E, Kaaks R (2006) Serum C-peptide levels and breast cancer risk: results from the European Prospective Investigation into Cancer and Nutrition (EPIC). Int J Cancer 119:659–667
102. Malin A, Dai Q, Yu H, Shu XO, Jin F, Gao YT, Zheng W (2004) Evaluation of the synergistic effect of insulin resistance and insulin-like growth factors on the risk of breast carcinoma. Cancer 100:694–700
103. Yang G, Lu G, Jin F, Dai Q, Best R, Shu XO, Chen JR, Pan XY, Shrubsole M, Zheng W (2001) Population-based, case-control study of blood C-peptide level and breast cancer risk. Cancer Epidemiol Biomarkers Prev 10:1207–1211
104. Keinan-Boker L, Bueno De Mesquita HB, Kaaks R, Van Gils CH, van Noord PA, Rinaldi S, Riboli E, Seidell JC, Grobbee DE, Peeters PH (2003) Circulating levels of insulin-like growth factor I, its binding proteins -1,-2, -3, C peptide risk postmenopausal breast cancer. Int J Cancer 106:90–95
105. Schairer C, Hill D, Sturgeon SR, Fears T, Pollak M, Mies C, Ziegler RG, Hoover RN, Sherman ME (2004) Serum concentrations of IGF-I, IGFBP-3 and c-peptide and risk of hyperplasia and cancer of the breast in postmenopausal women. Int J Cancer 108:773–779
106. Toniolo P, Bruning PF, Akhmedkhanov A, Bonfrer JM, Koenig KL, Lukanova A, Shore RE, Zeleniuch-Jacquotte A (2000) Serum insulin-like growth factor-I and breast cancer. Int J Cancer 88:828–832
107. Pisani P (2008) Hyper-insulinaemia and cancer, meta-analyses of epidemiological studies. Arch Physiol Biochem 114:63–70
108. Williams CL, Hayman LL, Daniels SR, Robinson TN, Steinberger J, Paridon S, Bazzarre T (2002) Cardiovascular health in childhood: A statement for health professionals from the Committee on Atherosclerosis, Hypertension, and Obesity in the Young (AHOY) of the Council on Cardiovascular Disease in the Young, American Heart Association. Circulation 106:143–160
109. Warburg O (1956) On the origin of cancer cells. Science 123:309–314
110. Zendehdel K, Nyren O, Ostenson CG, Adami HO, Ekbom A, Ye W (2003) Cancer incidence in patients with type 1 diabetes mellitus: a population-based cohort study in Sweden. J Natl Cancer Inst 95:1797–1800
111. Rapp K, Schroeder J, Klenk J, Ulmer H, Concin H, Diem G, Oberaigner W, Weiland SK (2006) Fasting blood glucose and cancer risk in a cohort of more than 140,000 adults in Austria. Diabetologia 49:945–952
112. Mathieu MC, Clark GM, Allred DC, Goldfine ID, Vigneri R (1997) Insulin receptor expression and clinical outcome in node-negative breast cancer. Proc Assoc Am Physicians 109:565–571
113. Frasca F, Pandini G, Scalia P, Sciacca L, Mineo R, Costantino A, Goldfine ID, Belfiore A, Vigneri R (1999) Insulin receptor isoform A, a newly recognized, high-affinity insulin-like growth factor II receptor in fetal and cancer cells. Mol Cell Biol 19:3278–3288
114. Goodwin PJ, Ennis M, Pritchard KI, Trudeau ME, Koo J, Madarnas Y, Hartwick W, Hoffman B, Hood N (2002) Fasting insulin and outcome in early-stage breast cancer: results of a prospective cohort study. J Clin Oncol 20:42–51

115. Coughlin SS, Calle EE, Teras LR, Petrelli J, Thun MJ (2004) Diabetes mellitus as a predictor of cancer mortality in a large cohort of US adults. Am J Epidemiol 159:1160–1167
116. Verlato G, Zoppini G, Bonora E, Muggeo M (2003) Mortality from site-specific malignancies in type 2 diabetic patients from verona. Diabetes Care 26:1047–1051
117. Kessler II (1970) Cancer mortality among diabetics. J Natl Cancer Inst 44:673–686
118. Du W, Simon MS (2005) Racial disparities in treatment and survival of women with stage I-III breast cancer at a large academic medical center in metropolitan Detroit. Breast Cancer Res Treat 91:243–248
119. Lipscombe LL, Goodwin PJ, Zinman B, McLaughlin JR, Hux JE (2008) The impact of diabetes on survival following breast cancer. Breast Cancer Res Treat 109:389–395
120. Tammemagi CM, Nerenz D, Neslund-Dudas C, Feldkamp C, Nathanson D (2005) Comorbidity and survival disparities among black and white patients with breast cancer. JAMA 294:1765–1772
121. van de Poll-Franse LV, Houterman S, Janssen-Heijnen ML, Dercksen MW, Coebergh JW, Haak HR (2007) Less aggressive treatment and worse overall survival in cancer patients with diabetes: a large population based analysis. Int J Cancer 120:1986–1992
122. Yancik R, Wesley MN, Ries LA, Havlik RJ, Edwards BK, Yates JW (2001) Effect of age and comorbidity in postmenopausal breast cancer patients aged 55 years and older. JAMA 285:885–892
123. Barone BB, Yeh HC, Snyder CF, Peairs KS, Stein KB, Derr RL, Wolff AC, Brancati FL (2008) Long-term all-cause mortality in cancer patients with preexisting diabetes mellitus: a systematic review and meta-analysis. JAMA 300:2754–2764
124. Louwman WJ, Janssen-Heijnen ML, Houterman S, Voogd AC, van der Sangen MJ, Nieuwenhuijzen GA, Coebergh JW (2005) Less extensive treatment and inferior prognosis for breast cancer patient with comorbidity: A population-based study. Eur J Cancer 41:779–785
125. Lipscombe LL, Hux JE, Booth GL (2005) Reduced screening mammography among women with diabetes. Arch Intern Med 165:2090–2095
126. Giovannucci E, Michaud D (2007) The role of obesity and related metabolic disturbances in cancers of the colon, prostate, and pancreas. Gastroenterology 132:2208–2225
127. Pischon T, Lahmann PH, Boeing H, Friedenreich C, Norat T, Tjonneland A, Halkjaer J, Overvad K, Clavel-Chapelon F, Boutron-Ruault MC, Guernec G, Bergmann MM, Linseisen J, Becker N, Trichopoulou A, Trichopoulos D, Sieri S, Palli D, Tumino R, Vineis P, Panico S, Peeters PH, Bueno-de-Mesquita HB, Boshuizen HC, Van GB, Palmqvist R, Berglund G, Gonzalez CA, Dorronsoro M, Barricarte A, Navarro C, Martinez C, Quiros JR, Roddam A, Allen N, Bingham S, Khaw KT, Ferrari P, Kaaks R, Slimani N, Riboli E (2006) Body size and risk of colon and rectal cancer in the European Prospective Investigation Into Cancer and Nutrition (EPIC). J Natl Cancer Inst 98:920–931
128. Schoen RE, Tangen CM, Kuller LH, Burke GL, Cushman M, Tracy RP, Dobs A, Savage PJ (1999) Increased blood glucose and insulin, body size, and incident colorectal cancer. J Natl Cancer Inst 91:1147–1154
129. Giovannucci E, Ascherio A, Rimm EB, Colditz GA, Stampfer MJ, Willett WC (1995) Physical activity, obesity, and risk for colon cancer and adenoma in men. Ann Intern Med 122:327–334
130. Bostick RM, Potter JD, Kushi LH, Sellers TA, Steinmetz KA, McKenzie DR, Gapstur SM, Folsom AR (1994) Sugar, meat, and fat intake, and non-dietary risk factors for colon cancer incidence in Iowa women (United States). Cancer Causes Control 5:38–52
131. Russo A, Franceschi S, La VC, Dal ML, Montella M, Conti E, Giacosa A, Falcini F, Negri E (1998) Body size and colorectal-cancer risk. Int J Cancer 78:161–165
132. Martinez ME, Giovannucci E, Spiegelman D, Stampfeer MJ, Hunter DJ, Speizer FE, Willett WC, Colditz GA (1996) Physical activity, body size, and colorectal cancer in women. Am J Epidemiol 143:S73
133. Giovannucci E, Colditz GA, Stampfer MJ, Willett WC (1996) Physical activity, obesity, and risk of colorectal adenoma in women (United States). Cancer Causes Control 7:253–263

134. Trevisan M, Liu J, Muti P, Misciagna G, Menotti A, Fucci F (2001) Markers of insulin resistance and colorectal cancer mortality. Cancer Epidemiol Biomarkers Prev 10:937–941
135. Colangelo LA, Gapstur SM, Gann PH, Dyer AR, Liu K (2002) Colorectal cancer mortality and factors related to the insulin resistance syndrome. Cancer Epidemiol Biomarkers Prev 11:385–391
136. Ahmed RL, Schmitz KH, Anderson KE, Rosamond WD, Folsom AR (2006) The metabolic syndrome and risk of incident colorectal cancer. Cancer 107:28–36
137. Bowers K, Albanes D, Limburg P, Pietinen P, Taylor PR, Virtamo J, Stolzenberg-Solomon R (2006) A prospective study of anthropometric and clinical measurements associated with insulin resistance syndrome and colorectal cancer in male smokers. Am J Epidemiol 164:652–664
138. Yamada K, Araki S, Tamura M, Sakai I, Takahashi Y, Kashihara H, Kono S (1998) Relation of serum total cholesterol, serum triglycerides and fasting plasma glucose to colorectal carcinoma in situ. Int J Epidemiol 27:794–798
139. Saydah SH, Platz EA, Rifai N, Pollak MN, Brancati FL, Helzlsouer KJ (2003) Association of markers of insulin and glucose control with subsequent colorectal cancer risk. Cancer Epidemiol Biomarkers Prev 12:412–418
140. Tsushima M, Nomura AM, Lee J, Stemmermann GN (2005) Prospective study of the association of serum triglyceride and glucose with colorectal cancer. Dig Dis Sci 50:499–505
141. Saydah SH, Loria CM, Eberhardt MS, Brancati FL (2003) Abnormal glucose tolerance and the risk of cancer death in the United States. Am J Epidemiol 157:1092–1100
142. Bayerdorffer E, Mannes GA, Richter WO, Ochsenkuhn T, Seeholzer G, Kopcke W, Wiebecke B, Paumgartner G (1993) Decreased high-density lipoprotein cholesterol and increased low-density cholesterol levels in patients with colorectal adenomas. Ann Intern Med 118:481–487
143. Park SK, Joo JS, Kim DH, Kim YE, Kang D, Yoo KY (2000) Association of serum lipids and glucose with the risk of colorectal adenomatous polyp in men: a case-control study in Korea. J Korean Med Sci 15:690–695
144. Tabuchi M, Kitayama J, Nagawa H (2006) Hypertriglyceridemia is positively correlated with the development of colorectal tubular adenoma in Japanese men. World J Gastroenterol 12:1261–1264
145. Wang YY, Lin SY, Lai WA, Liu PH, Sheu WH (2005) Association between adenomas of rectosigmoid colon and metabolic syndrome features in a Chinese population. J Gastroenterol Hepatol 20:1410–1415
146. Yang YX, Hennessy S, Lewis JD (2005) Type 2 diabetes mellitus and the risk of colorectal cancer. Clin Gastroenterol Hepatol 3:587–594
147. Kune GA, Kune S, Watson LF (1988) Colorectal cancer risk, chronic illnesses, operations, and medications: case control results from the Melbourne Colorectal Cancer Study. Cancer Res 48:4399–4404
148. Le Marchand L, Wilkens LR, Kolonel LN, Hankin JH, Lyu LC (1997) Associations of sedentary lifestyle, obesity, smoking, alcohol use, and diabetes with the risk of colorectal cancer. Cancer Res 57:4787–4794
149. La Vecchia C, Negri E, Decarli A, Franceschi S (1997) Diabetes mellitus and colorectal cancer risk. Cancer Epidemiol Biomarkers Prev 6:1007–1010
150. Levi F, Pasche C, Lucchini F, La VC (2002) Diabetes mellitus, family history, and colorectal cancer. J Epidemiol Community Health 56:479–480
151. Hu FB, Manson JE, Liu S, Hunter D, Colditz GA, Michels KB, Speizer FE, Giovannucci E (1999) Prospective study of adult onset diabetes mellitus (type 2) and risk of colorectal cancer in women. J Natl Cancer Inst 91:542–547
152. Weiderpass E, Gridley G, Nyren O, Ekbom A, Persson I, Adami HO (1997) Diabetes mellitus and risk of large bowel cancer. J Natl Cancer Inst 89:660–661
153. Steenland K, Hu S, Walker J (2004) All-cause and cause-specific mortality by socioeconomic status among employed persons in 27 US states, 1984–1997. Am J Public Health 94:1037–1042

154. Will JC, Galuska DA, Vinicor F, Calle EE (1998) Colorectal cancer: another complication of diabetes mellitus? Am J Epidemiol 147:816–825
155. Nilsen TI, Vatten LJ (2001) Prospective study of colorectal cancer risk and physical activity, diabetes, blood glucose and BMI: exploring the hyperinsulinaemia hypothesis. Br J Cancer 84:417–422
156. Seow A, Yuan JM, Koh WP, Lee HP, Yu MC (2006) Diabetes mellitus and risk of colorectal cancer in the Singapore Chinese Health Study. J Natl Cancer Inst 98:135–138
157. Khaw KT, Wareham N, Bingham S, Luben R, Welch A, Day N (2004) Preliminary communication: glycated hemoglobin, diabetes, and incident colorectal cancer in men and women: a prospective analysis from the European prospective investigation into cancer-Norfolk study. Cancer Epidemiol Biomarkers Prev 13:915–919
158. Limburg PJ, Anderson KE, Johnson TW, Jacobs DR Jr, Lazovich D, Hong CP, Nicodemus KK, Folsom AR (2005) Diabetes mellitus and subsite-specific colorectal cancer risks in the Iowa Women's Health Study. Cancer Epidemiol Biomarkers Prev 14:133–137
159. Larsson SC, Giovannucci E, Wolk A (2005) Diabetes and colorectal cancer incidence in the cohort of Swedish men. Diabetes Care 28:1805–1807
160. Palmqvist R, Stattin P, Rinaldi S, Biessy C, Stenling R, Riboli E, Hallmans G, Kaaks R (2003) Plasma insulin, IGF-binding proteins-1 and -2 and risk of colorectal cancer: a prospective study in northern Sweden. Int J Cancer 107:89–93
161. Bonser AM, Garcia-Webb P (1984) C-peptide measurement: methods and clinical utility. Crit Rev Clin Lab Sci 19:297–352
162. Kaaks R, Toniolo P, Akhmedkhanov A, Lukanova A, Biessy C, Dechaud H, Rinaldi S, Zeleniuch-Jacquotte A, Shore RE, Riboli E (2000) Serum C-peptide, insulin-like growth factor (IGF)-I, IGF-binding proteins, and colorectal cancer risk in women. J Natl Cancer Inst 92:1592–1600
163. Ma J, Giovannucci E, Pollak M, Leavitt A, Tao Y, Gaziano JM, Stampfer MJ (2004) A prospective study of plasma C-peptide and colorectal cancer risk in men. J Natl Cancer Inst 96:546–553
164. Wei EK, Ma J, Pollak MN, Rifai N, Fuchs CS, Hankinson SE, Giovannucci E (2005) A prospective study of C-peptide, insulin-like growth factor-I, insulin-like growth factor binding protein-1, and the risk of colorectal cancer in women. Cancer Epidemiol Biomarkers Prev 14:850–855
165. Yang YX, Hennessy S, Lewis JD (2004) Insulin therapy and colorectal cancer risk among type 2 diabetes mellitus patients. Gastroenterology 127:1044–1050
166. Platz EA, Hankinson SE, Rifai N, Colditz GA, Speizer FE, Giovannucci E (1999) Glycosylated hemoglobin and risk of colorectal cancer and adenoma (United States). Cancer Causes Control 10:379–386
167. Smith GD, Egger M, Shipley MJ, Marmot MG (1992) Post-challenge glucose concentration, impaired glucose tolerance, diabetes, and cancer mortality in men. Am J Epidemiol 136:1110–1114
168. Shonka NA, Anderson JR, Panwalkar AW, Reed EC, Steen PD, Ganti AK (2006) Effect of diabetes mellitus on the epidemiology and outcomes of colon cancer. Med Oncol 23:515–519
169. Gross CP, Guo Z, McAvay GJ, Allore HG, Young M, Tinetti ME (2006) Multimorbidity and survival in older persons with colorectal cancer. J Am Geriatr Soc 54:1898–1904
170. Polednak AP (2006) Comorbid diabetes mellitus and risk of death after diagnosis of colorectal cancer: a population-based study. Cancer Detect Prev 30:466–472
171. Park SM, Lim MK, Shin SA, Yun YH (2006) Impact of prediagnosis smoking, alcohol, obesity, and insulin resistance on survival in male cancer patients: National Health Insurance Corporation Study. J Clin Oncol 24:5017–5024
172. Meyerhardt JA, Catalano PJ, Haller DG, Mayer RJ, Macdonald JS, Benson AB III, Fuchs CS (2003) Impact of diabetes mellitus on outcomes in patients with colon cancer. J Clin Oncol 21:433–440
173. Bardeesy N, DePinho RA (2002) Pancreatic cancer biology and genetics. Nat Rev Cancer 2:897–909

174. Bueno De Mesquita HB, Moerman CJ, Runia S, Maisonneuve P (1990) Are energy and energy-providing nutrients related to exocrine carcinoma of the pancreas? Int J Cancer 46:435–444
175. Ghadirian P, Simard A, Baillargeon J, Maisonneuve P, Boyle P (1991) Nutritional factors and pancreatic cancer in the francophone community in Montreal, Canada. Int J Cancer 47:1–6
176. Howe GR, Ghadirian P, Bueno De Mesquita HB, Zatonski WA, Baghurst PA, Miller AB, Simard A, Baillargeon J, de Waard F, Przewozniak K (1992) A collaborative case-control study of nutrient intake and pancreatic cancer within the search programme. Int J Cancer 51:365–372
177. Michaud DS, Giovannucci E, Willett WC, Colditz GA, Stampfer MJ, Fuchs CS (2001) Physical activity, obesity, height, and the risk of pancreatic cancer. JAMA 286:921–929
178. Coughlin SS, Calle EE, Patel AV, Thun MJ (2000) Predictors of pancreatic cancer mortality among a large cohort of United States adults. Cancer Causes Control 11:915–923
179. Samanic C, Gridley G, Chow WH, Lubin J, Hoover RN, Fraumeni JF Jr (2004) Obesity and cancer risk among white and black United States veterans. Cancer Causes Control 15:35–43
180. Moller H, Mellemgaard A, Lindvig K, Olsen JH (1994) Obesity and cancer risk: a Danish record-linkage study. Eur J Cancer 30A:344–350
181. Wolk A, Gridley G, Svensson M, Nyren O, McLaughlin JK, Fraumeni JF, Adam HO (2001) A prospective study of obesity and cancer risk (Sweden). Cancer Causes Control 12:13–21
182. Larsson SC, Permert J, Hakansson N, Naslund I, Bergkvist L, Wolk A (2005) Overall obesity, abdominal adiposity, diabetes and cigarette smoking in relation to the risk of pancreatic cancer in two Swedish population-based cohorts. Br J Cancer 93:1310–1315
183. Rapp K, Schroeder J, Klenk J, Stoehr S, Ulmer H, Concin H, Diem G, Oberaigner W, Weiland SK (2005) Obesity and incidence of cancer: a large cohort study of over 145,000 adults in Austria. Br J Cancer 93:1062–1067
184. Gapstur SM, Gann PH, Lowe W, Liu K, Colangelo L, Dyer A (2000) Abnormal glucose metabolism and pancreatic cancer mortality. JAMA 283:2552–2558
185. Calle EE, Rodriguez C, Walker-Thurmond K, Thun MJ (2003) Overweight, obesity, and mortality from cancer in a prospectively studied cohort of U.S. adults. N Engl J Med 348:1625–1638
186. Patel AV, Rodriguez C, Bernstein L, Chao A, Thun MJ, Calle EE (2004) Obesity, location of weight gain, and risk of pancreatic cancer in a large United States cohort. Am J Epidemiol 159:S67
187. Silverman DT, Swanson CA, Gridley G, Wacholder S, Greenberg RS, Brown LM, Hayes RB, Swanson GM, Schoenberg JB, Pottern LM, Schwartz AG, Fraumeni JF Jr, Hoover RN (1998) Dietary and nutritional factors and pancreatic cancer: a case-control study based on direct interviews. J Natl Cancer Inst 90:1710–1719
188. Hanley AJ, Johnson KC, Villeneuve PJ, Mao Y (2001) Physical activity, anthropometric factors and risk of pancreatic cancer: results from the Canadian enhanced cancer surveillance system. Int J Cancer 94:140–147
189. Eberle CA, Bracci PM, Holly EA (2005) Anthropometric factors and pancreatic cancer in a population-based case-control study in the San Francisco Bay area. Cancer Causes Control 16:1235–1244
190. Pan SY, Johnson KC, Ugnat AM, Wen SW, Mao Y (2004) Association of obesity and cancer risk in Canada. Am J Epidemiol 159:259–268
191. Stolzenberg-Solomon RZ, Pietinen P, Taylor PR, Virtamo J, Albanes D (2002) A prospective study of medical conditions, anthropometry, physical activity, and pancreatic cancer in male smokers (Finland). Cancer Causes Control 13:417–426
192. Sinner PJ, Schmitz KH, Anderson KE, Folsom AR (2005) Lack of association of physical activity and obesity with incident pancreatic cancer in elderly women. Cancer Epidemiol Biomarkers Prev 14:1571–1573
193. de Berrington GA, Spencer EA, Bueno-de-Mesquita HB, Roddam A, Stolzenberg-Solomon R, Halkjaer J, Tjonneland A, Overvad K, Clavel-Chapelon F, Boutron-Ruault MC, Boeing H,

Pischon T, Linseisen J, Rohrmann S, Trichopoulou A, Benetou V, Papadimitriou A, Pala V, Palli D, Panico S, Tumino R, Vineis P, Boshuizen HC, Ocke MC, Peeters PH, Lund E, Gonzalez CA, Larranaga N, Martinez-Garcia C, Mendez M, Navarro C, Quiros JR, Tormo MJ, Hallmans G, Ye W, Bingham SA, Khaw KT, Allen N, Key TJ, Jenab M, Norat T, Ferrari P, Riboli E (2006) Anthropometry, physical activity, and the risk of pancreatic cancer in the European prospective investigation into cancer and nutrition. Cancer Epidemiol Biomarkers Prev 15:879–885

194. Isaksson B, Jonsson F, Pedersen NL, Larsson J, Feychting M, Permert J (2002) Lifestyle factors and pancreatic cancer risk: a cohort study from the Swedish Twin Registry. Int J Cancer 98:480–482
195. de Berrington GA, Sweetland S, Spencer E (2003) A meta-analysis of obesity and the risk of pancreatic cancer. Br J Cancer 89:519–523
196. Everhart J, Wright D (1995) Diabetes mellitus as a risk factor for pancreatic cancer. A meta-analysis. JAMA 273:1605–1609
197. Huxley R, Ansary-Moghaddam A, de GA Berrington, Barzi F, Woodward M (2005) Type-II diabetes and pancreatic cancer: a meta-analysis of 36 studies. Br J Cancer 92:2076–2083
198. Fisher WE, Muscarella P, Boros LG, Schirmer WJ (1998) Variable effect of streptozotocin-diabetes on the growth of hamster pancreatic cancer (H2T) in the Syrian hamster and nude mouse. Surgery 123:315–320
199. Fisher WE, Boros LG, Schirmer WJ (1996) Insulin promotes pancreatic cancer: evidence for endocrine influence on exocrine pancreatic tumors. J Surg Res 63:310–313
200. Pour PM, Stepan K (1984) Modification of pancreatic carcinogenesis in the hamster model. VIII. Inhibitory effect of exogenous insulin. J Natl Cancer Inst 72:1205–1208
201. Stolzenberg-Solomon RZ, Graubard BI, Chari S, Limburg P, Taylor PR, Virtamo J, Albanes D (2005) Insulin, glucose, insulin resistance, and pancreatic cancer in male smokers. JAMA 294:2872–2878
202. Michaud DS, Wolpin B, Giovannucci E, Liu S, Cochrane B, Manson JE, Pollak MN, Ma J, Fuchs CS (2007) Prediagnostic plasma C-peptide and pancreatic cancer risk in men and women. Cancer Epidemiol Biomarkers Prev 16:2101–2109
203. Pour PM, Kazakoff K (1996) Stimulation of islet cell proliferation enhances pancreatic ductal carcinogenesis in the hamster model. Am J Pathol 149:1017–1025
204. Schneider MB, Matsuzaki H, Haorah J, Ulrich A, Standop J, Ding XZ, Adrian TE, Pour PM (2001) Prevention of pancreatic cancer induction in hamsters by metformin. Gastroenterology 120:1263–1270
205. Pour PM, Donnelly K, Stepan K (1983) Modification of pancreatic carcinogenesis in the hamster model. 3. Inhibitory effect of alloxan. Am J Pathol 110:310–314
206. Nishikawa T, Edelstein D, Du XL, Yamagishi S, Matsumura T, Kaneda Y, Yorek MA, Beebe D, Oates PJ, Hammes HP, Giardino I, Brownlee M (2000) Normalizing mitochondrial superoxide production blocks three pathways of hyperglycaemic damage. Nature 404:787–790
207. Cullen JJ, Weydert C, Hinkhouse MM, Ritchie J, Domann FE, Spitz D, Oberley LW (2003) The role of manganese superoxide dismutase in the growth of pancreatic adenocarcinoma. Cancer Res 63:1297–1303
208. Cullen JJ, Mitros FA, Oberley LW (2003) Expression of antioxidant enzymes in diseases of the human pancreas: another link between chronic pancreatitis and pancreatic cancer. Pancreas 26:23–27
209. Batty GD, Shipley MJ, Marmot M, Smith GD (2004) Diabetes status and post-load plasma glucose concentration in relation to site-specific cancer mortality: findings from the original Whitehall study. Cancer Causes Control 15:873–881
210. Lew EA, Garfinkel L (1979) Variations in mortality by weight among 750,000 men and women. J Chron Dis 32:563–576
211. Snowdon DA, Phillips RL, Choi W (1984) Diet, obesity, and risk of fatal prostate cancer. Am J Epidemiol 120:244–250

212. Chyou PH, Nomura AM, Stemmermann GN (1994) A prospective study of weight, body mass index and other anthropometric measurements in relation to site-specific cancers. Int J Cancer 57:313–317
213. Thune I, Lund E (1994) Physical activity and the risk of prostate and testicular cancer: a cohort study of 53,000 Norwegian men. Cancer Causes Control 5:549–556
214. Cerhan JR, Torner JC, Lynch CF, Rubenstein LM, Lemke JH, Cohen MB, Lubaroff DM, Wallace RB (1997) Association of smoking, body mass, and physical activity with risk of prostate cancer in the Iowa 65+ Rural Health Study (United States). Cancer Causes Control 8:229–238
215. Veierod MB, Laake P, Thelle DS (1997) Dietary fat intake and risk of prostate cancer: a prospective study of 25,708 Norwegian men. Int J Cancer 73:634–638
216. Thompson MM, Garland C, Barrett-Connor E, Khaw KT, Friedlander NJ, Wingard DL (1989) Heart disease risk factors, diabetes, and prostatic cancer in an adult community. Am J Epidemiol 129:511–517
217. Whittemore AS, Paffenbarger RS Jr, Anderson K, Lee JE (1985) Early precursors of site-specific cancers in college men and women. J Natl Cancer Inst 74:43–51
218. Greenwald P, Damon A, Kirmss V, Polan AK (1974) Physical and demographic features of men before developing cancer of the prostate. J Natl Cancer Inst 53:341–346
219. Le ML, Kolonel LN, Wilkens LR, Myers BC, Hirohata T (1994) Animal fat consumption and prostate cancer: a prospective study in Hawaii. Epidemiology 5:276–282
220. Mills PK, Beeson WL, Phillips RL, Fraser GE (1989) Cohort study of diet, lifestyle, and prostate cancer in Adventist men. Cancer 64:598–604
221. Giovannucci E, Rimm EB, Stampfer MJ, Colditz GA, Willett WC (1997) Height, body weight, and risk of prostate cancer. Cancer Epidemiol Biomarkers Prev 6:557–563
222. Putnam SD, Cerhan JR, Parker AS, Bianchi GD, Wallace RB, Cantor KP, Lynch CF (2000) Lifestyle and anthropometric risk factors for prostate cancer in a cohort of Iowa men. Ann Epidemiol 10:361–369
223. Habel LA, Van Den Eeden SK, Friedman GD (2000) Body size, age at shaving initiation, and prostate cancer in a large, multiracial cohort. Prostate 43:136–143
224. Nilsen TI, Vatten LJ (1999) Anthropometry and prostate cancer risk: a prospective study of 22,248 Norwegian men. Cancer Causes Control 10:269–275
225. Gapstur SM, Gann PH, Colangelo LA, Barron-Simpson R, Kopp P, Dyer A, Liu K (2001) Postload plasma glucose concentration and 27-year prostate cancer mortality (United States). Cancer Causes Control 12:763–772
226. Macinnis RJ, English DR (2006) Body size and composition and prostate cancer risk: systematic review and meta-regression analysis. Cancer Causes Control 17:989–1003
227. Macinnis RJ, English DR, Gertig DM, Hopper JL, Giles GG (2003) Body size and composition and prostate cancer risk. Cancer Epidemiol Biomarkers Prev 12:1417–1421
228. Gong Z, Neuhouser ML, Goodman PJ, Albanes D, Chi C, Hsing AW, Lippman SM, Platz EA, Pollak MN, Thompson IM, Kristal AR (2006) Obesity, diabetes, and risk of prostate cancer: results from the prostate cancer prevention trial. Cancer Epidemiol Biomarkers Prev 15:1977–1983
229. Bradbury BD, Wilk JB, Kaye JA (2005) Obesity and the risk of prostate cancer (United States). Cancer Causes Control 16:637–641
230. Robinson WR, Stevens J, Gammon MD, John EM (2005) Obesity before age 30 years and risk of advanced prostate cancer. Am J Epidemiol 161:1107–1114
231. Porter MP, Stanford JL (2005) Obesity and the risk of prostate cancer. Prostate 62:316–321
232. Giovannucci E, Rimm EB, Liu Y, Leitzmann M, Wu K, Stampfer MJ, Willett WC (2003) Body mass index and risk of prostate cancer in U.S. health professionals. J Natl Cancer Inst 95:1240–1244
233. Schuurman AG, Goldbohm RA, Dorant E, van den Brandt PA (2000) Anthropometry in relation to prostate cancer risk in the Netherlands Cohort Study. Am J Epidemiol 151:541–549
234. Tan RS, Pu SJ (2002) Impact of obesity on hypogonadism in the andropause. Int J Androl 25:195–201

235. Thompson IM, Goodman PJ, Tangen CM, Lucia MS, Miller GJ, Ford LG, Lieber MM, Cespedes RD, Atkins JN, Lippman SM, Carlin SM, Ryan A, Szczepanek CM, Crowley JJ, Coltman CA Jr (2003) The influence of finasteride on the development of prostate cancer. N Engl J Med 349:215–224
236. Schatzl G, Madersbacher S, Thurridl T, Waldmuller J, Kramer G, Haitel A, Marberger M (2001) High-grade prostate cancer is associated with low serum testosterone levels. Prostate 47:52–58
237. Platz EA, Leitzmann MF, Rifai N, Kantoff PW, Chen YC, Stampfer MJ, Willett WC, Giovannucci E (2005) Sex steroid hormones and the androgen receptor gene CAG repeat and subsequent risk of prostate cancer in the prostate-specific antigen era. Cancer Epidemiol Biomarkers Prev 14:1262–1269
238. Severi G, Morris HA, Macinnis RJ, English DR, Tilley W, Hopper JL, Boyle P, Giles GG (2006) Circulating steroid hormones and the risk of prostate cancer. Cancer Epidemiol Biomarkers Prev 15:86–91
239. Adami HO, McLaughlin J, Ekbom A, Berne C, Silverman D, Hacker D, Persson I (1991) Cancer risk in patients with diabetes mellitus. Cancer Causes Control 2:307–314
240. Giovannucci E, Rimm EB, Stampfer MJ, Colditz GA, Willett WC (1998) Diabetes mellitus and risk of prostate cancer (United States). Cancer Causes Control 9:3–9
241. Weiderpass E, Ye W, Vainio H, Kaaks R, Adami HO (2002) Reduced risk of prostate cancer among patients with diabetes mellitus. Int J Cancer 102:258–261
242. Kasper JS, Giovannucci E (2006) A meta-analysis of diabetes mellitus and the risk of prostate cancer. Cancer Epidemiol Biomarkers Prev 15:2056–2062
243. Ando S, Rubens R, Rottiers R (1984) Androgen plasma levels in male diabetics. J Endocrinol Invest 7:21–24
244. Tavani A, Gallus S, Bosetti C, Tzonou A, Lagiou P, Negri E, Trichopoulos D, La VC (2002) Diabetes and the risk of prostate cancer. Eur J Cancer Prev 11:125–128
245. Rodriguez C, Patel AV, Mondul AM, Jacobs EJ, Thun MJ, Calle EE (2005) Diabetes and risk of prostate cancer in a prospective cohort of US men. Am J Epidemiol 161:147–152
246. Lund HL, Wisloff TF, Holme I, Nafstad P (2006) Metabolic syndrome predicts prostate cancer in a cohort of middle-aged Norwegian men followed for 27 years. Am J Epidemiol 164:769–774
247. Laukkanen JA, Laaksonen DE, Niskanen L, Pukkala E, Hakkarainen A, Salonen JT (2004) Metabolic syndrome and the risk of prostate cancer in Finnish men: a population-based study. Cancer Epidemiol Biomarkers Prev 13:1646–1650
248. Hsing AW, Chua S Jr, Gao YT, Gentzschein E, Chang L, Deng J, Stanczyk FZ (2001) Prostate cancer risk and serum levels of insulin and leptin: a population-based study. J Natl Cancer Inst 93:783–789
249. Hammarsten J, Hogstedt B (2005) Hyperinsulinaemia: a prospective risk factor for lethal clinical prostate cancer. Eur J Cancer 41:2887–2895
250. Lehrer S, Diamond EJ, Stagger S, Stone NN, Stock RG (2002) Increased serum insulin associated with increased risk of prostate cancer recurrence. Prostate 50:1–3
251. Stattin P, Bylund A, Rinaldi S, Biessy C, Dechaud H, Stenman UH, Egevad L, Riboli E, Hallmans G, Kaaks R (2000) Plasma insulin-like growth factor-I, insulin-like growth factor-binding proteins, and prostate cancer risk: a prospective study. J Natl Cancer Inst 92:1910–1917
252. Tande AJ, Platz EA, Folsom AR (2006) The metabolic syndrome is associated with reduced risk of prostate cancer. Am J Epidemiol 164:1094–1102
253. Larsson SC, Orsini N, Brismar K, Wolk A (2006) Diabetes mellitus and risk of bladder cancer: a meta-analysis. Diabetologia 49:2819–2823
254. Dunn SE, Kari FW, French J, Leininger JR, Travlos G, Wilson R, Barrett JC (1997) Dietary restriction reduces insulin-like growth factor I levels, which modulates apoptosis, cell proliferation, and tumor progression in p53-deficient mice. Cancer Res 57:4667–4672
255. Zhao H, Grossman HB, Spitz MR, Lerner SP, Zhang K, Wu X (2003) Plasma levels of insulin-like growth factor-1 and binding protein-3, and their association with bladder cancer risk. J Urol 169:714–717

256. Tripathi A, Folsom AR, Anderson KE (2002) Risk factors for urinary bladder carcinoma in postmenopausal women. The Iowa Women's Health Study. Cancer 95:2316–2323
257. Joshi N, Caputo GM, Weitekamp MR, Karchmer AW (1999) Infections in patients with diabetes mellitus. N Engl J Med 341:1906–1912
258. Kravchick S, Gal R, Cytron S, Peled R, Weissman Y, Mukamel E, Koren R (2001) Increased incidence of diabetes mellitus in the patients with transitional cell carcinoma of urinary bladder. Pathol Oncol Res 7:56–59
259. Friberg E, Orsini N, Mantzoros CS, Wolk A (2007) Diabetes mellitus and risk of endometrial cancer: a meta-analysis. Diabetologia 50:1365–1374
260. Key TJ, Pike MC (1988) The dose-effect relationship between 'unopposed' oestrogens and endometrial mitotic rate: its central role in explaining and predicting endometrial cancer risk. Br J Cancer 57:205–212
261. Ferenczy A, Bertrand G, Gelfand MM (1979) Proliferation kinetics of human endometrium during the normal menstrual cycle. Am J Obstet Gynecol 133:859–867
262. Lukanova A, Zeleniuch-Jacquotte A, Lundin E, Micheli A, Arslan AA, Rinaldi S, Muti P, Lenner P, Koenig KL, Biessy C, Krogh V, Riboli E, Shore RE, Stattin P, Berrino F, Hallmans G, Toniolo P, Kaaks R (2004) Prediagnostic levels of C-peptide, IGF-I, IGFBP -1, -2 and -3 and risk of endometrial cancer. Int J Cancer 108:262–268

Chapter 6
Animal Models of Hyperinsulinemia, Insulin Resistance, and Cancer

Ruslan Novosyadlyy, Archana Vijayakumar, Yvonne Fierz, and Derek LeRoith

Numerous lines of evidence indicate that insulin and its receptor regulate cell proliferation, survival and transformation, and thus, tumorigenesis [52]. Indeed, the fact that insulin has a potent tumor-promoting activity has been known for a long time. In wild-type animals, administration of exogenous insulin markedly enhances development of experimental breast and colon tumors [34, 68, 117]. In contrast, insulinopenia in animals with chemically-induced type 1 diabetes (T1D) results in a significantly reduced tumor growth, which is restored after insulin administration [29, 67, 112, 113]. Moreover, intraportal implantation of pancreatic islets in rats with T1D creates an insulin-enriched microenvironment, which promotes hepatocarcinogenesis [43]. The aforementioned studies thus link insulin and cancer mechanistically, and indicate that insulin plays the role of both a tumor initiator and promoter.

Growing evidence also suggests that insulin, in the setting of insulin resistance and hyperinsulinemia, has a potent tumor-promoting effect in type 2 diabetes (T2D). This activitiy of insulin has been observed in a broad range of experimental murine models that have been developed to study the pathophysiology of insulin resistance. The most common models include diet- and genetically-induced obesity. However, during the last decade several genetically engineered mouse models have been generated in which insulin resistance and hyperinsulinemia develop in the absence of obesity.

Numerous epidemiological studies suggest a positive relationship between obesity, T2D, and cancer. Moreover, most studies implicate hyperinsulinemia as the most likely factor underlying the tumor-promoting activity of obesity and T2D, although the role of other mechanisms cannot be neglected. Indeed, multiple pathophysiological mechanisms can be attributed to the tumor-promoting effects of obesity, including increased influx of nutrients, elevated circulating levels of IGF-I, adipokines, lipids,

D. LeRoith (✉)
Division of Endocrinology, Diabetes and Bone Diseases, Department of Medicine, Mount Sinai School of Medicine, New York, NY 10029, USA
e-mail: derek.leroith@mssm.edu

I.G. Fantus (ed.), *Insulin Resistance and Cancer: Epidemiology, Cellular and Molecular Mechanisms and Clinical Implications*, Energy Balance and Cancer 1,
DOI 10.1007/978-1-4419-9911-5_6,

proinflammatory cytokines, chemokines, and/or adipocyte-derived sex steroids [120]. Hyperglycemia, resulting from diabetes, can also affect both normal and transformed cells [86]. Therefore, obesity- and T2D-related effects on tumor development and growth can be attributed to insulin, although the factors discussed earlier may also play an important role.

In the following sections of this chapter, we will summarize the results of cancer studies conducted in rodent models of genetically-induced and diet-induced obesity (DIO) and T2D. Moreover, we will provide data obtained from cancer studies in models of obesity-independent T2D.

Genetically-Induced Obesity and Cancer

Monogenetic obesity syndromes in humans and rodents are mainly caused by a disruption of the leptin-melanocortin pathway [49]. The hormone leptin is secreted by adipocytes, in proportion to body fat content, and interacts with hypothalamic neurons to ultimately decrease appetite, and regulate energy homeostasis and thermogenesis. The central effects of leptin are primarily mediated via stimulation of the anorexigenic neurons (pro-opiomelacortin (POMC)) and inhibition of the orexigenic neurons (NPY, AgRP) [111]. Rodent models of monogenetic obesity have been widely used to study the relationship between excess body weight and/or insulin resistance and cancer. However, in the human population genetic alterations leading to obesity appear to be much more complex than single-gene mutations and only few cases of single gene mutations in obese human subjects have been identified. In the following section we will discuss the most common rodent models of monogenic obesity that were used to identify the role of obesity and insulin resistance on cancer.

Yellow Mice

The spontaneously occurring lethal yellow, or yellow agouti (A^Y), mouse strain was discovered in 1927 [36], and is one of the earliest rodent models in which a correlation between increased body weight and a higher susceptibility to tumor formation has been observed [64, 65]. Subsequently, several dominant yellow mutations have been identified, such as the viable yellow (A^{vy}) mutation, which unlike the A^y mutation, is not lethal when inherited in a homozygous manner. The yellow mice (both A^y, A^{vy}) develop a pleiotropic syndrome which includes obesity, insulin resistance, enhanced linear growth and increased susceptibility to tumor formation [129, 130, 135]. The obese phenotype of the yellow mouse is caused by ectopic expression of the agouti signaling protein resulting in blockade of hypothalamic melanocortin-4 receptors, which are involved in regulating feeding behavior and energy homeostasis [10, 48]. However, while the factors related to obesity may contribute to the increased predisposition to carcinogenesis in these mice, there is also growing evidence suggesting that ectopic expression of agouti per se may promote carcinogenesis [85, 131]. Therefore, the yellow obese mice, although a useful experimental model for obesity and diabetes research, are not very suitable to study the impact of obesity and insulin resistance on cancer growth and progression.

ob/ob Mouse

The *Lep*^{ob}/*Lep*^{ob} (*ob/ob*) mice, first described in 1950 by Ingalls et al. at Jackson Laboratories, harbor a naturally occurring autosomal recessive mutation in the *obese* (*ob*) gene [73]. It was later identified that these mice bear a mutation in the leptin gene which renders them leptin-deficient [137]. The *ob/ob* mice are obese, hyperglycemic, hyperinsulinemic, and infertile [32, 55]. The *ob* mutation has been described in two genetic strains (C57BL/6 (BL/6) and C57BL/KsJ (BL/Ks)), each with slightly different phenotypes [32, 55].

The *ob/ob* mouse model has been used to determine the role of obesity, hyperinsulinemia, hyperglycemia, and insulin resistance on tumor development, progression, and metastasis. The first experiments describing cancer growth in *ob/ob* mice involved subcutaneous inoculation of B16 melanoma cells into female *ob/ob* and lean mice. Interestingly, tumor growth was either *at par* or retarded in the *ob/ob* mice, when compared to the lean controls. Moreover, irrespective of age, tumor metastasis was suppressed in the *ob/ob* mice [5, 116]. However, intravenous (tail vein) injection of the B16 melanoma cells resulted in increased lung metastasis in the *ob/ob* mice [95]. This ambiguity was attributed to the different route of cell injection in the two studies. A recent study also reported that *ob/ob* mice developed carcinogen-induced skin papillomas and spontaneous p53-deficient malignancies (mostly lymphomas) in a manner similar to lean controls, whereas lipodystrophic and hyperinsulemic A-ZIP mice (described later) had increased susceptibility to carcinogenesis. Since both mouse models develop hyperphagia, hyperinsulinemia, and hyperglycemia, the authors of the study suggested that insulin resistance may not be a critical determinant of tumor development and progression in these models [2].

ob/ob mice had an increased incidence of premalignant lesions in the colon compared to lean controls when treated with the carcinogens azoxymethane (AOM) and *N*-methyl-*N*-nitrosourea (NMU). These findings were attributed to the hyperinsulinemia, hypertriglyceridemia, and hyperglycemia observed in the *ob/ob* mice and not in the lean controls [45]. In an attempt to study mammary carcinogenesis in these mice, Cleary *et al* crossed *ob/ob* mice with MMTV-TGF-α mice which overexpress transforming growth factor-α (TGF-α) specifically in the mammary epithelium. Reduced incidence of breast cancer in MMTV-TGF-α/*ob/ob* mice compared to lean controls (MMTV-TGF-α) was observed [20, 94]. However, the *ob/ob* mice also demonstrate severely impaired mammary gland development, suggesting that leptin is indispensable for mouse mammary gland development [71].

db/db Mouse

About 16 years after the description of the *ob/ob* mice, Hummel et al. at Jackson Laboratories described another obesity-prone mouse with an autosomal recessive mutation in the *diabetes* (*db*) gene which was later mapped to the leptin receptor (*LepR*) gene locus [61, 72]. Through the use of elegant parabiosis experiments it was shown that the *ob* and *db* mutations were not synonymous and that, in fact, they may represent the impairment of a common metabolic pathway [30, 31]. However, it took several years to understand that the *db* mouse is leptin resistant owing to a mutation in the long form of the leptin receptor which is expressed primarily in the brain. Thus, the *db* mouse has high circulating levels of leptin, in contrast to the leptin-deficient *ob* mouse [61, 72]. The $LepR^{db}/LepR^{db}$ (*db/db*) mouse is also obese, hyperglycemic, hyperinsulinemic, and infertile, like the *ob/ob* mouse [33].

The *db/db* mouse has also been used to study the effect of obesity and insulin resistance on cancer. The *db/db* mice display a higher incidence of lung metastasis when injected with B16 melanoma cells intravenously (tail vein) [95]. They also demonstrate greater susceptibility to carcinogen-induced premalignant lesions of the colon under energy restriction and *ad libitum* feeding conditions. However, while energy restriction normalized body weights and glucose levels in the *db/db* mice, the hyperinsulinemia and hyperleptinemia persisted, suggesting that either of these factors might be mediating the increased tumor growth [45, 70]. $APC^{1638N/+}$ mice have a mutation in the tumor suppressor APC and have been used as a model for genetically-induced colon carcinogenesis [51]. $APC^{1638N/+}$ mice, when crossed with *db/db* mice, have a higher number of tumors in the small intestine than $APC^{1638N/+}$ mice. Moreover, tumors were also observed in the stomach and large intestine of the double mutants ($APC^{1638N/+}$/*db/db*) but not in the $APC^{1638N/+}$ mice [58]. These findings support the link between obesity, insulin resistance, and gastrointestinal carcinogenesis previously reported in *ob/ob* mice. Similar to the *ob/ob* mouse, the *db/db* mice also have reduced incidence of mammary tumors when crossed with MMTV-TGF-α mice [19]. Moreover, *db/db* mice also have severely impaired mammary gland development owing to nonfunctional leptin receptors [71].

Taken together, the data obtained in *ob/ob* and *db/db* mice suggest that obesity and/or insulin resistance promote colon carcinogenesis. However, the studies performed on skin carcinogenesis have been inconclusive. Moreover, a critical role of leptin in mouse mammary gland development renders *ob/ob* and *db/db* models unsuitable to study breast carcinogenesis.

Zucker Fatty Rats

$LepR^{fa}/LepR^{fa}$ Zucker fatty rats (*fa/fa rat*) are the best known and most widely used rat model of genetically-induced obesity. Originally described in 1961, these rats inherit the autosomal recessive *fatty* (*fa*) mutation which has since been mapped to the *LepR* gene locus [16, 118, 138]. Similar to the *db/db* mice, the Zucker rats also harbor a mutation in the long form of the leptin receptor, and are leptin resistant [100].

Rats homozygous for the *fa* mutation are obese, insulin resistant, and hyperinsulinemic and display higher leptin levels compared to lean controls [8, 62]

The *fa/fa* rats are more susceptible to carcinogen-induced colon carcinogenesis when compared to lean controls, similar to the *db/db* and *ob/ob* mice [87, 125]. Moreover, when subjected to moderate energy restriction, that does not affect the body weight, the appearance of advanced crypt foci in the colon is significantly reduced in the *fa/fa* rats [102]. Accordingly, pair feeding of *fa/fa* rats with lean rats results in reduced body weight and decreased number of aberrant crypt foci (ACF) in the *fa/fa* rats [82]. However, these dietary interventions do not significantly affect circulating insulin levels, thus suggesting that hyperinsulinemia is not implicated in the promoting action on colon carcinogenesis in *fa/fa* rats.

The *fa/fa* rats have also been used to study the role of obesity and hyperinsulinemia in breast cancer progression. Interestingly, in contrast to *ob/ob* and *db/db* mice, leptin receptor signaling appears to be dispensable for mammary gland development in *fa/fa* rats [38]. The development of NMU-induced breast cancer is suppressed in female *fa/fa* rats [87], whereas 7,12-dimethylbenz(a)anthracene (DMBA)-induced mammary tumors exhibit a shorter latency period and a more aggressive phenotype [59, 60]. The authors attribute this discrepancy to the different modes of action of NMU and DMBA. However, since NMU-induced tumor growth is enhanced in rats fed a high-fat diet (HFD) (as described later), it is equally possible that the leptin receptor may be essential for the carcinogenic activity of NMU in the mammary gland of *fa/fa* rats. Interestingly, in contrast to DIO as described later, ovariectomy results in a reduced incidence of DMBA-induced mammary tumors in *fa/fa* rats despite increased total body weight [60]. These findings suggest that ovarian hormones play an important role in DMBA-induced carcinogenesis in this model. Although not addressed in these studies, hyperinsulinemia may also be involved in the estrogen-mediated breast tumor promotion by repressing sex hormone binding globulin and stimulating steroidogenesis, which results in increased levels of bioavaiable estrogen [11, 101].

LA/N-cp (Corpulent) Rat

The LA/N-cp rat is another model of genetically-induced obesity that has been used to study the impact of obesity and insulin resistance on mammary carcinogenesis. Homozygous inheritance of a recessive mutation in the *corpulent* gene (*cp/cp*) (mapped to the *LepR* gene locus) results in obesity, hyperlipidemia, and hyperinsulinemia [74, 110]. Similar to the *fa/fa* rats, female LA/N-cp rats develop DMBA-induced mammary tumors with a shorter latency and higher incidence compared to lean controls. Moreover, when these rats are subjected to energy restriction, mammary tumor incidence is reduced to the level of lean mice; a finding that has been correlated with a significant reduction of body weight and circulating insulin levels [80].

Taken together, studies in genetically obese *fa/fa* and LA/N-cp rats indicate that obesity promotes mammary and colon carcinogenesis. However, the role of insulin resistance in mediating these effects remains elusive.

The models of monogenic obesity discussed thus far have been valuable tools to establish a connection between obesity/insulin resistance and cancer. Nevertheless, as mentioned previously, monogenic obesity is rarely found in humans and most of the human obesity syndromes are polygenic in nature. Thus, studies investigating the tumor development and growth in models of DIO, which are more heterogeneous in nature, would be far more relevant to humans.

Diet-Induced Obesity and Cancer

Experimental models of DIO have been commonly used in cancer research and provide significant insight into the influence of different diets, excess weight, and secondary pathophysiological abnormalities on tumorigenesis. Numerous approaches have been undertaken to induce obesity by dietary modifications in rodents. They include high calorie diets, which result in high energy intake, or isocaloric diets, which provide a normal daily amount of calories but substantially change the ratio between major constituents of the diet such as carbohydrates, proteins, and fat. Different types of HFD, in which up to 60% calories are coming from fat, have been extensively employed in research. Animal models utilizing HFD are particularly helpful in corroborating a positive relationship between obesity, insulin resistance, and tumor development. The major drawback of these models, similar to models of genetically-induced obesity, is that in most cases they fail to identify a specific pathophysiological mechanism of obesity-mediated tumor progression. Herein, we present the experimental data available for different types of cancers (primarily breast, prostate and colon cancer) studied in the setting of DIO, and discuss a possible role for insulin resistance, hyperinsulinemia, and other related factors on tumor growth.

Breast Cancer

In most experimental models of breast cancer including NMU- and DMBA-induced models of chemically-induced carcinogenesis as well as transgenic and implantation breast cancer models, DIO results in enhanced tumor development and progression. However, HFD also affects mammary gland development. Corn oil diet significantly enhances the effects of exogenous estrogen and progesterone on mammary gland development [126], while fish oil diet rich in ω-3 polyunsaturated fatty acids (PUFA) has an inhibitory effect in intact mammary glands [127].

HFD promotes NMU-induced mammary carcinogenesis as demonstrated by shortened latency and increased multiplicity of tumors in Sprague–Dawley and Fischer 344 (F344) rats [14]. Studies conducted in both Sprague–Dawley and F344 rats suggest that dietary fat does not enhance NMU-induced mammary tumorigenesis in a dose-dependent manner [3, 24]. In addition, supplementation of HFD with cholesterol does not affect NMU-induced mammary carcinogenesis in F344 rats [21]. However, caloric restriction, voluntary exercise, and dietary fibers inhibit the stimulatory effect of HFD on NMU-induced tumor development [25, 26]. HFD also does not affect the growth and metastasis of the 13,762 transplantable mammary tumors in F344 rats [7]. The incidence and multiplicity of DMBA-induced mammary tumors in Sprague–Dawley rats, however, increases in animals fed a HFD [12], and ovariectomy further enhances this effect [22]. In C3H mice, obesity induced by a single injection of gold thioglucose, which induces necrosis in the venromedial portion of hypothalamus [40], results in accelerated development of spontaneous mammary tumors [124]. However, HFD (10% wt/wt) further enhances the incidence of mammary tumors in gold thioglucose-treated C3H mice [122]. Moreover, while ovariectomized lean C3H female mice fail to develop mammary tumors, ovariectomized obese mice have a significantly higher rate of tumor incidence than non-ovariectomized obese controls [123]. These results have also been reproduced in the syngeneic Wnt-1 model of breast cancer. Ovariectomy results in suppressed growth of tumors developed after orthotopic inoculation of estrogen-sensitive Wnt-1 breast cancer cells in syngeneic C57Bl/6 mice fed with regular chow, whereas ovariectomized mice fed on high calorie diet further gained weight and demonstrated accelerated tumor growth [98]. These data indicate the following: (1) ovarian hormones affect tumor growth in lean and obese animals differently; (2) the tumor-promoting activity of obesity is exacerbated in the absence of ovarian hormones. However, it has also been shown that obese rats have elevated levels of prolactin and estrogens [13]; adequate circulating levels of estrogens and prolactin are required to achieve the optimal effect of HFD on DMBA-induced tumor growth in Sprague–Dawley rats [4, 115]. The cause for ambiguity in these data is not fully understood but could be explained, at least in part, by the existence of different pools of sex steroids (ovarian vs. adipose tissue-derived), which were surgically or pharmacologically ablated in these studies. Interestingly, in Noble female rats, HFD does not affect mammary carcinogenesis induced by 17β-estradiol suggesting a potent tumor-promoting activity of exogenous estrogen, which cannot be potentiated by HFD in this specific model [88].

HFD containing primarily ω-6 PUFA enhances DMBA-induced breast cancer progression only in pregnant Sprague–Dawley rats, indicating an important role for pregnancy-related hormones in this activity [69]. HFD also has an additive effect on obesity and tumor incidence in DMBA-exposed Zucker rats with mimicked pregnancy [38].Interestingly, exposure of pregnant Sprague–Dawley rats to HFD substantially increased the susceptibility of their offspring to DMBA-induced mammary carcinogenesis [37]. The authors attribute this phenomenon to the increased leptin levels, although gestational diabetes and hyperinsulinemia could also mediate this effect.

The tumor-promoting effects of HFD in breast tissue depend on the composition of the fat in the diet. F344 rats fed on seed oils rich in monosaturated fatty acids exhibit accelerated NMU-induced breast cancer development, demonstrated by shortened tumor latency and increased tumor incidence and multiplicity, whereas fruit oils, such as olive and coconut oils, rich in oleic acid fail to enhance tumor growth [27]. Furthermore, the tumor-promoting effect of HFD in NMU-induced breast carcinogenesis was alleviated when longer-unsaturated-chain triglycerides or ω-3 PUFA were included in the diet [23, 28].

In xenograft models of breast cancer, growth of human ER^+/PR^+ MCF-7 cells and ER^-/PR^- MDA-MB-231 cells was enhanced in athymic nude mice fed with corn oil diet (20% fat wt/wt) and reduced in animals fed a fish oil diet rich in ω-3 PUFA [56]. The growth of MDA-MB-231 tumors was also retarded in mice fed canola oil containing high levels of linolenic acid, which can convert to ω-3 PUFA in vivo [63]. Rag1−/− immunodeficient mice inoculated with MCF-7 or MDA-MB-231 cells do not display HFD-induced change in tumor latency, burden, and grade [104]. However, the mammary tissue in these animals exhibits elevated levels of leptin receptors, IGF-I receptors (IGF-IR), and Bcl-2, each of which is an important regulator of cell survival.

DIO has been shown to mediate tumor progression in several transgenic mouse models of breast cancer. In the transgenic MMTV-v-Ha-ras model (on an FVB/N background, which is relatively resistant to obesity), HFD (0, 5, 25% calories from corn oil) increased the incidence of breast tumors increased in a dose-dependent manner [41]. Similarly, transgenic MMTV-TGF-α mice (on obesity-prone C57Bl/6 background) fed a HFD (11% fat calories) also demonstrated increased incidence of breast cancer [18]. HFD significantly enhances mammary tumor growth, and development of pulmonary metastases, when MMTV-driven polyoma virus middle T antigen (PyVmT) was introduced into M16i mice, which represent a model of polygenic obesity [57].

The effect of HFD on Neu/ErbB2-induced mammary tumorigenesis is not completely understood. HFD (32.5% fat calories) does not affect breast tumor latency, incidence, burden, and metastasis in FVB/N mice overexpressing wild-type Neu in mammary epithelium [17]. However, HFD (20% wt/wt) increases tumor burden in MMTV-c-Neu mice (also on FVB/N background) that overexpress a constitutively active form of Neu [91]. In contrast, MMTV-c-Neu mice fed a fish oil diet demonstrate delayed latency of mammary tumors compared to mice fed a corn oil diet [92] suggesting an important role of individual dietary components.

Therefore, taken together, DIO has tumor-promoting effects in the majority of the breast cancer models as described earlier. Dietary constituents such as fatty acids, along with sex steroids, appear to be important determinants of this activity. It remains unclear, however, whether insulin resistance and hyperinsulinemia are essential for these effects; this question was not addressed in any of the referred studies.

Prostate Cancer

In the xenograft DU-145 model of prostate cancer, a diet rich in ω-3 PUFA significantly decreases tumor growth [75, 105]. HFD also does not affect sex hormone-induced prostate carcinogenesis in Noble male rates [88]. However, subcutaneous inoculation of human prostate carcinoma LNCaP cells into athymic mice fed on a high carbohydrate/HFD results in increased tumor growth. These mice also demonstrate significantly elevated serum insulin and IGF-I levels. Furthermore, tumor tissues obtained from these animals exhibit elevated insulin receptor (IR) levels and increased phosphorylation of Akt [119]. In another study employing the LNCaP xenograft model, mice fed a HFD demonstrates marked upregulation of the IGF-IR in the tumor tissue [96]. In accordance with these findings, transgenic Hi-Myc mice fed a low-fat diet demonstrates decreased incidence of prostate cancer, higher circulating IGF binding protein 1 levels, and reduced Akt activation, suggesting a suppression of IR signaling [81]. Taken together, these results indicate a potential role of insulin resistance and hyperinsulinemia in the HFD-related effects on prostate tumor growth, although a cause-and-effect relationship has not been demonstrated in any of the aforementioned studies.

Colon Cancer

Sprague–Dawley rats treated with the carcinogen 1,2-dimethylhydrazine (DMH) and fed graded levels of dietary fat, demonstrated an increased number of ACFs that has been correlated to circulating leptin levels. The role of hyperinsulinemia and insulin resistance was not addressed in this study [89]. However, another study employing high-energy diet (15% energy as protein, 33% as fat, and 52% as carbohydrate) feeding of Sprague–Dawley rats did not demonstrate accelerated development of DMH-induced precancerous lesions despite increased fat mass and elevated levels of insulin, leptin, and triglycerides in the circulation [44]

In a model of AOM-induced colon carcinogenesis, HFD (59% fat calories) enhanced ACF formation in F344 rats [83]. HFD also increased the number of AOM-induced colon polyps in adiponectin and adiponectin receptor knockout mice compared to wild-type controls [53]. These data suggest that the effects of obesity on tumor growth can be attributed to hypoadiponectinemia, which is one of the characteristics of obesity.

As seen in breast cancer, the effect of HFD on colon carcinogenesis also depends on the fat composition in the diet. Compared to a low fat corn oil diet or a high fat fish oil diet, a HFD enriched in saturated fatty acids, significantly accelerates AOM-induced colon tumorigenesis in F344 rats [103]. In line with these data, Sprague–Dawley rats that receive intraperitoneal injections of AOM supplemented with 10% corn and beef tallow, but not olive or fish oils, also demonstrated increased ACF, tumor incidence, and multiplicity [54]. In the xenograft colon carcinoma WiDr model, dietary supplementation with ω-3 PUFA results in marked suppression of tumor growth. Recipient BALB/c nu/+ mice fed with golden algae oil rich in a single ω-3 fatty acid (docosahexaenoic acid) also demonstrated a 90% reduction in tumor size compared to corn oil fed animals [76]. Taken together, these data further support the hypothesis that saturated and ω-6 PUFA promote tumorigenesis whereas, oleic and ω-3 fatty acids exert neutral or inhibitory effects.

In the APC/Min mouse model of intestinal tumorigenesis, HFD does not affect polyp formation, although a diet rich in olive oil and supplemented with dry fruit and vegetable extracts has an inhibitory effect on polyp formation [93]. However, a Western style diet containing high fat and phosphate but low calcium and vitamin D, enhances intestinal tumorigenesis in this model [134]. The same diet induces adenoma formation in wild-type mice and significantly increases incidence, frequency, and size of small and large intestinal adenomas in $p27^{kip}$–/– mice. Moreover, the genetic and dietary combination in the $p27^{kip}$–/– mice also results in the development of malignant tumors [133].

In the syngeneic colon carcinoma MC38 model, C57Bl/6 mice fed a HFD demonstrated increased tumor growth and metastasis [46, 97]. Furthermore, the growth of MC38 tumors in obese mice is potentiated by ovariectomy [97]. In line with the aforementioned data obtained in different breast cancer models, this study thus strongly supports the hypothesis that ovarian hormones protect against diet- and obesity-induced tumor growth ([132] – PMID: 16959846).

Other Cancers

ω-3 PUFA significantly inhibits the growth of human lung mucoepidermoid carcinoma cells in athymic mice [39]. HFD also enhances growth of Lewis lung carcinoma (LLC) cells in C57Bl/6 mice [97]. In addition to HFD, high sucrose (HSD) and high cholesterol diets (HCD) also stimulate LLC growth and metastasis in recipient C57Bl/6 mice [79]. However, only HFD led to the development of obesity, insulin resistance, and hyperinsulinemia suggesting that factors other than insulin mediate tumor-stimulating effects of HSD and HCD. HFD also promoted the development of spontaneous hepatomas and diethylnitrosamine-induced hepatocarcinogenesis in C3H mice and Sprague–Dawley rats, respectively [114, 121, 124].

A diet with 30% fat and protein led to increases in the incidence of DMBA-induced pancreatic cancer in Sprague–Dawley rats [136]. In Syrian hamsters, in the model of *N*-nitrosobis-2-oxopropylamine-induced pancreatic cancer, the incidence of liver metastasis was significantly decreased in animals fed on fish oil rich in ω-3 PUFA [66, 136]. In mice of the "Rockland strain," HFD promotes benzpyrene-induced skin tumorigenesis [6]. Rapid body weight gain also increases the risk of UV radiation-induced skin carcinogenesis in SKH-1 hairless mice [42], while voluntary exercise and partial lipectomy stimulates apoptosis of UV-induced tumors in tumor-bearing mice [90].

NMRI nude mice subjected to subcutaneous inoculation of gastric adenocarcinoma 23132/87 cells and fed a ketogenic diet (high in fat enriched with ω-3 PUFA and medium-chain triglycerides), demonstrated suppressed tumor growth [99]. However, nude mice demonstrates enhanced growth and metastasis of inoculated MDA-MB-435 tumor cells, which are of melanocytic origin, when fed on corn oil diet (23% wt/wt) [47], and delayed tumor growth, reduced recurrence rates, and pulmonary metastasis when fed a diet rich in ω-3 PUFA [106–109].

Taken together, these data, despite some discrepancies, support a tumor-promoting role of obesity and clearly point to antitumor effects of ω-3 PUFA. One possible mechanism for the antitumor effect of ω-3 PUFA has been attributed to the suppression of tumor eicosanoid biosynthesis [109]. However, the drawback of these studies is that they do not identify specific pathophysiological mechanisms implicated in these activities.

Hyperinsulinemia, Insulin Resistance, and Cancer: Lessons from Nonobese Models of Type 2 Diabetes

An attempt to uncouple the tumor-promoting effect of body adiposity from diabetes was performed in transgenic A-ZIP/F-1 mice that develop lipoatrophic diabetes [2, 97]. A-ZIP/F-1 mice demonstrate markedly accelerated skin and mammary tumor formation suggesting a direct role of the diabetic milieu in tumor development. This study, however, has several limitations: (1) fatless mice represent lipoatrophic form of T2D which is rare in humans; (2) these mice have severely impaired mammary gland development [35]; (3) the mice develop multiple hormonal and metabolic abnormalities including hyperinsulinemia, severe hyperglycemia, hyperlipidemia, elevated levels of circulating IGF-I, and proinflammatory cytokines, each of which can potentially enhance tumorigenesis; and (4) tumor tissue in A-ZIP mice that has increased levels of phosphorylated ERK1/2 and Akt in the face of decreased IR phosphorylation suggesting that factors other than the IR drive activation of the PI3K and MAPK pathways in this diabetic model.

Our laboratory developed a unique transgenic MKR model of T2D [50]. In this model, a dominant-negative form of the human insulin-like growth factor I (IGF-I) receptor with a point mutation $K^{1003} \rightarrow R^{1003}$ is expressed in the skeletal muscle under the control of a muscle creatine kinase promoter resulting in the inactivation of endogenous insulin and IGF-IR in skeletal muscle. Female MKR mice display a mild diabetic phenotype; they develop severe insulin resistance and hyperinsulinemia in the setting of moderately reduced body adiposity and mild dysglycemia and hyperlipidemia. Therefore, it is a valuable model for studying the role of hyperinsulinemia and insulin resistance in tumor development and progression. MKR female mice demonstrate a more aggressive phenotype and enhanced tumor growth in transgenic PyVmT and Neu/ErbB2 models, syngeneic Met-1 and MCNeuA orthograft models, and in the model of DMBA-induced breast cancer. Tumor tissue extracted from MKR mice displays markedly increased phosphorylation of the IR/IGF-IR and Akt that strongly suggests a pathophysiological role of hyperinsulinemia in the enhanced tumor development.

A broad range of other related models of insulin resistance and T2D have been developed. They employ genetically engineered mice with a targeted disruption of genes encoding key components of insulin signaling including insulin receptor, insulin receptor substrates 1 and 2, Akt2, glucokinase, and Glut4 [1, 9, 15, 77, 78, 84, 128]. These mice also develop marked insulin resistance and hyperinsulinemia and have normal or reduced body adiposity. Application of these models in cancer studies would help to understand pathophysiological role of insulin resistance, hyperinsulinemia, and T2D in tumor development and progression.

References

1. Abel ED, Peroni O et al (2001) Adipose-selective targeting of the GLUT4 gene impairs insulin action in muscle and liver. Nature 409(6821):729–733
2. Ablamunits V, Cohen Y et al (2006) Susceptibility to induced and spontaneous carcinogenesis is increased in fatless A-ZIP/F-1 but not in obese ob/ob mice. Cancer Res 66(17):8897–8902
3. Aksoy M, Berger MR et al (1987) The influence of different levels of dietary fat on the incidence and growth of MNU-induced mammary carcinoma in rats. Nutr Cancer 9(4):227–235
4. Aylsworth CF, Van Vugt DA et al (1984) Role of estrogen and prolactin in stimulation of carcinogen-induced mammary tumor development by a high-fat diet. Cancer Res 44(7):2835–2840
5. Black PL, Holly M et al (1983) Enhanced tumor resistance and immunocompetence in obese (ob/ob) mice. Life Sci 33(Suppl 1):715–718
6. Boutwell RK, Brush MK et al (1949) The stimulating effect of dietary fat on carcinogenesis. Cancer Res 9(12):741–746
7. Boylan ES, Cohen LA (1986) The influence of dietary fat on mammary tumor metastasis in the rat. Nutr Cancer 8(3):193–200
8. Bray GA (1977) Experimental models for the study of obesity: introductory remarks. Fed Proc 36(2):137–138
9. Bruning JC, Winnay J et al (1997) Development of a novel polygenic model of NIDDM in mice heterozygous for IR and IRS-1 null alleles. Cell 88(4):561–572
10. Butler AA (2006) The melanocortin system and energy balance. Peptides 27(2):281–290
11. Calle EE, Kaaks R (2004) Overweight, obesity and cancer: epidemiological evidence and proposed mechanisms. Nat Rev Cancer 4(8):579–591
12. Carroll KK, Khor HT (1970) Effects of dietary fat and dose level of 7,12-dimethylbenz(alpha)-anthracene on mammary tumor incidence in rats. Cancer Res 30(8):2260–2264
13. Chan PC, Didato F et al (1975) High dietary fat, elevation of rat serum prolactin and mammary cancer. Proc Soc Exp Biol Med 149(1):133–135
14. Chan PC, Head JF et al (1977) Influence of dietary fat on the induction of mammary tumors by N-nitrosomethylurea: associated hormone changes and differences between Sprague–Dawley and F344 rats. J Natl Cancer Inst 59(4):1279–1283
15. Cho H, Mu J et al (2001) Insulin resistance and a diabetes mellitus-like syndrome in mice lacking the protein kinase Akt2 (PKB beta). Science 292(5522):1728–1731
16. Chua SC Jr, Chung WK et al (1996) Phenotypes of mouse diabetes and rat fatty due to mutations in the OB (leptin) receptor. Science 271(5251):994–996
17. Cleary MP, Grande JP et al (2004) Diet-induced obesity and mammary tumor development in MMTV-neu female mice. Nutr Cancer 50(2):174–180
18. Cleary MP, Grande JP et al (2004) Effect of high fat diet on body weight and mammary tumor latency in MMTV-TGF-alpha mice. Int J Obes Relat Metab Disord 28(8):956–962
19. Cleary MP, Juneja SC et al (2004) Leptin receptor-deficient MMTV-TGF-alpha/Lepr(db) Lepr(db) female mice do not develop oncogene-induced mammary tumors. Exp Biol Med (Maywood) 229(2):182–193
20. Cleary MP, Phillips FC et al (2003) Genetically obese MMTV-TGF-alpha/Lep(ob)Lep(ob) female mice do not develop mammary tumors. Breast Cancer Res Treat 77(3):205–215
21. Cohen LA, Chan PC (1982) Dietary cholesterol and experimental mammary cancer development. Nutr Cancer 4(2):99–106

22. Cohen LA, Chan PC et al (1981) The role of a high-fat diet in enhancing the development of mammary tumors in ovariectomized rats. Cancer 47(1):66–71
23. Cohen LA, Chen-Backlund JY et al (1993) Effect of varying proportions of dietary menhaden and corn oil on experimental rat mammary tumor promotion. Lipids 28(5):449–456
24. Cohen LA, Choi K et al (1986) Effect of varying proportions of dietary fat on the development of N-nitrosomethylurea-induced rat mammary tumors. Anticancer Res 6(2):215–218
25. Cohen LA, Choi KW et al (1988) Influence of dietary fat, caloric restriction, and voluntary exercise on N-nitrosomethylurea-induced mammary tumorigenesis in rats. Cancer Res 48(15):4276–4283
26. Cohen LA, Kendall ME et al (1991) Modulation of N-nitrosomethylurea-induced mammary tumor promotion by dietary fiber and fat. J Natl Cancer Inst 83(7):496–501
27. Cohen LA, Thompson DO et al (1986) Dietary fat and mammary cancer. I. Promoting effects of different dietary fats on N-nitrosomethylurea-induced rat mammary tumorigenesis. J Natl Cancer Inst 77(1):33–42
28. Cohen LA, Thompson DO et al (1984) Influence of dietary medium-chain triglycerides on the development of N-methylnitrosourea-induced rat mammary tumors. Cancer Res 44(11): 5023–5028
29. Cohen ND, Hilf R (1974) Influence of insulin on growth and metabolism of 7,12-dimethylbenz-(alpha)anthracene-induced mammary tumors. Cancer Res 34(12):3245–3252
30. Coleman DL (1973) Effects of parabiosis of obese with diabetes and normal mice. Diabetologia 9(4):294–298
31. Coleman DL, Hummel KP (1969) Effects of parabiosis of normal with genetically diabetic mice. Am J Physiol 217(5):1298–1304
32. Coleman DL, Hummel KP (1973) The influence of genetic background on the expression of the obese (Ob) gene in the mouse. Diabetologia 9(4):287–293
33. Coleman DL, Hummel KP (1974) Hyperinsulinemia in pre-weaning diabetes (db) mice. Diabetologia 10(Suppl):607–610
34. Corpet DE, Jacquinet C et al (1997) Insulin injections promote the growth of aberrant crypt foci in the colon of rats. Nutr Cancer 27(3):316–320
35. Couldrey C, Moitra J et al (2002) Adipose tissue: a vital in vivo role in mammary gland development but not differentiation. Dev Dyn 223(4):459–468
36. Danforth C (1927) Hereditary adiposity in mice. J Hered 18(4):153–162
37. de Assis S, Khan G et al (2006) High birth weight increases mammary tumorigenesis in rats. Int J Cancer 119(7):1537–1546
38. de Assis S, Wang M et al (2006) Excessive weight gain during pregnancy increases carcinogen-induced mammary tumorigenesis in Sprague–Dawley and lean and obese Zucker rats. J Nutr 136(4):998–1004
39. de Bravo MG, de Antueno RJ et al (1991) Effects of an eicosapentaenoic and docosahexaenoic acid concentrate on a human lung carcinoma grown in nude mice. Lipids 26(11):866–870
40. Debons AF, Krimsky I et al (1977) Gold thioglucose obesity syndrome. Fed Proc 36(2): 143–147
41. DeWille JW, Waddell K et al (1993) Dietary fat promotes mammary tumorigenesis in MMTV/v-Ha-ras transgenic mice. Cancer Lett 69(1):59–66
42. Dinkova-Kostova AT, Fahey JW et al (2008) Rapid body weight gain increases the risk of UV radiation-induced skin carcinogenesis in SKH-1 hairless mice. Nutr Res 28(8):539–543
43. Dombrowski F, Bannasch P et al (1997) Hepatocellular neoplasms induced by low-number pancreatic islet transplants in streptozotocin diabetic rats. Am J Pathol 150(3):1071–1087
44. Drew JE, Farquharson AJ et al (2007) Insulin, leptin, and adiponectin receptors in colon: regulation relative to differing body adiposity independent of diet and in response to dimethylhydrazine. Am J Physiol Gastrointest Liver Physiol 293(4):G682–G691
45. Ealey KN, Lu S et al (2008) Development of aberrant crypt foci in the colons of ob/ob and db/db mice: evidence that leptin is not a promoter. Mol Carcinog 47(9):667–677
46. Earl TM, Nicoud IB et al (2009) Silencing of TLR4 decreases liver tumor burden in a murine model of colorectal metastasis and hepatic steatosis. Ann Surg Oncol 16(4):1043–1050

47. Ellison G, Klinowska T et al (2002) Further evidence to support the melanocytic origin of MDA-MB-435. Mol Pathol 55(5):294–299
48. Fan W, Boston BA et al (1997) Role of melanocortinergic neurons in feeding and the agouti obesity syndrome. Nature 385(6612):165–168
49. Farooqi IS, O'Rahilly S (2005) Monogenic obesity in humans. Annu Rev Med 56:443–458
50. Fernandez AM, Kim JK et al (2001) Functional inactivation of the IGF-I and insulin receptors in skeletal muscle causes type 2 diabetes. Genes Dev 15(15):1926–1934
51. Fodde R, Edelmann W et al (1994) A targeted chain-termination mutation in the mouse Apc gene results in multiple intestinal tumors. Proc Natl Acad Sci USA 91(19):8969–8973
52. Frasca F, Pandini G et al (2008) The role of insulin receptors and IGF-I receptors in cancer and other diseases. Arch Physiol Biochem 114(1):23–37
53. Fujisawa T, Endo H et al (2008) Adiponectin suppresses colorectal carcinogenesis under the high-fat diet condition. Gut 57(11):1531–1538
54. Fujise T, Iwakiri R et al (2007) Long-term feeding of various fat diets modulates azoxymethane-induced colon carcinogenesis through Wnt/beta-catenin signaling in rats. Am J Physiol Gastrointest Liver Physiol 292(4):G1150–G1156
55. Genuth SM, Przybylski RJ et al (1971) Insulin resistance in genetically obese, hyperglycemic mice. Endocrinology 88(5):1230–1238
56. Gonzalez MJ, Schemmel RA et al (1991) Effect of dietary fat on growth of MCF-7 and MDA-MB231 human breast carcinomas in athymic nude mice: relationship between carcinoma growth and lipid peroxidation product levels. Carcinogenesis 12(7):1231–1235
57. Gordon RR, Hunter KW et al (2008) Genotype X diet interactions in mice predisposed to mammary cancer: II. Tumors and metastasis. Mamm Genome 19(3):179–189
58. Gravaghi C, Bo J et al (2008) Obesity enhances gastrointestinal tumorigenesis in Apc-mutant mice. Int J Obes (Lond) 32(11):1716–1719
59. Hakkak R, Holley AW et al (2005) Obesity promotes 7,12-dimethylbenz(a)anthracene-induced mammary tumor development in female zucker rats. Breast Cancer Res 7(5):R627–R633
60. Hakkak R, MacLeod S et al (2007) Obesity increases the incidence of 7,12-dimethylbenz(a) anthracene-induced mammary tumors in an ovariectomized Zucker rat model. Int J Oncol 30(3):557–563
61. Halaas JL, Gajiwala KS et al (1995) Weight-reducing effects of the plasma protein encoded by the obese gene. Science 269(5223):543–546
62. Hardie LJ, Rayner DV et al (1996) Circulating leptin levels are modulated by fasting, cold exposure and insulin administration in lean but not Zucker (fa/fa) rats as measured by ELISA. Biochem Biophys Res Commun 223(3):660–665
63. Hardman WE (2007) Dietary canola oil suppressed growth of implanted MDA-MB 231 human breast tumors in nude mice. Nutr Cancer 57(2):177–183
64. Heston WE (1942) Relationship between the lethal yellow (A(y)) gene of the mouse and susceptibility to induced pulmonary tumors. J Natl Cancer Inst 3(3):303–308
65. Heston WE, Deringer MK (1947) Relationship between the lethal yellow (Ay) gene of the mouse and susceptibility to spontaneous pulmonary tumors. J Natl Cancer Inst 7(6):463–465
66. Heukamp I, Gregor JI et al (2006) Influence of different dietary fat intake on liver metastasis and hepatic lipid peroxidation in BOP-induced pancreatic cancer in Syrian hamsters. Pancreatology 6(1–2):96–102
67. Heuson JC, Legros N (1972) Influence of insulin deprivation on growth of the 7,12-dimethylbenz(a)anthracene-induced mammary carcinoma in rats subjected to alloxan diabetes and food restriction. Cancer Res 32(2):226–232
68. Heuson JC, Legros N et al (1972) Influence of insulin administration on growth of the 7,12-dimethylbenz(a)anthracene-induced mammary carcinoma in intact, oophorectomized, and hypophysectomized rats. Cancer Res 32(2):233–238
69. Hilakivi-Clarke L, Onojafe I et al (1996) Breast cancer risk in rats fed a diet high in n-6 polyunsaturated fatty acids during pregnancy. J Natl Cancer Inst 88(24):1821–1827
70. Hirose Y, Hata K et al (2004) Enhancement of development of azoxymethane-induced colonic premalignant lesions in C57BL/KsJ-db/db mice. Carcinogenesis 25(5):821–825

71. Hu X, Juneja SC et al (2002) Leptin–a growth factor in normal and malignant breast cells and for normal mammary gland development. J Natl Cancer Inst 94(22):1704–1711
72. Hummel KP, Dickie MM et al (1966) Diabetes, a new mutation in the mouse. Science 153(740):1127–1128
73. Ingalls AM, Dickie MM et al (1950) Obese, a new mutation in the house mouse. J Hered 41(12):317–318
74. Kahle EB, Butz KG et al (1997) The rat corpulent (cp) mutation maps to the same interval on (Pgm1-Glut1) rat chromosome 5 as the fatty (fa) mutation. Obes Res 5(2):142–145
75. Karmali RA, Reichel P et al (1987) The effects of dietary omega-3 fatty acids on the DU-145 transplantable human prostatic tumor. Anticancer Res 7(6):1173–1179
76. Kato T, Hancock RL et al (2002) Influence of omega-3 fatty acids on the growth of human colon carcinoma in nude mice. Cancer Lett 187(1–2):169–177
77. Katz EB, Stenbit AE et al (1995) Cardiac and adipose tissue abnormalities but not diabetes in mice deficient in GLUT4. Nature 377(6545):151–155
78. Kido Y, Burks DJ et al (2000) Tissue-specific insulin resistance in mice with mutations in the insulin receptor, IRS-1, and IRS-2. J Clin Invest 105(2):199–205
79. Kimura Y, Sumiyoshi M (2007) High-fat, high-sucrose, and high-cholesterol diets accelerate tumor growth and metastasis in tumor-bearing mice. Nutr Cancer 59(2):207–216
80. Klurfeld DM, Lloyd LM et al (1991) Reduction of enhanced mammary carcinogenesis in LA/N-cp (corpulent) rats by energy restriction. Proc Soc Exp Biol Med 196(4):381–384
81. Kobayashi N, Barnard RJ et al (2008) Effect of low-fat diet on development of prostate cancer and Akt phosphorylation in the Hi-Myc transgenic mouse model. Cancer Res 68(8):3066–3073
82. Koch TC, Briviba K et al (2008) Obesity-related promotion of aberrant crypt foci in DMH-treated obese Zucker rats correlates with dyslipidemia rather than hyperinsulinemia. Eur J Nutr 47(3):161–170
83. Koohestani N, Tran TT et al (1997) Insulin resistance and promotion of aberrant crypt foci in the colons of rats on a high-fat diet. Nutr Cancer 29(1):69–76
84. Kubota N, Tobe K et al (2000) Disruption of insulin receptor substrate 2 causes type 2 diabetes because of liver insulin resistance and lack of compensatory beta-cell hyperplasia. Diabetes 49(11):1880–1889
85. Kuklin AI, Mynatt RL et al (2004) Liver-specific expression of the agouti gene in transgenic mice promotes liver carcinogenesis in the absence of obesity and diabetes. Mol Cancer 3:17
86. Lann D, LeRoith D (2008) The role of endocrine insulin-like growth factor-I and insulin in breast cancer. J Mammary Gland Biol Neoplasia 13(4):371–379
87. Lee WM, Lu S et al (2001) Susceptibility of lean and obese Zucker rats to tumorigenesis induced by N-methyl-N-nitrosourea. Cancer Lett 162(2):155–160
88. Leung G, Benzie IF et al (2002) No effect of a high-fat diet on promotion of sex hormone-induced prostate and mammary carcinogenesis in the Noble rat model. Br J Nutr 88(4):399–409
89. Liu Z, Uesaka T et al (2001) High fat diet enhances colonic cell proliferation and carcinogenesis in rats by elevating serum leptin. Int J Oncol 19(5):1009–1014
90. Lu YP, Lou YR et al (2006) Stimulatory effect of voluntary exercise or fat removal (partial lipectomy) on apoptosis in the skin of UVB light-irradiated mice. Proc Natl Acad Sci USA 103(44):16301–16306
91. Luijten M, Thomsen AR et al (2004) Effects of soy-derived isoflavones and a high-fat diet on spontaneous mammary tumor development in Tg.NK (MMTV/c-neu) mice. Nutr Cancer 50(1):46–54
92. Luijten M, Verhoef A et al (2007) Modulation of mammary tumor development in Tg.NK (MMTV/c-neu) mice by dietary fatty acids and life stage-specific exposure to phytoestrogens. Reprod Toxicol 23(3):407–413
93. Mai V, Colbert LH et al (2003) Calorie restriction and diet composition modulate spontaneous intestinal tumorigenesis in Apc(Min) mice through different mechanisms. Cancer Res 63(8):1752–1755
94. Matsui Y, Halter SA et al (1990) Development of mammary hyperplasia and neoplasia in MMTV-TGF alpha transgenic mice. Cell 61(6):1147–1155

95. Mori A, Sakurai H et al (2006) Severe pulmonary metastasis in obese and diabetic mice. Int J Cancer 119(12):2760–2767
96. Narita S, Tsuchiya N et al (2008) Candidate genes involved in enhanced growth of human prostate cancer under high fat feeding identified by microarray analysis. Prostate 68(3): 321–335
97. Nunez NP, Oh WJ et al (2006) Accelerated tumor formation in a fatless mouse with type 2 diabetes and inflammation. Cancer Res 66(10):5469–5476
98. Nunez NP, Perkins SN et al (2008) Obesity accelerates mouse mammary tumor growth in the absence of ovarian hormones. Nutr Cancer 60(4):534–541
99. Otto C, Kaemmerer U et al (2008) Growth of human gastric cancer cells in nude mice is delayed by a ketogenic diet supplemented with omega-3 fatty acids and medium-chain triglycerides. BMC Cancer 8:122
100. Phillips MS, Liu Q et al (1996) Leptin receptor missense mutation in the fatty Zucker rat. Nat Genet 13(1):18–19
101. Poretsky L, Cataldo NA et al (1999) The insulin-related ovarian regulatory system in health and disease. Endocr Rev 20(4):535–582
102. Raju J, Bird RP (2003) Energy restriction reduces the number of advanced aberrant crypt foci and attenuates the expression of colonic transforming growth factor beta and cyclooxygenase isoforms in Zucker obese (fa/fa) rats. Cancer Res 63(20):6595–6601
103. Rao CV, Hirose Y et al (2001) Modulation of experimental colon tumorigenesis by types and amounts of dietary fatty acids. Cancer Res 61(5):1927–1933
104. Ray A, Nkhata KJ et al (2007) Diet-induced obesity and mammary tumor development in relation to estrogen receptor status. Cancer Lett 253(2):291–300
105. Rose DP, Cohen LA (1988) Effects of dietary menhaden oil and retinyl acetate on the growth of DU 145 human prostatic adenocarcinoma cells transplanted into athymic nude mice. Carcinogenesis 9(4):603–605
106. Rose DP, Connolly JM (1993) Effects of dietary omega-3 fatty acids on human breast cancer growth and metastases in nude mice. J Natl Cancer Inst 85(21):1743–1747
107. Rose DP, Connolly JM et al (1996) Effect of omega-3 fatty acids on the progression of metastases after the surgical excision of human breast cancer cell solid tumors growing in nude mice. Clin Cancer Res 2(10):1751–1756
108. Rose DP, Connolly JM et al (1991) Effect of dietary fat on human breast cancer growth and lung metastasis in nude mice. J Natl Cancer Inst 83(20):1491–1495
109. Rose DP, Connolly JM et al (1995) Influence of diets containing eicosapentaenoic or docosahexaenoic acid on growth and metastasis of breast cancer cells in nude mice. J Natl Cancer Inst 87(8):587–592
110. Russell JC, Ahuja SK et al (1987) Insulin resistance and impaired glucose tolerance in the atherosclerosis-prone LA/N corpulent rat. Arteriosclerosis 7(6):620–626
111. Schwartz MW, Woods SC et al (2000) Central nervous system control of food intake. Nature 404(6778):661–671
112. Shafie SM, Grantham FH (1981) Role of hormones in the growth and regression of human breast cancer cells (MCF-7) transplanted into athymic nude mice. J Natl Cancer Inst 67(1):51–56
113. Sharon R, Pillemer G et al (1993) Insulin dependence of murine T-cell lymphoma. II. Insulin-deficient diabetic mice and mice fed low-energy diet develop resistance to lymphoma growth. Int J Cancer 53(5):843–849
114. Silverstone H, Tannenbaum A (1951) The influence of dietary fat and riboflavin on the formation of spontaneous hepatomas in the mouse. Cancer Res 11(3):200–203
115. Sylvester PW, Ip C et al (1986) Effects of high dietary fat on the growth and development of ovarian-independent carcinogen-induced mammary tumors in rats. Cancer Res 46(2):763–769
116. Thompson CI, Kreider JW et al (1983) Genetically obese mice: resistance to metastasis of B16 melanoma and enhanced T-lymphocyte mitogenic responses. Science 220(4602):1183–1185
117. Tran TT, Medline A et al (1996) Insulin promotion of colon tumors in rats. Cancer Epidemiol Biomark Prev 5(12):1013–1015

118. Truett GE, Bahary N et al (1991) Rat obesity gene fatty (fa) maps to chromosome 5: evidence for homology with the mouse gene diabetes (db). Proc Natl Acad Sci USA 88(17): 7806–7809
119. Venkateswaran V, Haddad AQ et al (2007) Association of diet-induced hyperinsulinemia with accelerated growth of prostate cancer (LNCaP) xenografts. J Natl Cancer Inst 99(23):1793–1800
120. Vona-Davis L, Howard-McNatt M et al (2007) Adiposity, type 2 diabetes and the metabolic syndrome in breast cancer. Obes Rev 8(5):395–408
121. Wang Y, Ausman LM et al (2009) Nonalcoholic steatohepatitis induced by a high-fat diet promotes diethylnitrosamine-initiated early hepatocarcinogenesis in rats. Int J Cancer 124(3):540–546
122. Waxler SH, Brecher G et al (1979) The effect of fat-enriched diet on the incidence of spontaneous mammary tumors in obese mice. Proc Soc Exp Biol Med 162(2):365–368
123. Waxler SH, Leef MF (1966) Augmentation of mammary tumors in castrated obese C3H mice. Cancer Res 26(5):860–862
124. Waxler SH, Tabar P (1953) Appearance of hepatomas in obese C3H male mice. Stanford Med Bull 11(4):272–273
125. Weber RV, Stein DE et al (2000) Obesity potentiates AOM-induced colon cancer. Dig Dis Sci 45(5):890–895
126. Welsch CW, DeHoog JV et al (1985) Influence of dietary fat levels on development and hormone responsiveness of the mouse mammary gland. Cancer Res 45(12 Pt 1):6147–6154
127. Welsch CW, O'Connor DH (1989) Influence of the type of dietary fat on developmental growth of the mammary gland in immature and mature female BALB/c mice. Cancer Res 49(21):5999–6007
128. Withers DJ, Gutierrez JS et al (1998) Disruption of IRS-2 causes type 2 diabetes in mice. Nature 391(6670):900–904
129. Wolff GL (1987) Body weight and cancer. Am J Clin Nutr 45(1 Suppl):168–180
130. Wolff GL, Roberts DW et al (1986) Prenatal determination of obesity, tumor susceptibility, and coat color pattern in viable yellow (Avy/a) mice. The yellow mouse syndrome. J Hered 77(3):151–158
131. Wolff GL, Roberts DW et al (1987) Tumorigenic responses to lindane in mice: potentiation by a dominant mutation. Carcinogenesis 8(12):1889–1897
132. Yakar S, Nunez NP et al (2006) Increased tumor growth in mice with diet-induced obesity: impact of ovarian hormones. Endocrinology 147(12):5826–5834
133. Yang W, Bancroft L et al (2003) Targeted inactivation of p27kip1 is sufficient for large and small intestinal tumorigenesis in the mouse, which can be augmented by a Western-style high-risk diet. Cancer Res 63(16):4990–4996
134. Yang WC, Mathew J et al (2001) Targeted inactivation of the p21(WAF1/cip1) gene enhances Apc-initiated tumor formation and the tumor-promoting activity of a Western-style high-risk diet by altering cell maturation in the intestinal mucosal. Cancer Res 61(2):565–569
135. Yen TT, Gill AM et al (1994) Obesity, diabetes, and neoplasia in yellow A(vy)/- mice: ectopic expression of the agouti gene. FASEB J 8(8):479–488
136. Z'Graggen K, Warshaw AL et al (2001) Promoting effect of a high-fat/high-protein diet in DMBA-induced ductal pancreatic cancer in rats. Ann Surg 233(5):688–695
137. Zhang Y, Proenca R et al (1994) Positional cloning of the mouse obese gene and its human homologue. Nature 372(6505):425–432
138. Zucker LM, Zucker TF (1961) Fatty – new mutation in rat. J Hered 52(6):275–278

Chapter 7
Potential Mechanisms Linking Insulin to Cancer

Yael Babichev, Sarah Khalid, and I. George Fantus

Introduction

The association between obesity and the incidence of various forms of cancer is well established [11, 20, 86]. Although this association is present for several cancers in both men and women, at least three primary cancers of women show this link, namely uterine, ovarian, and mammary cancers [11]. Previous chapters have reviewed the epidemiological data in detail. The focus of this chapter is to review and discuss the potential pathophysiology and biological mechanisms, which could account for this relationship. It appears unlikely that an identical and unique mechanism will explain the impact of obesity on cancer development and progression in these different tumors. Some examples of effects on different tumors have been mentioned, which support specific mechanisms [11], the focus here will be on breast cancer (BC).

Many studies have documented using both cross-sectional and prospective data that obesity as well as type 2 diabetes mellitus (T2DM) are associated with an increased incidence and mortality of BC [84, 85, 93, 137, 145]. A number of mechanisms have been proposed. However, major questions remain regarding: (1) the most important contributing factor(s); and (2) whether similar or different obesity-related factors are involved in cancer initiation/development and progression. With regard to the second question, although it is likely that some common mediators may exist, it would not be surprising given the varied signals involved in tumor promotion, growth, and metastasis that different mechanisms will be predominant in each phase.

I.G. Fantus (✉)
Departments of Medicine and Physiology, University of Toronto, Toronto, ON, Canada

Division of Cellular and Molecular Biology, Toronto General Research Institute,
University Health Network and Banting and Best Diabetes Centre, Toronto, ON, Canada

Centre for Modeling Human Disease, Samuel Lunenfeld Research Institute,
Mount Sinai Hospital, Toronto, ON, Canada
e-mail: gfantus@mtsinai.on.ca

I.G. Fantus (ed.), *Insulin Resistance and Cancer: Epidemiology, Cellular and Molecular Mechanisms and Clinical Implications*, Energy Balance and Cancer 1,
DOI 10.1007/978-1-4419-9911-5_7,

Concomitants of Obesity: Candidate Factors

Nutrition and Lifestyle

Obesity has been increasing worldwide over the past several decades and has reached "epidemic" proportions in the Western world [37]. Although genetic factors certainly predispose some individuals, the major cause of the dramatic increase within a short period of 2–3 generations is environmental. Overnutrition, characterized for the most part by a high fat diet (HFD), and decreased physical activity are the critical determinants of this phenomenon [37, 111]. Along with the increased obesity, an increased incidence of T2DM, cardiovascular disease as well as BC has been observed [134]. An extensive amount of work has documented the hormonal and metabolic alterations that accompany obesity. These include hyperinsulinemia, resulting from insulin resistance of the classical metabolic target tissues, namely muscle, adipose tissue, and liver, elevated levels of lipids, e.g., triglycerides, free fatty acids (FFA), as well as the fat-derived satiety hormone, leptin, decreased circulating levels of the insulin sensitizing adipokine, adiponectin, and elevation of both fat- and macrophage-derived inflammatory mediators such as TNF-α, Il-6, Il-1, and MCP-1 [61, 113, 132] (Fig. 7.1). In addition to these and relevant to BC are the associations of elevated insulin levels with higher levels of estrogen as well as of free insulin-like growth factor-1 (IGF-1). Each of these changes may alter cell signaling directly, both in the mammary epithelial cell as well as in cells of the surrounding stromal tissue. While space limitation prevents a comprehensive review of each signaling system, several of these important factors and their potential contributions will be discussed.

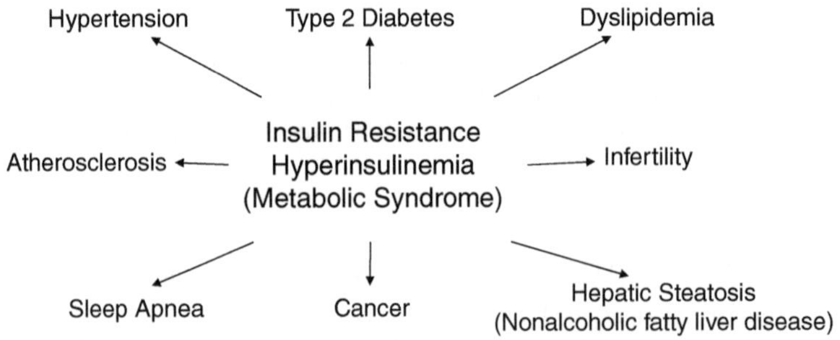

Fig. 7.1 Insulin resistance of metabolic target tissues, adipose, muscle, and liver, leads to hyperinsulinemia and the metabolic syndrome. This perturbation in metabolic regulation is associated with a wide range of adverse consequences including several cancers. The mechanisms by which cancer development and growth are promoted appear to be both direct and indirect

The Metabolic Syndrome

Prior to focusing on the individual factors and attempting to define the relative contributions of each to the pathophysiology of BC, it is important to note that these abnormalities very frequently coexist in individuals with obesity, in particular, "visceral" obesity. Visceral obesity has been identified clinically by a high waist/hip ratio [28, 61] and more recently, by elevated waist circumference [144] and appears to show a stronger association with insulin resistance than the traditional measure of obesity, i.e., the body mass index (BMI), weight (kg)/height (meters)^2. The term "metabolic syndrome" has been widely utilized to define a cluster of associated abnormalities. Although minor variations in definitions among American and European groups exist [2, 33], all agree that insulin resistance is the primary etiological factor and that the major concomitants include abnormal glucose tolerance, dyslipidemia (elevated triglycerides and low HDL cholesterol), and hypertension. The above mentioned BC-associated factors also associate with the metabolic syndrome which accounts, in part, for the difficulty of isolating a single mechanism and the requirement of multiple experimental approaches to identify the critical ones [124].

Diet and Cancer

A great deal of effort has been expended to identify the dietary components, which protect or predispose to malignancy. These have been reviewed elsewhere [143]. In this section, we focus on the macronutrient content and in the context of obesity and metabolic syndrome, specifically a HFD. HFDs, typical of Western societies, are associated in humans as well as in rodents with the development of obesity and insulin resistance [61, 113, 132, 134]. It is not surprising, therefore, that HFD has been identified as a risk for increased BC [13, 70, 80, 118]. One challenge has been to determine whether there is an independent effect of dietary fat from the insulin resistance and consequent abnormalities described above. Some in vitro and in vivo data, however, do indicate that dietary fat can influence BC independent of insulin resistance.

Feeding rodents equivalent amounts but different types of fat, which tend to elevate different circulating FFAs, had variable effects on BC development in the 7,12-dimethylbenz(a)anthracene (DMBA) chemical carcinogen-induced BC model. Thus, a 20% sunflower seed oil (polyunsaturated fat) diet promoted BC in comparison to saturated or a low fat diet [70]. Furthermore, switching and lowering fat after tumor onset to 10% saturated fat was associated within weeks with a risk reduction for subsequent tumors similar to that found with a 0% fat diet. Of interest, in the latter study, although the fat type and amount significantly influenced tumor development, there was no effect on tumor growth. In a model of transplanted tumors, namely MDA-MB-435 BC cells injected into mammary fat pads of nude mice, linoleic acid feeding resulted in a dose-dependent increase in tumor weight and size as well as an increase in pulmonary metastatic nodules [118]. While insulin resistance was not evaluated in these early studies, weight gain was not different and the diet fat contents were relatively low, 20% and 23%, respectively. In vitro studies have demonstrated opposing effects of oleic acid (monounsaturated) and palmitic acid (saturated). Exposure to oleic acid stimulated mammary epithelial cell and BC cell proliferation while palmitate induced apoptosis [55]. At the same time, oleate exposure of HER2/neu overexpressing BC cell lines (BT-474 and SKBR-3) resulted in a marked (~50%) reduction of Her-2/neu expression and an associated sensitization to trastuzumab (anti-Her-2/neu) induced cytotoxicity and apoptosis [91]. It is not clear whether these apparently opposite effects of oleic acid in vivo and in vitro are due to concentration-dependent effects or specific responses determined by inherent properties of different cancer cell lines.

More recent studies support both a tumor promoting and growth effect of HFD. In the mammary gland specific TGF-α overexpressing murine model of BC, a modest increase in dietary fat increased the number of tumors, shortened tumor latency, and resulted in somewhat larger tumors [21]. Although insulin resistance was not formally assessed in this study, an important observation was made when the HFD-fed cohort of mice were separated into 3 groups, obesity-resistant, obesity-sensitive, and obesity-prone, based on the extent of weight gain. Even in the obesity-resistant group which showed no weight gain, the HFD caused a shortened tumor latency and increased number of tumors but did not significantly alter tumor growth rates. These data suggest that a HFD has a tumor promoting action independent of significant obesity and insulin resistance and that HFD/obesity-associated insulin resistance and hyperinsulinemia may mediate the growth promoting and tumor progression effects. We have recently completed a study in HER2/neu mice. On a 45% HFD, the HER2/neu mice bred on a FVB background strain developed very mild obesity but did not manifest overt insulin resistance or hyperinsulinemia. In accord with this hypothesis, the HFD shortened the latency of appearance of a second mammary tumor and resulted in an overall increased incidence of tumors but no change in tumor growth rates [73].

The mechanism by which a HFD or elevated levels of specific circulating FFAs promote tumors independent of hyperinsulinemia remains unclear. A potential link is the well characterized association of inflammation with tumor formation [108, 150]. Polyunsaturated FFAs may be metabolized by cyclooxygenases to form inflammatory prostaglandins, which have been proposed as mediators of tumor promotion [117]. Indeed in some examples such as colon cancer, cyclooxygenase inhibitors such as indomethacin, acetylsalycilic acid (ASA), and other nonsteroidal antiinflammatory drugs (NSAIDs) have been found to decrease tumor formation [7, 14]. On the other hand, saturated FFAs such as palmitate, bind to TOLL-like receptors, mediators of innate immune responses [75]. Signaling via TOLL-like receptor 4 (TLR4) activates NF-kB and the synthesis and secretion of inflammatory cytokines [1]. While these actions are important and primarily found in lymphocytes, TLR4 signaling and inflammation have been documented to occur directly in the other cell types, e.g., adipocytes [123] and endothelial cells [76]. Although these have been associated with insulin resistance and suggested to contribute to atherosclerosis, tumor promotion may be stimulated in other tissues. A recent study has also implicated inflammation and TNF-α signaling via the TNFR1 in HFD-induced pancreatic neoplasm formation [74]. In this study, insulin sensitivity was maintained by increased FFA mitochondrial β-oxidation. Cancers have long been known to show dependence on anaerobic metabolism (Warburg effect) [57] and require fatty acids for development and growth (reviewed in [26]). Thus, the relative contribution of inflammation versus altered metabolism in the tumor promoting effects of HFD requires further evaluation.

Hyperinsulinemia

As outlined earlier, the primary hormonal change in obesity and the metabolic syndrome is the elevation of circulating levels of insulin, and both an increased risk of BC and a poorer prognosis have been correlated with elevated insulin [5, 27, 47, 51, 79, 136]. Increased concentrations of insulin are reflective of insulin resistance, but this "resistance" has been found to be selective, i.e., confined to specific pathways of insulin signaling, primarily the phosphatidylinositol 3′ kinase (PI3K) – protein kinase B (Akt/PKB) pathway, and may also be limited to specific target tissues, e.g., metabolic targets and endothelial cells [63, 81], but not epithelial and/or cancer cells. Although primarily a metabolic regulator, insulin is a "growth factor" ligand, which signals via its receptor, a member of the tyrosine (Tyr) kinase family of growth factor receptors. The insulin receptor (IR) is homologous to the insulin-like growth factor-1 receptor (IGF-1R) and shares common signaling pathways [40]. Thus, depending on context, insulin can have direct effects to stimulate cell growth and proliferation as well as indirect effects to promote cell growth and proliferation mediated by other factors/hormones. Both of these general mechanisms, specific examples, and supporting evidence are discussed later.

Direct Effects of Insulin

1. Direct stimulation of growth and proliferation
   The insulin signaling pathway has been reviewed in Chap. 2 (see [129]). The major pathways stimulating cell growth by Tyr kinase receptors are also stimulated by IR signaling. These include the PI3K-Akt and Ras-Raf-MEK-MAPK (mitogen activated protein kinase) pathways, as well as the enzyme target of rapamycin (mTOR), downstream of Akt, which in turn activates $p70^{s6k}$ and phosphorylates the 4E-binding proteins (4E-BPs) to stimulate translation, protein synthesis, and ribosome biogenesis [129]. The PI3K pathway mediates antiapoptosis and promotes cell survival, while the MAPK pathway alters several enzyme activities, transcription factors, and gene expression [40, 129]. Both of these pathways are also activated in many models of BC such as TGF-α and HER2/neu overexpression [59, 130]. Indeed, unregulated PI3K activity, e.g., seen in phosphatase and tensin homologue deleted on chromosome 10 (PTEN) deficient

mice and humans with Cowden's syndrome, is associated with a markedly increased incidence of breast and other cancers [29, 127]. Insulin stimulation of proliferation of MCF-7 BC cells (at low, 10 nM, concentrations) was blocked by the PI3-kinase inhibitor, wortmannin [94].

Of importance is that normal mammary epithelial cells (MECs) express IRs, and these are upregulated several-fold by transformation and in BC cells [39, 88, 107]. Thus, BC cells would be expected to and have been shown to respond to insulin [105]. Since these cells also express IGF-1R and insulin, at a high concentration, can bind to and activate the IGF-1R, there has been some controversy whether insulin mediates its growth promoting effect only via the IGF-1R or both receptors [63]. Complicating matter is the observation that in BC cells, in the context of upregulation of both receptors, there exist hybrid receptors made up of heterodimers [106]. In addition, the IR is expressed as two isoforms. The shorter isoform A (missing exon 11 which codes for 12 amino acids in the extracellular α subunit) is the fetal form and appears to be the predominant form upregulated in the "dedifferentiated" cancer cell state [38]. The heterodimeric IGF-1R/IR-A appears to bind IGF-1, insulin, and IGF-II with almost equal affinity [3]. This combination of cancer cell genetic and phenotypic alterations would explain how elevated circulating levels of any of the 3 growth factors could contribute to enhanced cell proliferation (see Chap. 11 for further details).

In the classical studies of hyperinsulinemia in obese individuals, IRs in target tissues demonstrate downregulation [104]. This would limit signaling, at least in part, by decreasing insulin sensitivity [138]. However, in human BC cells, we found a lack of correlation between IR expression and circulating insulin suggesting that physiologic downregulation does not occur or is limited in malignant cells [99]. Taken together, based on these data, there is a very strong biological argument for a direct effect of insulin to promote tumor growth and progression and a rationale to lower circulating levels of insulin in obese insulin resistant women with BC.

2. Enhancement of Growth and Proliferation
   While insulin can signal growth effects on its own, it has also been found to augment the proliferative signaling by other growth factors.

   (a) One example is via the activation of small G proteins, such as Ras and Rho, which are essential for growth factor signal transduction [116]. The G-proteins are activated when bound to GTP, which is exchanged for GDP by guanine nucleotide exchange factors such as the protein SOS, which is bound to Grb2 and activated upon Grb2 SH2-domain binding to Tyr phosphorylated residues of docking proteins such as IRS-1, Shc and Gab1 [129]. This G-protein activation mechanism is efficiently catalyzed at the plasma membrane (PM). Localization of G-proteins to membranes is regulated by lipidation, i.e. by the covalent addition of a 15–20 carbon isoprenoid lipid chain at the carboxy terminus. Depending on the lipid moiety either farnesyltransferase or geranylgeranyltransferase can catalyze this reaction [15].

Insulin stimulates the phosphorylation and activation of these two enzymes and promotes membrane localization of at least 2 small G-proteins, Ras and Rho-A, thereby sensitizing cells to proliferation stimulated by other growth factors, e.g., EGF, IGF-1, PDGF, and lysophosphatidic acid (LPA) [18, 19, 44, 45]. These effects appear to be mediated by Shc and, at least in part, by MAPK [46].

The downstream effects in MCF-7 BC cells by which insulin potentiates LPA-stimulated cell proliferation have been investigated. Thus, the activation of the prenyltransferase and Rho-A activation led to an increase in cyclin E and a decrease in the cyclin-dependent kinase (Cdk) inhibitor p27^{Kip1} [18]. These changes promote cell cycle progression and proliferation.

(b) A second more recently explored phenomenon is the interaction between and synergistic response mediated by combined growth factor signaling of the classical growth stimulating pathways [4, 155]. These interactions have been noted in HER2 positive tumors, which manifested or developed de novo resistance to inhibitory anti-HER2 antibodies (trastuzumab) or to EGFR/HER2 Tyr kinase inhibitors (e.g., lapatinib) [12, 67]. In these tumors, evidence for IGF-1R activation and signaling was found and dual inhibition of both EGFR/HER and IGF-1R restored responsiveness.

One mechanism of "crosstalk" between these two families of Tyr kinase receptors is a direct physical interaction or heterodimerization [68, 100]. Thus, IGF-1R has been found in some cancers to be associated with one or more of the 4 members of the EGFR family, namely EGFR, HER2, HER3, and HER4. Another noted mechanism is the upregulation of both the ligand, IGF-II, along with IGF-1R resulting in a transactivation of EGFR via IGF-1R signaling. The latter is mediated by a Src-dependent Tyr phosphorylation of EGFR Tyr 845, a Src target site (reviewed in [64]). Finally, an indirect receptor-signaling mechanism may contribute. Effective EGFR signaling may suppress IGF-1R action by EGFR binding and sequestration of the IGF-1R substrate, IRS-1, and by upregulating IGFBPs [77]. Conversely, it has been observed that inhibiting EGFR signaling results in the release of IRS-1, a downregulation of IGFBPs, as well as upregulation of the EGFR ligands, amphiregulin, heparin binding-EGF (HB-EGF), and/or TGF [64, 140]. These mechanisms serve to create an adaptive signaling platform promoting cancer cell survival and resistance to therapy [50]. Although the above studies involved IGF-1R, as discussed earlier, the IR is also overexpressed in BC, uses IRSs as substrates and can mediate growth effects similar to the IGF-1R.

Since inhibition of EGFR signaling may, in some tumors, be submaximal and anti-EGFR/HER2 agents may dampen but not completely inhibit signaling, the synergism of dual growth factor stimulation is another relevant cause of resistance to therapy. This has been explored by computer modeling and experimental data using a low concentration of EGF in the presence and absence of insulin [4, 155]. Thus, significant and synergistic potentiation of MAPK activation by insulin added to low EGF was found to be localized to two sites in the signaling pathways. First, the increased PI3-kinase and its lipid products, (PI 3,4,5-P_3), induced by insulin in the presence of EGF, served to recruit more of the docking protein GAB1, to the membrane and its subsequent Tyr phosphorylation. This, in turn, led to increased binding of the Grb2-SOS complex, the activator of Ras. In addition, although increased recruitment of Ras-GAP, the GTPase activating protein which, by accelerating GTP hydrolysis, decreases the active GTP bound form of Ras, would also be expected, the additional recruitment of the Tyr phosphatase, SHP2, resulted in the dephosphorylation of the Ras-GAP phosphotyrosine binding sites resulting ultimately in a net positive effect to augment and maintain Ras in its active GTP bound state. The second site of interaction is downstream of Ras-GTP, characterized by enhanced activity of the Ser/Thr kinase, Raf, secondary to more potent Src activation by EGF than by insulin.

It should be noted that synergism with insulin was best observed in the context of a low level of EGF stimulation, characterized by either low EGF, EGFR, or limiting levels of GAB1. In addition, it is important to note that insulin potentiation of signaling was demonstrated at concentrations (10 ng/mL), which did not activate IGF-1R, clearly implicating the IR as a key signaling molecule. Additional computer modeling has implicated these receptor signaling networks, i.e., EGFR with IR and/or with IGF-1R, in amplification of Akt, $p70^{s6k}$ and Jun N-terminal kinase (JNK), in addition to ERK1/2 [155].

(c) A third direct mechanism by which insulin/IGF signaling may enhance growth and proliferation of BC is via crosstalk with estrogen receptors. The estrogen sensitivity of BC development and growth is well documented [22]. The classical estrogen signaling pathway is that of the nuclear receptor family [49]. Upon ligand binding, these steroid hormone receptors homodimerize, translocate to the nucleus, and bind in combination with coactivators or corepressors to consensus DNA sequences to enhance or repress the expression of specific genes. While many of estrogen's effects largely depend on these events, there is increasing evidence for nonclassical signaling by these nuclear hormone receptors (reviewed in [53]). Apart from some acute effects of estrogen itself to activate enzymes, e.g., ERK1/2, via estrogen receptor (ER) interactions, there are two mechanisms which are relevant to insulin/IGF signaling. First, Ser/Thr phosphorylation of the ER has been observed, which has been found to promote classical nuclear ER signaling in the absence of ligand [121]. Thus, phosphorylation of the ER by both MAPK (ERK1/2) (e.g., Ser118 in the AF-1 region of human ER-α) and Akt (Ser 167 of ER-α), both activated by insulin, promote and/or enhance the alterations in gene expression in the absence or presence of estrogen [54, 72, 121, 148]. In this way, estrogen responsive tumors can be stimulated by growth factors, insulin/IGF1.

While classical ER signaling involves direct binding of the ER to cis-acting DNA sequences, indirect transactivation functions have also been documented. This is a function of heterodimerization with transcription factors such as Jun with the Jun DNA-binding domain serving as the direct DNA attachment factor. Since Jun and the Jun containing AP-1 transcriptional regulator are sensitive to growth factors such as insulin/IGFs, the gene regulation induced by ER-Jun complexes will also be sensitive to insulin [49, 53, 54, 72].

(d) A novel mechanism by which insulin could affect prognosis and response of BC to treatment was recently described. In ER+ BC cells which become resistant to hormone therapy, it was noted that there was an increased expression of the transcription factor T-bet (Tb×21). This factor negatively regulates two other transcription factors, namely GATA-3 and FOXA1. A proportion of estrogen responsive genes are coregulated by ER-α, GATA-3, and FOXA1, so that in the absence of GATA-3 and FOXA1, there was a decreased response. Insulin and IGF-1 induce T-bet expression in several BC cell lines, e.g., MCF7, associated with a decrease in GATA-3 and FOXA1. Thus in the presence of both E2 and tamoxifen, insulin was able to stimulate increased cell proliferation. This unresponsiveness to tamoxifen in the presence of insulin was even greater when T-bet was overexpressed [90]. Further studies in human subjects are required to determine the importance of these observations.

(e) Finally, although not as well understood, insulin/IGF signaling appears also to interact with other tumor promoting pathways. For example, polyoma virus middle T antigen (PyVMT) expressing mammary epithelial cells undergo rapid and aggressive tumor formation [52, 83]. It has been found that oncogene activation and in particular, MAPK activation, requires both insulin and IGF-1 and their cognate receptors. Both receptors appeared to physically interact with PyVMT and promote recruitment and activation of the nonreceptor Tyr kinase, Src [102]. Another tumor promoting pathway well documented in both colon and BC is the Wnt signaling pathway [56, 71]. Activation of the Wnt pathway results in inhibition of glycogen synthase kinase-3 (GSK-3), accumulation of β-catenin, and its translocation to the nucleus, in turn stimulating target gene expression, e.g., c-Myc [92, 95]. In addition, there is an increase in cellular cyclin D1, which is a cyclin-dependent kinase activator, (CDK4 and CDK6) [82]. Insulin has been found to also increase cyclin D1 [89], and interestingly metformin treatment, which inhibited cell proliferation, was associated with decreased cyclin D1 [154]. We have found that in high fat-diet-induced insulin resistance, there is β-catenin accumulation apparently caused by hyperinsulinemia in the colon [128]. This was also observed in cultured colon cancer cells [149]. Although insulin and Wnt both signal to inhibit GSK-3 activity, there is some evidence that each acts uniquely on GSK-3 to block specific substrate phosphorylation [31]. Indeed, our results indicate that β-catenin accumulation by insulin is not mediated by Akt mediated GSK-3 inhibition, but dependent on PI3-kinase and PAK1 (p21-activated kinase 1) [128]. Further work is necessary to understand the complexities of these signaling networks.

3. Genetic models

   Very recently, studies are emerging using genetic techniques, which clearly demonstrate a direct role for insulin signaling in breast and other cancers. Zhang et al. showed that knockdown of IR using shRNA in two cancer cell lines, LCC6 (metastatic cell line derived from MDA-MB-435) and T47D (BC), decreased insulin signaling but not that of IGF1 [152]. Furthermore, cells with IR knockdown formed fewer colonies in anchorage-independent conditions and xenografts manifested reduced growth, angiogenesis, and metastases. These findings were associated with decreased expression of vascular endothelial growth factor-A (VEGF-A), VEGF-D, and hypoxia-inducible factor (HIF-1α). In a mouse model of pancreatic neuroendocrine tumor, insulin receptors were found to be upregulated along with IGF-1 receptors. Responsiveness to IGF-1 inhibitor was enhanced by genetic deletion in the tumors of the IR, a maneuver that even without treatment reduced tumor number and growth and increased apoptosis [135]. In addition, the decreased growth rate of the BC cell line MDA-MB-231, in response to IGF-1R antibody treatment, was enhanced by insulin receptor knockdown using shRNA.

   The importance of insulin signaling in tumor development and progression in a hyperinsulinemic insulin resistant state has also been found in two genetic BC models in mice, the HER2/neu and PyVMT. When crossed with the muscle-specific dominant-negative IGF-1R expressing (MKR) mouse strain, in which both insulin and IGF-1 signaling are abrogated in skeletal muscle resulting in a nonobese, but markedly insulin resistant state, both cancers manifested more rapid growth and progression [103]. Treatment of these insulin resistant cancer-prone mice with a B_3-adrenergic agonist to sensitize the mice to insulin reversed this increase [35].

   Taken together, the data indicate that insulin has significant and multiple direct effects on BC cells and likely, normal precancerous MECs to signal growth and proliferation pathways. Apart from the proliferative signals downstream of the insulin receptor, insulin stimulates augmentation of these signals in response to other stimulators of Tyr kinase, G-protein-coupled and nuclear receptor growth stimulating ligands (Fig. 7.2a).

Indirect Effects of Insulin

Indirect effects of insulin to promote tumor development, growth, and metastasis are also mediated via the insulin receptor. However, in contrast to direct effects on the MECs and BC cells, they result from insulin action on other organs and tissues (Fig. 7.2b).

1. As mentioned earlier, IGF-1 signaling via IGF-1R and/or hybrid IGF-1R/IR is a well established BC cell stimulator. Circulating IGF-1 is bound to binding proteins (IGFBPs), of which multiple forms exist (reviewed in [36]). Thus the amount of "free" or active circulating IGF-1 will depend on both the total IGF-1

synthesized in the liver and the level of IGFBPs. Although the action of some IGFBPs is controversial, e.g., IGFBP-3 may promote growth [65], insulin suppresses the hepatic synthesis and secretion of the inhibitory IGFBP-1 and -2 [110, 115]. At the same time, insulin appears to provide a nutritional signal to augment IGF-1 synthesis, at least in part by upregulating growth hormone (GH) receptors [43]. GH is the major physiological stimulator of hepatic IGF-1 synthesis. In combination, these actions of insulin increase bioavailable IGF-1.

2. A similar phenomenon is mediated by insulin, particularly in the context of hyperinsulinemia and insulin resistance, in the case of estrogen. Estrogen levels are strongly associated with risk and progression of BC and are also bound to circulating sex hormone binding globulin (SHBG) [22, 49]. Synthesis and secretion of SHBG is suppressed by hyperinsulinemia resulting in increased free or bioavailable estrogen [10]. This would contribute to the increased risk of BC associated with obesity.
3. In the context of obesity, insulin promotes adipogenesis and the associated synthesis of multiple adipose tissue associated proteins. One of these is aromatase, an enzyme that converts androgens to estrogens [114]. In obese postmenopausal women, the increased adipose tissue aromatase contributes to higher levels of estrogen [147]. While circulating levels may be increased and are correlated with BMI, it has also been suggested that local mammary gland adipose tissue aromatase activity may be particularly important in elevating local estrogen levels and the risk of BC [10, 22, 114].
4. In addition to aromatase, adipose tissue is a source of several inflammatory proteins, referred to as adipokines [61, 132, 139, 147]. These include TNF-α, IL-1, IL-6, IL-8, MCP-1, leptin, and adiponectin. First, it is interesting that TNF-α, IL-6, and leptin induce aromatase (discussed earlier) [8, 114]. Importantly, inflammation has also been associated with the development of many cancers, likely because of the generation of reactive oxygen species (ROS), which can result in DNA, protein, and lipid oxidation, as well as effects on cell proliferation and apoptosis (reviewed in [10, 17, 112]). Similar to the effect of aromatase and local estrogen production, local mammary gland stromal adipose tissue release of these mediators may be most relevant. The effect of insulin to promote inflammatory signals may depend on the presence of "selective" insulin resistance. Thus, metabolic pathways, e.g., mediated by PI3-kinase, become resistant in the obese state, while stimulation of specific gene expression and protein synthesis, e.g., via MAPK signaling, may remain "inappropriately" elevated. We have recently demonstrated this phenomenon in colon cancer and intestinal epithelial cells [128, 149], but further studies are required.

In terms of leptin, the satiety factor synthesized and secreted by adipocytes, many in vitro studies observed cancer stimulatory growth effects [126]. However, epidemiological studies have not consistently revealed leptin as an independent prognostic factor [48]. In contrast, adiponectin, an insulin sensitizing factor, has been associated with decreased cancer risk [60, 87, 142]. Since adiponectin activates AMP-activated kinase (AMPK) [8, 69], a negative regulator of mTOR, which is an experimental target of BC therapy, there is a plausible protective

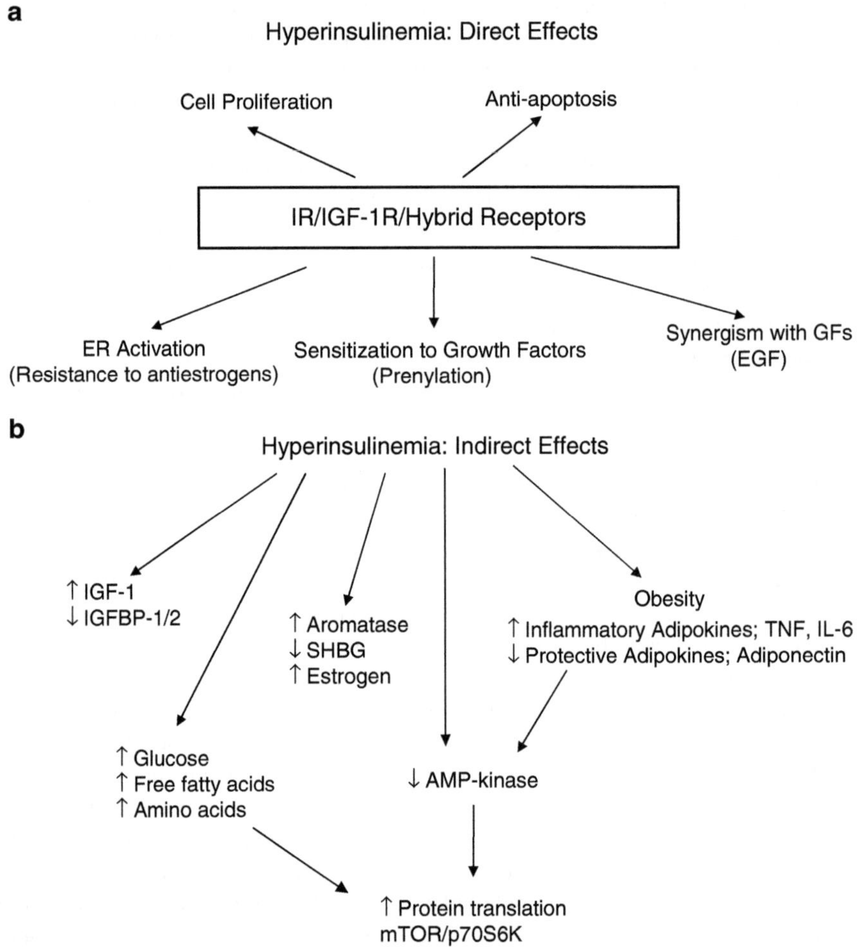

Fig. 7.2 (**a**) Direct effects of insulin which may promote cancer development and progression. Insulin binds to its cognate receptor (IR) as well as, at high concentrations, to the IGF-1 (insulin-like growth factor-1) receptor. In addition, in cancer cells the overexpression of IR and/or IGF-1R leads to the formation of hybrid receptors, which bind all three ligands, insulin, IGF-1, and IGF-II. Signaling via the IR can lead to cell proliferation and inhibition of apoptosis. Stimulation of the (1) Ser/Thr kinases, e.g., Akt/PKB and MAPK, can lead to ER (estrogen receptor) activation, (2) farnesyl and geranylgeranyltransferases to G-protein activation and sensitization to other GFs (growth factors), and (3) kinases, PI3-kinase, Akt/PKB and MAPK to synergism with other GFs such as EGF (epidermal growth factor). (**b**) Indirect effects of insulin which may promote cancer development and progression. The action of insulin on liver and adipose tissue regulates the expression of various genes encoding proteins, which alter growth factors, hormones, and inflammatory mediators. These in turn can influence mammary epithelial cell biology toward a malignant phenotype. Indirect effects mediated in insulin signaling in other tissues and by the metabolic insulin resistant state. Examples include (1) stimulation of IGF-1 and inhibition of IGFBP-1 and -2 synthesis in the liver resulting in elevated free "bioactive" IGF-1; (2) in adipose tissue, an increased expression of aromatase and in liver, suppression of sex hormone binding globulin (SHBG) resulting in elevated circulating levels of estrogen (most significant in postmenopausal women); and (3) by promoting obesity, inflammatory adipokines are synthesized and released by adipose tissue and

effect. There are data suggesting a direct action of adiponectin on cancer cells [30, 141] but further studies are needed to define whether its protective effects are direct or mostly indirect by enhancing metabolic sensitivity to insulin.

5. An area that has been well studied in the context of BC is the role of stromal cells surrounding the tumor and creating a growth supportive extracellular matrix environment (reviewed in [131]). However, the specific actions of insulin and/or IGF-1 on these cells and potential influence on cancer development and progression have not been well characterized. It is likely that insulin/IGF-1 will have stimulatory effects on these cells based on the ubiquitous expression of their receptors and their known actions. Mixed cell culture studies [109] and tissue specific knockout mice as exemplified by the effects of stromal cell PTEN deletion [133] will yield important information on the extent of insulin/IGF-1 actions on stromal cells in their contributions to BC growth and development.

Additional Considerations and Clinical Implications

Hyperinsulinemia, Insulin Therapy, and Cancer

As mentioned earlier and reviewed in Chap. 5, a number of epidemiological studies have linked higher circulating insulin concentrations with BC risk (reviewed in [24]). In studies of subjects with diabetes, elevated risk appears to correlate with the prediabetic insulin resistant/hyperinsulinemic phase consistent with a predominant role of insulin rather than hyperglycemia [84, 85]. Furthermore, subjects with type 2 diabetes treated with insulin and sulfonylureas, which elevate endogenous insulin secretion, had a higher cancer mortality rate than those treated with diet alone or metformin [6, 97]. Thus, exogenous insulin may confer the same increased risk as endogenous insulin. This has important implications for the treatment of diabetes since insulin is a most effective therapy, and excellent glycemic control is known to prevent the long-term complications of diabetes [101]. It is therefore presently not recommended to accept poor glycemic control (higher glucose levels) to avoid using insulin. To complicate matters, several recent studies have examined the risk of cancer in subjects with diabetes using human insulin or different insulin analogues

Fig. 7.2 (continued) adipose-localized macrophages, while the antiinflammatory and antitumor promoting adipokine, adiponectin, is decreased. Insulin resistance, hyperinsulinemia, and the metabolic syndrome are associated with impaired glucose metabolism and elevated levels of circulating fuels; glucose, fatty acids, and amino acids. The high rate of glucose metabolism by cancer cells and epidemiological correlations of increased cancer risk in hyperglycemic individuals [62] suggest that this may contribute. Fatty acids, particularly saturated fats, lead to inflammation via TOLL-like receptor signaling and are associated with tumor promotion. Finally, amino acids are activators of mTOR, a key regulator of protein translation and cell growth and a cancer therapeutic target. mTOR is also regulated (inhibited) by AMP-kinase. AMPK activity is suppressed by both excess fuels and a decrease in adiponectin, an AMPK activator

from large databases. In one report from Germany, the use of insulin glargine, one of the two new long acting, "24 h," insulin analogues, was associated with an increased risk of cancer compared with the use of human insulin [58]. Of interest, this increase was confined to those using insulin glargine alone, but not observed when glargine was used in combination with short-acting insulin. Whether this was due to the use of lower does in the multiple-injection combination insulin users was not clear; however, the effect of glargine itself did appear to be dose-dependent, 10 U (Units) increasing risk by 9% and 50 U by 31%. Another interesting aspect of this observation was the relatively short follow-up time of 3 years. This suggests that any effect, if confirmed (see below), appears to be on tumor growth, i.e., stimulation of the growth of small preexisting undiagnosed cancers. The time course was judged to be too rapid to invoke a tumor promoting effect. Further prospective studies will be required to specifically address this question.

Because of the important potential clinical implications of these findings, several other European countries organized similar studies of existing databases of subjects with diabetes. A Swedish Study found a twofold increased risk of BC in those using glargine alone versus those on other forms of insulin [66]. A study from Scotland found a small, but nonsignificant increased risk, also for BC [23]. In contrast, a UK study did not find any difference in the incidence of any cancers with the use of glargine [25]. The insulin analogue, glargine binds with higher affinity to the IGF-1 receptor than does native human insulin and has greater mitogenic potency on some BC cells in vitro [78, 146]. However, the lack of correlation with cancer in humans in all the studies taken together does not support a firm conclusion of a significant effect of glargine in comparison with other insulins [41, 119, 125]. In contrast, as noted above, the risk of cancer in subjects with type 2 diabetes is highest in those treated with insulin, followed by those on sulfonylureas (insulin secretagogues) and lowest in those on metformin alone [6, 34, 125]. In a more recent larger study of 62,809 patients, the frequency of four solid tumors was high enough for analysis. A significant positive effect was documented for colorectal and pancreatic cancer, but not for breast or prostate cancer for insulin and sulfonylureas compared with metformin [25]. Apart from the observation of the lowest risk of cancer in those treated with metformin, a biguanide that decreases hepatic insulin resistance and circulating levels of insulin and/or insulin requirements, a provocative observation in this study was that adding metformin to insulin therapy decreased the risk of development of cancer by ~50% (hazard ratio 0.54, 95% CI 0.43–0.66) and to sulfonylurea therapy by ~21% [25].

In summary, while cell culture, animal and many epidemiological studies have identified hyperinsulinemia as a risk factor and a stimulatory hormone for BC growth and development, it is important to recognize that these effects are context dependent. Thus, the associated metabolic and hormonal environment as well as tumor characteristics will likely influence the strength of this relationship. It appears, however, that in colon, pancreatic, endometrial and BCs, and perhaps other tumors, insulin has a significant effect. A second important clinical issue is the potential role of metformin, or other "insulin-sensitizing" or "insulin-sparing" agents in the prevention and/or treatment of cancer (see later).

Insulin Sensitization and Cancer

Although a detailed discussion of this topic is beyond the scope of this chapter, as outlined in the epidemiological observations above, and in many in vitro (cell culture) and several rodent studies, there is evidence indicating a beneficial effect of metformin to decrease cancer cell growth and in some cases metastases (reviewed in [42, 125]). These data have led to the initiation of clinical trials of metformin as adjuvant therapy for women with BC [16]. It should be noted that metformin has direct actions on cancer cells since it increases AMPK, which results in an inhibition of mTOR, a Ser/Thr kinase, which controls protein translation and is a recognized chemotherapeutic target [32, 98, 122, 151, 153]. However, whether metformin's action on cancer is related to its insulin lowering effect or direct AMPK action in vivo is not clear. For example, another insulin sensitizing agent, a β_3-adrenergic receptor agonist, used in a nonobese insulin-resistant, hyperinsulinemic model (the MKR mouse) in which BC growth is accelerated, lowered insulin levels and reversed the accelerated cancer growth [35]. Thus, the mechanism(s) of these actions by metformin and other potential agents, and importantly, the predictions of which tumors and/or tumor subtypes, will respond to these agents are critical issues to address in human studies. For example, the insulin-sensitizing anti-diabetic thiazolidinediones have not been associated with lowered cancer risk [96], and one clinical trial in BC has been negative [9]. These agents may in fact promote cancer under certain conditions [120]. Thus, until clinical studies are completed caution is warranted. Our abilities to dissect multiple signaling pathways and analyze tumor gene and protein expression in combination with metabolic and hormonal phenotyping of subjects now make these studies feasible. In the meantime, it is not unreasonable to use metformin in combination with insulin in the treatment of subjects with type 2 diabetes, who require high doses of insulin due to obesity and/or insulin resistance.

Conclusion

The data reviewed in this chapter, comprising cell culture, in vivo rodent models, and human epidemiological studies, together provide a convincing argument for a significant contribution of elevated levels of insulin to the development and growth of some cancers, including BC. Whether this is a graded phenomenon or a threshold effect is not clear. The mechanisms of tumor promotion and tumor growth by insulin may be different but likely overlap. Both direct actions via insulin receptor signaling in mammary gland as well as indirect actions appear to contribute. It is now most important to determine whether lowering circulating insulin levels is of benefit in those with BC (as well as colon and pancreas). These trials will require careful phenotyping of subjects, description of tumor characteristics, and measurement of biomarkers, as it is unlikely that this therapy will benefit all. Drugs such as metformin show promise, but similarly, the patients who will benefit need to be defined. Nevertheless, our increased understanding and appreciation of these apparently adverse effects of insulin raise the potential for more effective targeting of signaling pathways and improved outcomes for women with BC.

Acknowledgments This work was supported by a Translational Acceleration Grant from the CBCRA (Canadian Breast Cancer Research Alliance) and CIHR (Canada Institutes for Health Research) to IGF. (Grant # 016512). SK was supported in part by CBCRA and the Marvelle Koffler Breast Centre, Mount Sinai Hospital.

References

1. Akira S, Uematsu S, Takeuchi O (2006) Pathogen recognition and innate immunity. Cell 124:783–801
2. Alberti KG, Zimmet P, Shaw J, IDF Epidemiology Task Force Consensus (2005) The metabolic syndrome: a new worldwide definition. Lancet 366:1059–1062
3. Belfiore A (2007) The role of insulin receptor isoforms and hybrid insulin/IGF-I receptors in human cancer. Curr Pharm Des 13:671–686
4. Borisov N, Aksamitiene E, Kiyatkin A et al (2009) Systems-level interactions between insulin-EGF networks amplify mitogenic signaling. Mol Syst Biol 5:256. doi:10.1038/msb.2009.19
5. Borugian MJ, Sheps SB, Kim-Sing C et al (2004) Insulin, macronutrient intake, and physical activity: are potential indicators of insulin resistance associated with mortality from breast cancer? Cancer Epidemiol Biomarkers Prev 13:1163–1172
6. Bowker SL, Majumdar SR, Veugelers P et al (2006) Increased cancer-related mortality for patients with type 2 diabetes who use sulfonylureas or insulin. Diabetes Care 29:254–258
7. Brown JR, DuBois RN (2005) Cox-2: a molecular target for colorectal cancer prevention. J Clin Oncol 23:2840–2855
8. Brown KA, Simpson ER (2010) Obesity and breast cancer: progress to understanding the relationship. Cancer Res 70:4–7
9. Burstein HJ, Demetia GD, Mueller E et al (2003) Use of the peroxisome proliferators-activated receptor (PPAR) gamma ligand troglitazone as treatment for refractory breast cancer: a phase II study. Breast Cancer Res Treat 79:391–397
10. Calle EE, Kaaks R (2004) Overweight, obesity, and cancer: epidemiological evidence and proposed mechanisms. Nat Rev Cancer 4:579–591
11. Calle EE, Rodriguez C, Walker-Thurmond K et al (2003) Overweight, obesity, and mortality from cancer in a prospectively studied cohort of U.S. adults. N Engl J Med 348:1625–1638
12. Camirand A, Zakikhani M, Young F et al (2005) Inhibition of insulin-like growth factor-1 receptor signaling enhances growth-inhibitory and proapoptotic effects of gefitinib (Iressa) in human breast cancer cells. Breast Cancer Res 7:R570–R579
13. Carroll KK, Braden LM (1984) Dietary fat and mammary carcinogenesis. Nutr Cancer 6:254–259
14. Carter CA, Milholland RJ, Shea W et al (1983) Effect of the prostaglandin synthetase inhibitor indomethacin on 7,12-dimethylbenz(a)anthracene-induced mammary tumorigenesis in rats fed different levels of fat. Cancer Res 43:3559–3562
15. Casey PJ (1995) Protein lipidation in cell signaling. Science 268:221–225
16. Cazzaniga M, Bonanni B, Guerrieri-Gona A et al (2009) Is it time to test metformin in breast cancer clinical trials? Cancer Epidermiol Biomarkers Prev 18:701–705
17. Cejas P, Casado E, Belda-Iniesta C et al (2004) Implications of oxidative stress and cell membrane lipid peroxidation in human cancer (Spain). Cancer Causes Control 15:707–719

18. Chappell J, Golovchenko I, Wall K et al (2000) Potentiation of Rho-A-mediated lysophosphatidic acid activity by hyperinsulinemia. J Biol Chem 275:31792–31797
19. Chappell J, Leitner JW, Solomon S et al (2001) Effect of insulin on cell cycle progression in MCF-7 breast cancer cells. J Biol Chem 276:38023–38028
20. Cleary MP, Maihle NJ (1997) The role of body mass index in the relative risk of developing premenopausal versus postmenopausal breast cancer. Proc Soc Exp Biol Med 216:28–43
21. Cleary MP, Grande JP, Maihle NJ (2004) Effect of high fat diet on body weight and mammary tumor latency in MMTV-TGF-alpha mice. Int J Obes Relat Metab Disord 28:956–962
22. Clemons M, Goss P (2001) Estrogen and the risk of breast cancer. N Engl J Med 344:276–285
23. Colhoun H, SDRN Epidemiology Group (2009) Use of insulin glargine and cancer incidence in Scotland: a study from the Scottish Diabetes Network Epidemiology Group. Diabetologia 52:1755–1765
24. Cowey S, Hardy RW (2006) The metabolic syndrome: A high-risk state for cancer? Am J Pathol 169:1505–1522
25. Currie CJ, Poole CD, Gale EAM (2009) The influence of glucose-lowering therapies on cancer risk in type 2 diabetes. Diabetologia 52:1766–1777
26. DeBerardinis RJ, Lum JJ, Hatzivassiliou G et al (2008) The biology of cancer: metabolic reprogramming fuels cell growth and proliferation. Cell Metab 7:11–20
27. Del Giudice ME, Fantus IG, Ezzat S et al (1998) Insulin and related factors in premenopausal breast cancer risk. Breast Cancer Res Treat 47:111–120
28. Despres JP (2001) Health consequences of visceral obesity. Ann Med 33:534–541
29. DiCristofanoA PPP (2000) The multiple roles of PTEN in tumor suppression. Cell 100:387–390
30. Dieudonne MD, Bussiere M, Dos Santos E et al (2006) Adiponectin mediates antiproliferative and apoptotic responses in human MCF7 breast cancer cells. Biochem Biophys Res Commun 345:271–279
31. Ding VW, Chen RH, McCormick F (2000) Differential regulation of glycogen synthase kinase 3B by insulin and Wnt signaling. J Biol Chem 275:32475–32481
32. Dowling RJ, Zakikhani M, Fantus IG et al (2007) Metformin inhibits mammalian target of rapamycin-dependent translation initiation in breast cancer cells. Cancer Res 67:10804–10812
33. Eckel RH, Grundy SM, Zimmet PZ (2005) The metabolic syndrome. Lancet 365:1415–1428
34. Evans JM, Donnelly LA, Emslie-Smith AM et al (2005) Metformin and reduced risk of cancer in diabetic patients. BMJ 330:1304–1305
35. Fierz Y, Novosyadlyy R, Vijayakumar A et al (2010) Insulin-sensitizing therapy attenuates type 2 diabetes-mediated mammary tumor progression. Diabetes 59:686–693
36. Firth SM, Baxter RC (2002) Cellular actions of the insulin-like growth factor binding proteins. Endocr Rev 23:824–854
37. Flegal KM, Carroll MD, Ogden CL et al (2010) Prevalence and trends in obesity among US adults, 1999–2008. JAMA 303:235–241
38. Frasca F, Pandini G, Scalia P et al (1999) Insulin receptor isoform A, a newly recognized, high-affinity insulin-like growth factor II receptor in fetal and cancer cells. Mol Cell Biol 19:3278–3288
39. Frittitta L, Cerrato A, Sacco MG et al (1997) The insulin receptor content is increased in breast cancers initiated by three different oncogenes in transgenic mice. Breast Cancer Res Treat 45:141–147
40. Gallagher EJ, LeRoith D (2010) The proliferating role of insulin and insulin-like growth factors in cancer. Trends Endocrinol Metab 21:610–618
41. Gerstein HC (2010) Does insulin therapy promote, reduce or have a neutral effect on cancers. JAMA 303:446–447
42. Giovannucci E, Harlan DM, Archer MC et al (2010) Diabetes and cancer: A consensus report. Diabetes Care 33:1674–1685
43. Giovanucci E (2001) Insulin, insulin-like growth factors and colon cancer: a review of the evidence. J Nutri 131:3109S–3120S

44. Goalstone ML, Leitner JW, Wall K et al (1998) Effect of insulin on farnesyltransferase. Specificity of insulin action and potentiation of nuclear effects of insulin-like growth factor-1, epidermal growth factor, and platelet-derived growth factor. J Biol Chem 273:23892–23896
45. Goalstone ML, Leitner JW, Golovchenko I et al (1999) Insulin promotes phosphorylation and activation of geranyulgeranyltransferase II. J Biol Chem 274:2880–2884
46. Goalstone ML, Leitner JW, Berhanu P et al (2001) Insulin signals to prenyltransferases via the Shc branch of intracellular signaling. J Biol Chem 276:12805–12812
47. Goodwin PJ, Ennis M, Pritchard KI et al (2002) Fasting insulin and outcome in early-stage breast cancer: results of a prospective cohort study. J Clin Oncol 20:42–51
48. Goodwin PJ, Ennis M, Fantus IG et al (2005) Is leptin a mediator of adverse prognostic effects of obesity in breast cancer? J Clin Oncol 23:6037–6042
49. Gruber CJ, Tschugguel W, Schneeberger C et al (2002) Production and actions of estrogens. N Engl J Med 346:340–352
50. Guix M, Faber AC, Wang SE et al (2008) Acquired resistance to EGFR tyrosine kinase inhibitors in cancer cells is mediated by loss of IGF-binding proteins. J Clin Invest 118: 2609–2619
51. Gunter MJ, Hoover DR, Yu H et al (2009) Insulin, insulin-like growth factor-I, and risk of breast cancer in postmenopausal women. J Natl Cancer Inst 101:48–60
52. Guy CT, Cardiff RD, Muller WJ (1992) Induction of mammary tumors by expression of polyomavirus middle T oncogene: a transgenic mouse model for metastatic disease. Mol Cell Biol 12:954–961
53. Hall JM, Couse JF, Korach KS (2001) The multifaceted mechanisms of estradiol and estrogen receptor signaling. J Biol Chem 276:36869–36872
54. Hamelers IHL, Steenbergh PH (2003) Interactions between estrogen and insulin-like growth factor signaling pathways in human breast tumor cells. Endocr Relat Cancer 10:331–345
55. Hardy S, Langelier Y, Prentki M (2000) Oleate activates phosphatidylinositol 3-kinase and promotes proliferation and reduces apoptosis of MDA-MB-231 breast cancer cells, whereas palmitate has opposite effects. Cancer Res 60:6353–6358
56. Hatsell S, Rowlands T, Hiremath M et al (2003) B-catenin and Tcfs in mammary development and cancer. J Mammary Gland Biol Neoplasia 8:145–158
57. Heiden MG, Cantley CC, Thompson CB (2009) Understanding the Warburg effect: the metabolic requirements of cell proliferation. Science 324:1029–1033
58. Hemkens LG, Grouven U, Bender R et al (2009) Risk of malignancies in patients with diabetes treated with human insulin or insulin analogues: a cohort study. Diabetologia 52:1732–1744
59. Hynes NE, Lane HA (2005) ERBB receptors and cancer: the complexity of targeted inhibitors. Nat Rev Cancer 5:341–354
60. Ishikawa M, Kitayaama J, Kazama S et al (2005) Plasma adiponectin and gastric cancer. Clin Cancer Res 11:466–472
61. Iyer A, Fairlie DP, Prins JB et al (2010) Inflammatory lipid mediators in adipocytes function and obesity. Nat Rev Endocrinol 5:71–82
62. Jee SH, Ohrr H, Sull JW et al (2010) Associations of hyperglycemia and insulin usage with the risk of cancer in type 2 diabetes: the Hong Kong Diabetes Registry. Diabetes 59:1254–1260
63. Jiang ZY, Lin YW, Clemont A et al (1999) Characterization of selective resistance to insulin signaling in the vasculative of obese Zucker (fa/fa) rats. J Clin Invest 104:447–457
64. Jin Q, Esteva FJ (2008) Cross-talk between the ErbB/HER family and the type I insulin-like growth factor receptor signaling pathway in breast cancer. J Mammary Gland Biol Neoplasia 13:485–498
65. Jogie-Brahim S, Feldman D, Oh Y (2009) Unraveling insulin-like growth factor binding protein-3 actions in human disease. Endocr Rev 30:417–437
66. Jonasson JM, Ljung R, Talback M et al (2009) Insulin glargine use and short-term incidence of malignancies – a population-based follow-up study in Sweden. Diabetologia 52:1745–1754
67. Jones HE, Goddard L, Gee JM et al (2004) Insulin-like growth factor-I receptor signaling and acquired resistance to gefitinib (ZD1839; Iressa) in human breast and prostate cancer cells. Endocr Relat Cancer 11:793–814

68. Jones HE, Gee JM, Hutchenson IR et al (2006) Growth factor receptor interplay and resistance in cancer. Endocr Relat Cancer 13(Suppl 1):S45–S51
69. Kadowaki T, Yamauchi T (2005) Adiponectin and adiponectin receptors. Endocr Rev 26: 439–451
70. Kalamegham R, Carroll KK (1984) Reversal of the promotional effect of high-fat diet on mammary tumorigenesis by subsequent lowering of dietary fat. Nutr Cancer 6:22–31
71. Karim R, Tse G, Putti T et al (2004) The significance of the Wnt pathway in the pathology of human cancers. Pathology 36:120–128
72. Kato S (2001) Estrogen receptor-mediated cross-talk with growth factor signaling pathways. Breast Cancer 8:3–9
73. Khalid S, Hwang D, Babichev Y et al (2009) Evidence for a tumor promoting effect of high-fat diet independent of insulin resistance in HER2/Neu mammary carcinogenesis. Breast Cancer Res Treat 122:647–659
74. Khasawneh J, Schulz MD, Walch A et al (2009) Inflammation and mitochondrial fatty acid beta-oxidation link obesity to early tumor promotion. Proc Natl Acad Sci USA 106:3354–3359
75. Kim JK (2006) Fat uses a TOLL-road to connect inflammation and diabetes. Cell Metab 4:417–419
76. Kim F, Pham M, Luttrell I et al (2007) Toll-like receptor-4 mediates vascular inflammation and insulin resistance in diet-induced obesity. Circ Res 100:1589–1596
77. Knowlden JM, Jones JE, Barrow D et al (2008) Insulin receptor substrate-1 involvement in epidermal growth factor and insulin-like growth factor receptor signaling: implication for Getitinib (Iressa) response and resistance. Breast Cancer Res Treat 111:79–91
78. Kurtzhals P, Schaffer L, Sorensen A et al (2000) Correlations of receptor binding and metabolic and mitogenic potencies of insulin analogs designed form clinical use. Diabetes 49:999–1005
79. Lawlor DA, Smith GD, Ebrahim S (2004) Hyperinsulinaemia and increased risk of breast cancer: findings from the British Women's Heart and Health Study. Cancer Causes Control 15:267–275
80. Lee MM, Lin SS (2000) Dietary fat and breast cancer. Annu Rev Nutr 20:221–248
81. Li S, Brown MS, Goldstein JL (2010) Bifurcation of insulin signaling pathway in rat liver: mTORC1 required for stimulation of lipogenesis, but not inhibition of gluconeogenesis. Proc Natl Acad Sci USA 23:3281–3282
82. Lin SY, Xia W, Wang TC et al (2000) B-catenin, a novel prognostic marker for breast cancer: its roles in cyclin D1 expression and cancer progression. Proc Natl Acad Sci USA 87:4262–4266
83. Lin EY, Jones JG, Li P et al (2003) Progression to malignancy in the polyoma middle T oncoprotein mouse breast cancer model provides a reliable model for human diseases. Am J Pathol 163:2113–2126
84. Lipscombe LL, Goodwin PJ, Zinman B et al (2006) Increased prevalence of prior breast cancer in women with newly diagnosed diabetes. Breast Cancer Res Treat 98:303–309
85. Lipscombe LL, Goodwin PJ, Zinman B et al (2006) Diabetes mellitus and breast cancer: a retrospective population-based cohort study. Breast Cancer Res Treat 98:349–356
86. Manjer J, Kaaks R, Riboli E et al (2001) Risk of breast cancer in relation to anthropometry, blood pressure, blood lipids and glucose metabolism: a prospective study within the Malmo Preventive Project. Eur J Cancer Prev 10:33–42
87. Mantzoros C, Petridou E, Dessypris N et al (2004) Adiponectin and breast cancer risk. J Clin Endocrinol Metab 89:1102–1107
88. Mathieu MC, Clark GM, Allred DC et al (1997) Insulin receptor expression and clinical outcome in node-negative breast cancer. Proc Assoc Am Physicians 109:565–571
89. Mawson A, Lai A, Carroll JS et al (2005) Estrogen and insulin/IGF/1 cooperatively stimulates cell cycle progression in MCF-7 breast cancer cells through differential regulation of c-cyc and cyclin D1. Mol Cell Endocrinol 729:161–173
90. McCune K et al (2010) Prognosis of hormone-dependent breast cancers: implications of the presence of dysfunctional transcriptional networks activated by insulin via the immune transcription factor T-bet. Cancer Res 70:685–696

91. Menendez JA, Vellon L, Colomer R et al (2005) Oleic acid, the main monounsaturated fatty acid of olive oil, suppresses Her-2/neu (erbB-2) expression and synergistically enhances the growth inhibitory effects of trastuzumab (Herceptin) in breast cancer cells with Her-2/neu oncogene amplification. Ann Oncol 16:359–371
92. Michaelson JS, Leder P (2001) B-catenin is a downstream effector of Wnt-mediated tumorigenesis in the mammary gland. Oncogene 20:5093–5099
93. Michels KB, Solomon CG, Hu FB et al (2003) Type 2 Diabetes and subsequent incidence of breast cancer in the nurses' health study. Diabetes Care 26:1752–1758
94. Milazzo G, Giorgino MG, Damante G et al (1992) Insulin receptor expression and function in human breast cancer cell lines. Cancer Res 52:3924–3930
95. Miyoshi K, Hennighausen L (2003) B-catenin: a transforming actor on many stages. Breast Cancer Res 5:63–68
96. Monami M, Lamanna C, Marchionni N et al (2008) Rosiglitazone and risk of cancer: a meta-analysis of randomized clinical trials. Diabetes Care 31:1455–1460
97. Monami M, Lamanna C, Balzi D et al (2009) Sulphonylureas and cancer: a case-control study. Acta Diabetol 46:279–284
98. Motoshima H, Goldstein BJ, Igata M et al (2006) AMPK and cell proliferation–AMPK as a therapeutic target for atherosclerosis and cancer. J Physiol 574:63–71
99. Mulligan AM, O'Malley FP, Ennis M et al (2007) Insulin receptor is an independent predictor of a favorable outcome in early stage breast cancer. Breast Cancer Res Treat 106:39–47
100. Nahta R, Yuan LX, Zhang B et al (2005) Insulin-like growth factor-I receptor/human epidermal growth factor receptor 2 heterodimerization contributes to trastuzumab resistance of breast cancer cells. Cancer Res 65:11118–11128
101. Nathan DM, Cleary PA, Backlund BJ et al Diabetes Control and Complications Trial/Epidermiology of Diabetes Interventions and Complications (DCCT/EDIC) Study Research Group (2005) Intensive diabetes treatment and cardiovascular disease in patients with type 1 diabetes. N Engl J Med 353:2643–2653
102. Novosyadlyy R, Vijayakumar A, Lann D et al (2009) Physical and functional interaction between polyoma virus middle T antigen and insulin and IGF-I receptors is required for oncogene activation and tumour initiation. Oncogene 28:3477–3486
103. Novosyadlyy R, Lann DE, Vijayakumar A et al (2010) Insulin-mediated acceleration of breast cancer development and progeression in a nonobese model of type 2 diabetes. Cancer Res 70:741–751
104. Olefsky JM, Kolterman OG (1981) Mechanisms of insulin resistance in obesity and noninsulin-dependent (type II) diabetes. Am J Med 70:151–168
105. Osborne CK, Monaco ME, Lippman ME et al (1978) Correlation among insulin binding, degradation, and biological activity in human breast cancer cells in long-term tissue culture. Cancer Res 38:94–102
106. Papa V, Belfiore A (1996) Insulin receptors in breast cancer: biological and clinical role. J Endocrinol Invest 19:324–333
107. Papa V, PezzinoV CA et al (1990) Elevated insulin receptor content in human breast cancer. J Clin Invest 86:1503–1510
108. Park EJ, Lee JH, Yu GY et al (2010) Dietary and genetic obesity promote liver inflammation and tumorigenesis by enhancing Il-6 and TNF expression. Cell 140:197–208
109. Pontiggia O, Rodriguez V, Fabris V et al (2009) Establishment of an in vitro estrogen-dependent mouse mammary tumor model: a new tool to understand estrogen responsiveness and development of tamoxifen resistance in the context of stromal-epithelial interactions. Breast Cancer Res Treat 116:247–255
110. Powell DR, Suwanichkul A, Cubbage ML et al (1991) Insulin inhibits transcription of the human gene for insulin-like growth factor-binding protein-1. J Biol Chem 266:18868–18876
111. Prentice AM, Jebb SA (2003) Fast foods, energy density and obesity: a possible mechanistic link. Obes Rev 4:187–194
112. Rajala MW, Scherer PE (2003) Mini review: The adipocytes at the crossroads of energy homeostasis, inflammation, and atherosclerosis. Endocrinology 144:3765–3773

113. Reaven GM (2004) Insulin resistance and its consequences. In: LeRoith D, Taylor SI (eds) Diabetes mellitus: a fundamental and clinical text. Lippincott, Williams & Wilkins, Philadelphia, pp 899–915
114. Reed MJ, Purohit A (2001) Aromatase regulation and breast cancer. Clin Endocrinol (Oxf) 54:563–571
115. Renehan AG, Frystyk J, Flyvbjerg A (2006) Obesity and cancer risk: the role of the insulin-IGF axis. Trends Endocrinol Metab 17:328–336
116. Ridley AJ (1996) Rho: theme and variations. Curr Biol 6:1256–1264
117. Rose DP, Connolly JM (2000) Regulation of tumor angiogenesis by dietary fatty acids and eicosanoids. Nutr Cancer 37:119–127
118. Rose DP, Hatala MA, Connolly JM et al (1993) Effect of diets containing different levels of linoleic acid on human breast cancer growth and lung metastasis in nude mice. Cancer Res 53:4686–4690
119. Rosenstock J, Fonseca V, McGill JB et al (2009) Similar risk of malignancy with insulin glargine and neutral protamine Hagedorn (NPH) insulin in patients with type 2 diabetes: findings from a 5 year randomized, open-label study. Diabetologia 52:1971–1973
120. Rubenstrunk A, Hanf R, Hum DW et al (2007) Safety issues and prospects for future generations of PPAR modulators. Biochim Biophys Acta 1771:1065–1081
121. Shao D, Lazar MA (1999) Modulating nuclear receptor function: may the phos be with you. J Clin Invest 103:1617–1618
122. Shaw RJ, Lamia KA, Vasquez D et al (2005) The kinase LKB1 mediates glucose homeostasis in liver and therapeutic effects of metformin. Science 310:1642–1646
123. Shi H, Kokoeva V, Inouye K et al (2006) TLR4 links innate immunity and fatty acid-induced insulin resistance. J Clin Invest 116:3015–3025
124. Sinagra D, Amato C, Scarpilta AM et al (2002) Metabolic syndrome and breast cancer risk. Eur Rev Med Pharmacol Sci 6:55–59
125. Smith U, Gale EAM (2009) Does diabetes therapy influence the risk of cancer? Diabetologia 52:1699–1708
126. Somasundar P, McFadden DW, Hileman SM et al (2004) Leptin as a growth factor in cancer. J Surg Res 116:337–349
127. Stambolic V, Suzuki A, de la Pompa JL et al (1998) Negative regulation of PKB/Akt-dependent cell survival by the tumor suppressor PTEN. Cell 95:29–39
128. Sun J, Khalid S, Rozakis-Adcock M et al (2009) p-21 activated protein kinase-1 function as a linker between insulin and Wnt signaling pathways in the intestine. Oncogene 28:3132–3144
129. Taniguchi CM, Emanuelli B, Kahn CR (2006) Critical nodes in signaling pathways: insights into insulin action. Nat Rev Mol Cell Biol 7:85–96
130. Thompson JE, Thompson CB (2004) Putting the rap on Akt. J Clin Oncol 22:4217–4226
131. Tlsty TD, Coussens LM (2006) Tumor stroma and regulation of cancer development. Annu Rev Pathol 1:119–150
132. Trayhum P, Woods IS (2004) Adipokines: inflammation and the pleiotropic role of white adipose tissue. Br J Nutr 92:347–355
133. Trimboli AJ, Cantemir-Stone CZ, Li F et al (2009) PTEN in stromal fibroblasts suppresses mammary epithelial tumours. Nature 461:1084–1091
134. Uauy R, Diaz E (2005) Consequences of food energy excess and positive energy balance. Public Health Nutr 8:1077–1099
135. Ulanet DB, Ludwig DL, Kahn CR et al (2009) Insulin receptor functionally enhances multistage tumor progression and conveys instrinsic resistance to IGF-R targeted therapy. Proc Natl Acad Sci USA 107:10791–10798
136. Verheus M, Peeters PH, Rinaldi S et al (2006) Serum C-peptide levels and breast cancer risk: results from the European Prospective Investigation into Cancer and Nutrition (EPIC). Int J Cancer 119:659–667
137. Vigneri P, Frasca F, Sciacca L et al (2009) Diabetes and Cancer. Endocr Relat Cancer 16:1103–1123

138. Virkamaki A, Ueki K, Kahn CR (1999) Protein-protein interaction in insulin signaling and the molecular mechanisms of insulin resistance. J Clin Invest 103:931–943
139. Vona-Davis L, Rose DP (2007) Adipokines as endocrine, paracrine, and autocrine factors in breast cancer risk and progression. Endocr Relat Cancer 14:189–206
140. Wang D, Patel S, Li W et al (2002) Activation of the TGF-alpha autocrine loop in downstream of IGF-1 receptor activation during mitogenesis in growth factor dependent human colon carcinoma cells. Oncogene 21:2785–2796
141. Wang Y, Lam JB, Lam KSL et al (2006) Adiponectin modulates the glycogen synthase kinase-3beta/beta-catenin signaling pathway and attenuates mammary tumorigenesis of MDA-MB-231 cells in nude mice. Cancer Res 66:11462–11470
142. Wang Y, Lam KS, Xu A (2007) Adiponectin as a negative regulator in obesity-related mammary carcinogenesis. Cell Res 17:280–282
143. WCRF/AICR. Food, nutrition, physical activity, and the prevention of cancer: a global perspective (report online). World Cancer Research Fund, American Institute for Cancer Research, London. http://www.dietandcancerreport.org
144. Wei M, Gaskill SP, Haffner SM et al (1997) Waist circumference as the best predictor of noninsulin dependent diabetes mellitus (NIDDM) compared to body mass index, waist/hip ratio and other anthropometric measurements in Mexican Americans – a 7-year prospective study. Obes Res 5:16–23
145. Weiderpass E, Gridley G, Persson I et al (1997) Risk of endometrial and breast cancer in patients with diabetes mellitus. Int J Cancer 71:360–363
146. Weinstein D, Simon M, Yehezkel E et al (2009) Insulin analogues display IGFD-1-like mitogenic and anti-apoptotic activities in cultured cancer cells. Diabetes Metab Res Rev 25:41–49
147. Wellen KE, Hotamisligil GS (2003) Obesity-induced inflammatory changes in adipose tissue. J Clin Invest 112:1785–1788
148. Yee D, Lee AV (2000) Crosstalk between the insulin-like growth factors and estrogens in breast cancer. J Mammary Gland Biol Neoplasia 5:107–115
149. Yi F, Sun J, Lim GE et al (2008) Crosst6alk between the insulin and Wnt signaling pathways: evidence from intestinal endocrine L cells. Endocrinology 149:2341–2351
150. Yu H, Pardoll D, Jove R (2009) Stats in cancer inflammation and immunity: a leading role for STAT3. Nat Rev Cancer 9:798–809
151. Zakikhani M, Dowling R, Fantus IG et al (2006) Metformin is an AMP kinase-dependent growth inhibitor for breast cancer cells. Cancer Res 66:10269–10273
152. Zhang H, Fagan DH, Zeng X et al (2010) Inhibition of cancer cell proliferation and metastasis by insulin receptor downregulation. Oncogene 29:2517l–2527l
153. Zhou G, Myers R, Li Y et al (2001) Role of AMP-activated protein kinase in mechanism of metformin action. J Clin Invest 108:1167–1174
154. Zhuang Y, Miskimins WK (2008) Cell cycle arrest in metformin treated breast cancer cells involves activation of AMPK, downregulation of cyclin D1, and requires p27Kip1 or p21Cip1. J Mol Signal 3:18. doi:10.1186/1750-2187-3-18
155. Zielinski R, Przytycki PF, Zheng J et al (2009) The crosstalk between EGF, IGF, and Insulin cell signaling pathways – computational and experimental analysis. BMC Syst Biol 3:88. doi:10.1186/1752-0509-3-88

Chapter 8
Actions of Insulin As a Survival and Growth Factor: Akt, mTOR, and Regulation of Translation*

Luc Furic, Mark Livingstone, Ivan Topisirovic, and Nahum Sonenberg

Binding of insulin to the insulin receptor (IR) stimulates the receptor's tyrosine kinase activity. IR activation leads to the recruitment of key activators of downstream pathways via the insulin receptor substrate (IRS) proteins. In a similar fashion, the insulin growth factor-1 receptor (IGF1R) transduces signals to downstream effectors via the PI3K and MAPK pathways.

Insulin-Induced Survival Signals: Akt

Three *Akt* genes exist in mammals (*Akt1*, *Akt2*, and *Akt3*), the products of which appear to be subject to similar posttranslational regulatory mechanisms, despite differential phenotypic consequences of single and double *Akt* gene knockout in mice [1, 2]. Insulin binding to its receptor results in potent activation of the PI3K signaling pathway (Fig. 8.1), promoting Akt activity via phosphorylation on Thr308 by phosphoinositide-dependent kinase-1 (PDK1) and recruitment to the plasma membrane via an amino terminal pleckstrin homology (PH) domain. Full activation of Akt requires additional phosphorylation at Ser473 by the mTOR complex 2 (see later) [3], which is activated in response to insulin by yet-to-be elucidated mechanisms, although recent observations point to an involvement of PI3K or PKCα [4, 5]. mTORC2-dependent phosphorylation of Akt on Ser473 affects only a subset of Akt substrates in vivo, including FoxO1/3a, whereas it does not affect the phosphorylation status of TSC2 [6]. Accordingly, Ser473 phosphorylation of Akt is necessary for the prosurvival role of mTORC2, but is dispensable for Akt-dependent activation of mTORC1 [6].

*The authors Luc Furic and Mark Livingstone contributed equally to this chapter.

N. Sonenberg (✉)
Department of Biochemistry and Goodman Cancer Centre, McGill University, 1160 Avenue des Pins Ouest, Montréal, Québec, Canada H3A 1A3
e-mail: Nahum.Sonenberg@mcgill.ca

I.G. Fantus (ed.), *Insulin Resistance and Cancer: Epidemiology, Cellular and Molecular Mechanisms and Clinical Implications*, Energy Balance and Cancer 1, DOI 10.1007/978-1-4419-9911-5_8, © Springer Science+Business Media, LLC 2011

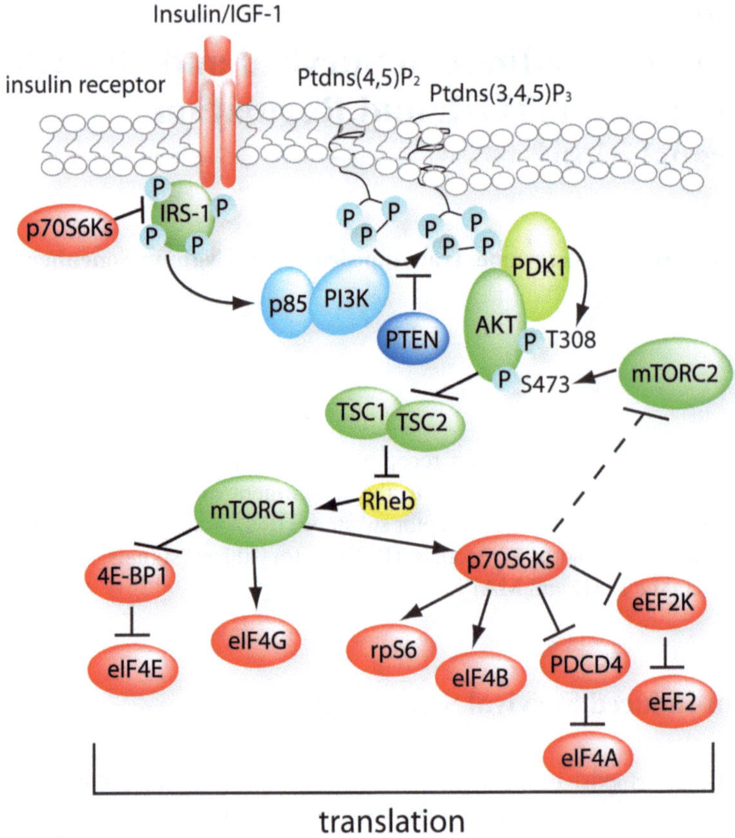

Fig. 8.1 Insulin activates the PI3K signaling pathway. The activated insulin receptor phosphorylates IRS-1, which in turn recruits and activates the PI3K. Following synthesis of phosphatidylinositol-(3,4,5)-triphosphate, Akt and PDK1 are recruited at the plasma membrane via their PH domain. Activation of Akt leads to the inhibition of the tuberous sclerosis complex (TSC1/TSC2), derepression of Rheb, and activation of mTORC1 and its downstream effectors. See text for details

The initial discoveries linking Akt activity to survival [7–9] have been followed up by the identification of a myriad of effectors, which together promote a concerted wave of prosurvival responses (Fig. 8.2). Downstream targets of Akt comprise canonical regulators of cell survival, which are involved in the acute response to proapototic stimuli, as well as the transcription factors and posttranscriptional regulators, which modulate gene expression to establish sustained survival responses [10].

mTOR

mTOR is the mammalian target of rapamycin. Mammals possess a single TOR gene when compared with two genes present in yeast (TOR1 and TOR2). Nonetheless, as in yeast there are two distinct mTOR protein complexes in mammals, named

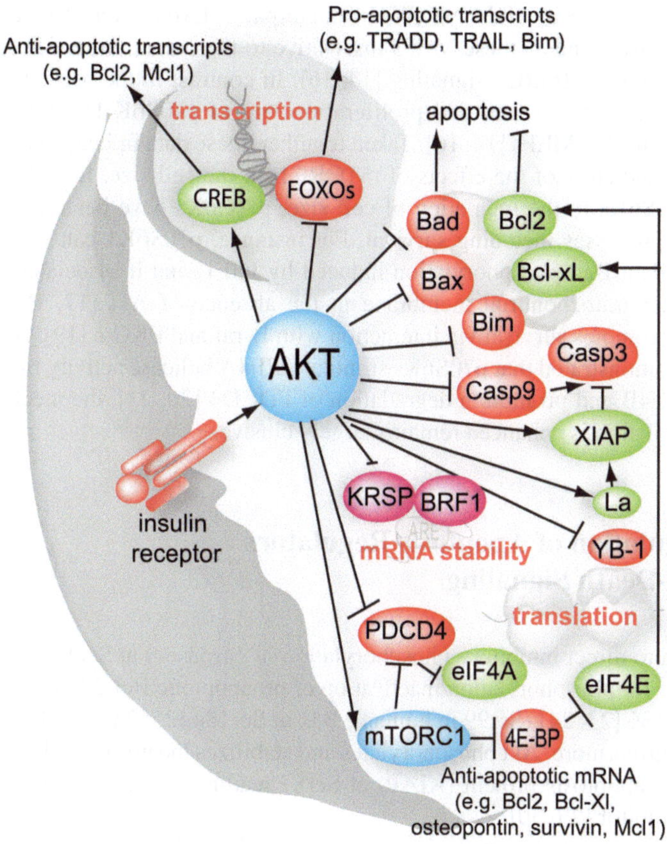

Fig. 8.2 Prosurvival signaling mediated by Akt. See text for details

mTORC1 and mTORC2. mTORC1 is the rapamycin sensitive complex. The two best known targets of mTORC1 are p70S6 kinase (p70S6K) and the eukaryotic translation initiation factor 4E (eIF4E) binding proteins (4E-BPs). 4E-BP1 was first identified as PHAS-I (phosphorylated heat- and acid-stable protein regulated by insulin), whose phosphorylation is induced by insulin treatment [11].

p70S6K has multiple reported substrates, including ribosomal protein S6 (rpS6), eukaryotic translation initiation factor 4B (eIF4B), programmed cell death protein 4 (PDCD4), eukaryotic translation elongation factor 2 kinase (eEF2K), cap-binding protein 80 kDa (CBP80), S6K1 Aly/REF-like substrate (SKAR), IRS1, mTOR, Bcl-2-associated death promoter (BAD), mouse double minute 2 (MDM2), and cAMP response element-binding (CREB) [12]. The link between p70S6K and growth was clearly demonstrated using genetically engineered animals. p70S6K1 knock-out (KO) mice are leaner and smaller and this phenotype is not due to a decreased number of cells but rather the consequence of smaller size cells [13]. p70S6K1/p70S6K2 double KO (DKO) murine embryonic fibroblasts (MEFs) and myoblasts are smaller than their wild-type (WT) counterparts. Expression of constitutively active p70S6K1 renders these MEFs insensitive to the reduction in size caused by the inhibition of mTORC1 signaling [14–16]. In contrast to the reduction in their size, cell cycle progression and proliferation rate of p70S6K DKO MEFs were comparable to WT MEFs [14, 16]. Taken together, these data indicate that p70S6Ks are major mediators of the effects of mTORC1 on the cell size. In addition to the role of p70S6Ks in the regulation of cell size, p70S6Ks have been implicated in numerous processes including survival. For instance, p70S6K1 can substitute for Akt-dependent Bad phosphorylation induced by IGF1, and it associates with Bad on the outer mitochondrial membrane in the absence of Akt [17, 18]. In turn, p70S6K2 promotes survival via interaction with B-raf and PKC-ε [19]. Although it has been demonstrated that p70S6Ks stimulate eIF4A helicase activity by phosphorylating eIF4B and promoting degradation of PDCD4 [20, 21], the mechanism by which translation is enhanced remains largely elusive.

Akt Regulation of Apoptosis Regulators and Pro-Death Signaling

In addition to direct inhibitory phosphorylation of caspase-9 at Ser196 [22], Akt is responsible for phosphorylation/inactivation of proapoptotic Bcl-2 family members: Bad at Ser136 [23, 24] (Ser99 in human), Bax at Ser184 [25, 26], and Bim at Ser87 [27, 28]. Furthermore, Akt phosphorylates and stabilizes the mitochondrial X-linked inhibitor of apoptosis protein (XIAP) at Ser87 leading to increased levels of this caspase inhibitor [29, 30].

Not all acutely acting apoptosis regulators, which are directly phosphorylated by Akt, are associated with control of mitochondrial (intrinsic pathway) apoptosis, however. Acinus phosphorylation at Ser1180, for example, prevents apoptosis-induced chromatin condensation, which together with fragmentation is among the key criteria in the identification of apoptotic cells [31]. Similarly, pro-death signaling transduction pathways, each with multiple effector substrates, are often antagonized by insulin-induced Akt signaling. Examples of this phenomenon include the G2/M cell cycle checkpoint inducing kinase Chk1 (Ser280) [32, 33] and both ASK1 (Ser83) [34] and MLK3 (Ser674): upstream activators of SAPK/JNK [35]. Akt also phosphorylates members of the Forkhead box transcription factor, class O family (FOXO1 and 3A) resulting in their relocalization to the cytoplasm. This reduces the ability of FOXO1 and 3A to transcriptionally activate the expression of apoptosis-promoting genes [36–38].

Insulin-stimulated activation of Akt also leads to the phosphorylation of glycogen synthase kinase-3 (GSK-3) (Ser21: α isoform and Ser9: β-isoform) and its inhibition. GSK-3 is a known regulator of glycogen synthesis in major insulin-responsive tissues [39]. GSK-3 itself elicits multiple signals promoting proapoptotic transcription, mitochondrial proapoptotic signals, and structural proapoptotic rearrangements (reviewed in [40]). GSK-3 phosphorylation of β-catenin leads to the degradation of this crucial regulator of cell fate, including that of pancreatic β-cells (reviewed in [41]). Similarly, GSK-3β interacts with p53 in the nucleus and promotes p53-dependent apoptosis [42–44]. Nonetheless, in contrast to its proapoptotic activity, it has been reported that GSK-3β exerts a prosurvival role by stimulating the activity of NFκB and consequently inhibiting TNF-induced apoptosis [45].

Akt Regulation of mRNA Translation Via mTOR-Dependent Signaling Pathways to Promote Survival

While Akt signaling controls cell survival via direct regulation of canonical apoptosis regulators and engenders a sustained survival environment by activating the transcription of the mRNA encoding these proteins, this important insulin-activated signaling protein also regulates translation. Insulin-activated Akt primarily enhances the translation of a subset of mRNAs via mTOR activation. This essential, evolutionarily-conserved (yeast to man), Ser/Thr protein kinase integrates inputs from ATP availability, amino acid abundance, oxygen status, and growth factor/IR activation to control cell proliferation, growth, survival, and metabolism.

The mTOR-dependent control of cell survival via regulation of mRNA translation occurs primarily through controlling the availability of eIF4E, which binds the 5′ cap of cellular mRNAs to facilitate their translation. eIF4E is the limiting component of the eIF4F complex. This complex also contains eIF4A (an ATP-dependent helicase) and eIF4G (a large adaptor protein), which serves as a docking scaffold for the other proteins. eIF4F is directed to the 5′ end of the mRNA via eIF4E, and acts through eIF4A (along with eIF4B and eIF4H) to unwind the mRNA 5′ secondary structure to facilitate ribosome binding [46]. mTORC1 modulates the availability and thus the activity of eIF4E by phosphorylation of the eIF4E-binding proteins (4E-BP1, 4E-BP2, and 4E-BP3), which prevent the binding of eIF4E to eIF4G and thus the assembly of the eIF4F preinitiation complex. The mTOR-dependent phosphorylation and inactivation of 4E-BP1 in response to insulin has been well characterized and occurs in a hierarchical manner wherein phosphorylation at Thr37 and Thr46 is required for subsequent phosphorylation at Thr70 and Ser65, thus dissociating it from eIF4E [47].

eIF4E controls cell survival as overexpression of eIF4E rescues MEFs from Myc-induced apoptosis [48]. In addition, eIF4E overexpression inhibits apoptosis induced by the mTOR inhibitor rapamycin in combination with doxorubicin in a murine lymphoma chemoresistance model [49, 50]. Inhibition of eIF4E activity by expressing a constitutively active nonphosphorylable mutant of 4E-BP1 or by using antisense RNA induces apoptosis in fibroblasts and HeLa cells, respectively [51, 52]. Furthermore, rapid apoptosis is induced by cell permeable peptides or small molecules that mimic the inhibitory binding of 4E-BP1 to eIF4E [53, 54]. Finally, antisense oligonucleotides used to knockdown eIF4E induce apoptosis in human tissue culture and xenograft models [55].

Overexpression of eIF4E does not result in uniform increase in translation. It rather leads to a selective upregulation of translation efficiencies of a subset of mRNAs, which are referred to as "eIF4E-sensitive." Since all nuclear transcribed eukaryotic mRNAs carry an mRNA 5′ cap, other features determine whether a particular mRNA is "eIF4E-sensitive" [56]. mRNAs with extensive 5′ UTR secondary structures have a higher demand for the unwinding activity of the eIF4F complex for efficient translation. Because eIF4E is the most limiting factor for the assembly of the eIF4F complex, mRNAs with excessive secondary structure critically depend on its availability. For example, the mRNAs of Bcl-Xl, survivin, Mcl-1, ODC, cyclins, and VEGF comprising long and complex 5′ UTRs are highly dependent on eIF4E for efficient translation and as such can be induced by insulin signaling (reviewed in [57]). In contrast, translation of mRNAs encoding housekeeping proteins (e.g., actin, GAPDH) which have short, unstructured 5′ UTRs does not tightly rely on eIF4E levels. By modulating the activity of eIF4E, 4E-BPs preferentially regulate translation of proliferation- and survival-promoting mRNAs, which at the cellular level is illustrated by the finding that 4E-BPs act as critical effectors of mTORC1 signaling to cell proliferation [14].

Akt Regulation of mRNA Translation Via mTOR-Independent Signaling Pathways to Regulate Survival

Acute inhibition of Akt signaling results in translation inhibition, although not having a major impact on the transcriptional activity in the cell [58]. The major effects of Akt on the regulation of mRNA translation appear to be mediated downstream via mTORC1. However, it was suggested that Akt can control translation of mRNAs encoding prosurvival factors independently of mTORC1. The lupus autoantigen (La) RNA binding protein is a known regulator of XIAP [59] and BiP [60] mRNA translation and is phosphorylated on Thr301 by Akt; an event that controls nuclear export of multiple mRNAs and recruitment of La to polysomes [61]. Similarly, YB-1 Ser102 phosphorylation by Akt blocks its ability to bind to many progrowth mRNAs, thus freeing them for eIF4E-mediated cap-dependent translation [62]. Programmed cell death 4 (Pdcd4), a known suppressor of eIF4A activity, in addition to its phosphorylation via the mTORC1/S6K pathway (see later) is phosphorylated by Akt at Ser67 and Ser457, causing nuclear translocation [63]. Mutation of Ser457, however, does not alter the Pdcd4/eIF4A interaction [64]. Another mRNA binding protein, BRF1, specifically binds targets with AU-rich elements (AREs) for mRNA decay, and Akt phosphorylation on Ser92 and Ser203 inhibits BRF1 mRNA decay activity by causing binding to 14-3-3 proteins [65]. Moreover, β-catenin (discussed earlier) mRNA stability is itself regulated by Akt phosphorylation of KSRP at Ser193 [66]. These findings were further corroborated by a recent study, which demonstrates that the inhibition of the PI3K-pathway decreases the stability of a multitude of transcripts, largely in a BRF1- and KSRP-dependent manner [67]. Additional Akt substrates that directly bind mRNA are likely numerous and include the calcium regulated heat stable protein 1 (CaRHSP1), identified as an Akt substrate in liver extracts [68], although the importance of this site (Ser52) remains to be elucidated.

eIF2

eIF2 is a trimeric protein consisting of α, β, and γ subunits, which when bound to GTP transfers the methionine-tRNA to the 40S ribosome to form the 43S ribosome complex. GTP hydrolysis leads to the release of eIF2-GDP, which is recycled to eIF2-GTP by the guanine nucleotide exchange factor, eIF2B [69]. Phosphorylation of eIF2α at Ser51 results in translation inhibition as phosphorylated eIF2α fails to release eIF2B upon nucleotide exchange, thus preventing further activity [70]. Paradoxically, eIF2α promotes translation of a subset of mRNAs, which contain upstream open reading frames, including the apoptosis regulator ATF-4 [71], in response to various stimuli. Four kinases heme-regulated inhibitor kinase (HRI), protein kinase R (PKR), protein kinase RNA-like endoplasmic reticulum kinase (PERK), and general control nonrepressed 2 (GCN2) phosphorylate Ser51 in response to heme-deficiency, double-stranded mRNA, endoplasmic reticulum stress, or amino acid deficiency, respectively. Although insulin fails to modulate eIF2α phosphorylation itself, there exists strong genetic evidence implicating this pathway in insulin-related disease. For example, loss-of-function mutations of the eIF2α kinase PERK in humans causes early onset diabetes [72], and genetically modified mice carrying homozygous Ser51Ala mutation die shortly after birth due to glucose homeostasis problems [73].

The GEF activity of eIF2B is negatively regulated by phosphorylation of its ε subunit by GSK-3 [74]. Under normal conditions, glycogen synthase kinase 3 (GSK-3) phosphorylates eIF2Bε on Ser^{540} [75]. Activated Akt phosphorylates and inactivates GSK-3 [76], thereby relieving the inhibitory effect of eIF2Bε phosphorylation on the rate of translation initiation. It has been reported that in tumor growth conditions in cells lacking the mTOR regulator, TSC2, a feedback loop that exist to attenuate Akt signaling is inefficient in inhibiting GSK-3 phosphorylation. This is explained by the fact that under these conditions GSK-3 is a direct substrate of S6K [77]. Specific inhibitors of GSK3 activity have revealed, however, that Ser540 dephosphorylation alone is insufficient to activate eIF2B [78], suggesting that other modifications on eIF2Bε and/or on other subunits are required.

Insulin and Elongation Factor eEF2K

Insulin not only impacts the rate of translation initiation, but also regulates translation elongation via the control of eEF2K activity. Insulin stimulates the dephosphorylation of eEF2 at Thr56 and the inhibitory phosphorylation of eEF2 kinase at Ser366, both events stimulating the rate of translation elongation [79, 80].

Conclusion

Insulin signaling to the PI3K pathway is of paramount importance for survival and growth. The IGF receptor relies mainly on the PI3K pathway to transduce its signal. Upon activation, Akt phosphorylates a bevy of effector substrates to promote survival and growth. The understanding of the concerted stimulation and inhibition of multiple cellular pathways by insulin is important for better treatment of pathologies, including cancers, diabetes, and obesity. Elucidating the mechanisms responsible for the regulation of the activity of multiple proteins involved in insulin signaling is an active field of research.

Acknowledgments This work was funded by Canadian Cancer Society grant 016208 to NS. LF is a Research Fellow of The Terry Fox Foundation through an award from the National Cancer Institute of Canada (Award #019676) and also received support from the USARMY PCRP Award#W81XWH-10-1-0357. M.L. is a Research Student of the Terry Fox Foundation (Award #700029).

References

1. Dummler B, Tschopp O, Hynx D, Yang ZZ, Dirnhofer S, Hemmings BA (2006) Life with a single isoform of Akt: mice lacking Akt2 and Akt3 are viable but display impaired glucose homeostasis and growth deficiencies. Mol Cell Biol 26:8042–8051
2. Yang ZZ, Tschopp O, Di-Poi N, Bruder E, Baudry A, Dummler B, Wahli W, Hemmings BA (2005) Dosage-dependent effects of Akt1/protein kinase Balpha (PKBalpha) and Akt3/PKBgamma on thymus, skin, and cardiovascular and nervous system development in mice. Mol Cell Biol 25:10407–10418
3. Sarbassov DD, Guertin DA, Ali SM, Sabatini DM (2005) Phosphorylation and regulation of Akt/PKB by the rictor-mTOR complex. Science 307:1098–1101
4. Cybulski N, Hall MN (2009) TOR complex 2: a signaling pathway of its own. Trends Biochem Sci 34:620–627
5. Partovian C, Ju R, Zhuang ZW, Martin KA, Simons M (2008) Syndecan-4 regulates subcellular localization of mTOR Complex2 and Akt activation in a PKCalpha-dependent manner in endothelial cells. Mol Cell 32:140–149
6. Jacinto E, Facchinetti V, Liu D, Soto N, Wei S, Jung SY, Huang Q, Qin J, Su B (2006) SIN1/MIP1 maintains rictor-mTOR complex integrity and regulates Akt phosphorylation and substrate specificity. Cell 127:125–137
7. Dudek H, Datta SR, Franke TF, Birnbaum MJ, Yao R, Cooper GM, Segal RA, Kaplan DR, Greenberg ME (1997) Regulation of neuronal survival by the serine-threonine protein kinase Akt. Science 275:661–665
8. Kauffmann-Zeh A, Rodriguez-Viciana P, Ulrich E, Gilbert C, Coffer P, Downward J, Evan G (1997) Suppression of c-Myc-induced apoptosis by Ras signalling through PI(3)K and PKB. Nature 385:544–548
9. Kennedy SG, Wagner AJ, Conzen SD, Jordan J, Bellacosa A, Tsichlis PN, Hay N (1997) The PI 3-kinase/Akt signaling pathway delivers an anti-apoptotic signal. Genes Dev 11:701–713
10. Bellacosa A, Kumar CC, Di Cristofano A, Testa JR (2005) Activation of AKT kinases in cancer: implications for therapeutic targeting. Adv Cancer Res 94:29–86
11. Hu C, Pang S, Kong X, Velleca M, Lawrence JC Jr (1994) Molecular cloning and tissue distribution of PHAS-I, an intracellular target for insulin and growth factors. Proc Natl Acad Sci U S A 91:3730–3734

12. Jastrzebski K, Hannan KM, Tchoubrieva EB, Hannan RD, Pearson RB (2007) Coordinate regulation of ribosome biogenesis and function by the ribosomal protein S6 kinase, a key mediator of mTOR function. Growth Factors 25:209–226
13. Pende M, Kozma SC, Jaquet M, Oorschot V, Burcelin R, Le Marchand-Brustel Y, Klumperman J, Thorens B, Thomas G (2000) Hypoinsulinaemia, glucose intolerance and diminished beta-cell size in S6K1-deficient mice. Nature 408:994–997
14. Dowling RJ, Topisirovic I, Alain T, Bidinosti M, Fonseca BD, Petroulakis E, Wang X, Larsson O, Selvaraj A, Liu Y, Kozma SC, Thomas G, Sonenberg N (2010) mTORC1-mediated cell proliferation, but not cell growth, controlled by the 4E-BPs. Science 328:1172–1176
15. Ohanna M, Sobering AK, Lapointe T, Lorenzo L, Praud C, Petroulakis E, Sonenberg N, Kelly PA, Sotiropoulos A, Pende M (2005) Atrophy of S6K1(–/–) skeletal muscle cells reveals distinct mTOR effectors for cell cycle and size control. Nat Cell Biol 7:286–294
16. Pende M, Um SH, Mieulet V, Sticker M, Goss VL, Mestan J, Mueller M, Fumagalli S, Kozma SC, Thomas G (2004) S6K1(–/–)/S6K2(–/–) mice exhibit perinatal lethality and rapamycin-sensitive 5′-terminal oligopyrimidine mRNA translation and reveal a mitogen-activated protein kinase-dependent S6 kinase pathway. Mol Cell Biol 24:3112–3124
17. Harada H, Andersen JS, Mann M, Terada N, Korsmeyer SJ (2001) p70S6 kinase signals cell survival as well as growth, inactivating the pro-apoptotic molecule BAD. Proc Natl Acad Sci U S A 98:9666–9670
18. Liu S, Okada T, Assmann A, Soto J, Liew CW, Bugger H, Shirihai OS, Abel ED, Kulkarni RN (2009) Insulin signaling regulates mitochondrial function in pancreatic beta-cells. PLoS ONE 4:e7983
19. Pardo OE, Wellbrock C, Khanzada UK, Aubert M, Arozarena I, Davidson S, Bowen F, Parker PJ, Filonenko VV, Gout IT, Sebire N, Marais R, Downward J, Seckl MJ (2006) FGF-2 protects small cell lung cancer cells from apoptosis through a complex involving PKCepsilon, B-Raf and S6K2. EMBO J 25:3078–3088
20. Dorrello NV, Peschiaroli A, Guardavaccaro D, Colburn NH, Sherman NE, Pagano M (2006) S6K1- and betaTRCP-mediated degradation of PDCD4 promotes protein translation and cell growth. Science 314:467–471
21. Raught B, Peiretti F, Gingras AC, Livingstone M, Shahbazian D, Mayeur GL, Polakiewicz RD, Sonenberg N, Hershey JW (2004) Phosphorylation of eucaryotic translation initiation factor 4B Ser422 is modulated by S6 kinases. EMBO J 23:1761–1769
22. Cardone MH, Roy N, Stennicke HR, Salvesen GS, Franke TF, Stanbridge E, Frisch S, Reed JC (1998) Regulation of cell death protease caspase-9 by phosphorylation. Science 282:1318–1321
23. Datta SR, Dudek H, Tao X, Masters S, Fu H, Gotoh Y, Greenberg ME (1997) Akt phosphorylation of BAD couples survival signals to the cell-intrinsic death machinery. Cell 91:231–241
24. del Peso L, Gonzalez-Garcia M, Page C, Herrera R, Nunez G (1997) Interleukin-3-induced phosphorylation of BAD through the protein kinase Akt. Science 278:687–689
25. Adams JM, Cory S (2007) The Bcl-2 apoptotic switch in cancer development and therapy. Oncogene 26:1324–1337
26. Gardai SJ, Hildeman DA, Frankel SK, Whitlock BB, Frasch SC, Borregaard N, Marrack P, Bratton DL, Henson PM (2004) Phosphorylation of Bax Ser184 by Akt regulates its activity and apoptosis in neutrophils. J Biol Chem 279:21085–21095
27. Grant S (2008) Cotargeting survival signaling pathways in cancer. J Clin Invest 118:3003–3006
28. Qi XJ, Wildey GM, Howe PH (2006) Evidence that Ser87 of BimEL is phosphorylated by Akt and regulates BimEL apoptotic function. J Biol Chem 281:813–823
29. Dan HC, Sun M, Kaneko S, Feldman RI, Nicosia SV, Wang HG, Tsang BK, Cheng JQ (2004) Akt phosphorylation and stabilization of X-linked inhibitor of apoptosis protein (XIAP). J Biol Chem 279:5405–5412
30. Fesik SW (2005) Promoting apoptosis as a strategy for cancer drug discovery. Nat Rev Cancer 5:876–885
31. Hu Y, Yao J, Liu Z, Liu X, Fu H, Ye K (2005) Akt phosphorylates acinus and inhibits its proteolytic cleavage, preventing chromatin condensation. EMBO J 24:3543–3554

32. King FW, Skeen J, Hay N, Shtivelman E (2004) Inhibition of Chk1 by activated PKB/Akt. Cell Cycle 3:634–637
33. Shtivelman E, Sussman J, Stokoe D (2002) A role for PI 3-kinase and PKB activity in the G2/M phase of the cell cycle. Curr Biol 12:919–924
34. Kim AH, Khursigara G, Sun X, Franke TF, Chao MV (2001) Akt phosphorylates and negatively regulates apoptosis signal-regulating kinase 1. Mol Cell Biol 21:893–901
35. Barthwal MK, Sathyanarayana P, Kundu CN, Rana B, Pradeep A, Sharma C, Woodgett JR, Rana A (2003) Negative regulation of mixed lineage kinase 3 by protein kinase B/AKT leads to cell survival. J Biol Chem 278:3897–3902
36. Biggs WH III, Meisenhelder J, Hunter T, Cavenee WK, Arden KC (1999) Protein kinase B/Akt-mediated phosphorylation promotes nuclear exclusion of the winged helix transcription factor FKHR1. Proc Natl Acad Sci U S A 96:7421–7426
37. Brunet A, Bonni A, Zigmond MJ, Lin MZ, Juo P, Hu LS, Anderson MJ, Arden KC, Blenis J, Greenberg ME (1999) Akt promotes cell survival by phosphorylating and inhibiting a Forkhead transcription factor. Cell 96:857–868
38. Kops GJ, de Ruiter ND, De Vries-Smits AM, Powell DR, Bos JL, Burgering BM (1999) Direct control of the Forkhead transcription factor AFX by protein kinase B. Nature 398:630–634
39. Pugazhenthi S, Khandelwal RL (1995) Regulation of glycogen synthase activation in isolated hepatocytes. Mol Cell Biochem 149–150:95–101
40. Beurel E, Jope RS (2006) The paradoxical pro- and anti-apoptotic actions of GSK3 in the intrinsic and extrinsic apoptosis signaling pathways. Prog Neurobiol 79:173–189
41. Rulifson IC, Karnik SK, Heiser PW, ten Berge D, Chen H, Gu X, Taketo MM, Nusse R, Hebrok M, Kim SK (2007) Wnt signaling regulates pancreatic beta cell proliferation. Proc Natl Acad Sci U S A 104:6247–6252
42. Beurel E, Kornprobst M, Blivet-Van Eggelpoel MJ, Ruiz-Ruiz C, Cadoret A, Capeau J, Desbois-Mouthon C (2004) GSK-3beta inhibition by lithium confers resistance to chemotherapy-induced apoptosis through the repression of CD95 (Fas/APO-1) expression. Exp Cell Res 300:354–364
43. Watcharasit P, Bijur GN, Song L, Zhu J, Chen X, Jope RS (2003) Glycogen synthase kinase-3beta (GSK3beta) binds to and promotes the actions of p53. J Biol Chem 278:48872–48879
44. Watcharasit P, Bijur GN, Zmijewski JW, Song L, Zmijewska A, Chen X, Johnson GV, Jope RS (2002) Direct, activating interaction between glycogen synthase kinase-3beta and p53 after DNA damage. Proc Natl Acad Sci U S A 99:7951–7955
45. Hoeflich KP, Luo J, Rubie EA, Tsao MS, Jin O, Woodgett JR (2000) Requirement for glycogen synthase kinase-3beta in cell survival and NF-kappaB activation. Nature 406:86–90
46. Gingras AC, Raught B, Sonenberg N (1999) eIF4 initiation factors: effectors of mRNA recruitment to ribosomes and regulators of translation. Annu Rev Biochem 68:913–963
47. Gingras AC, Raught B, Gygi SP, Niedzwiecka A, Miron M, Burley SK, Polakiewicz RD, Wyslouch-Cieszynska A, Aebersold R, Sonenberg N (2001) Hierarchical phosphorylation of the translation inhibitor 4E-BP1. Genes Dev 15:2852–2864
48. Polunovsky VA, Rosenwald IB, Tan AT, White J, Chiang L, Sonenberg N, Bitterman PB (1996) Translational control of programmed cell death: eukaryotic translation initiation factor 4E blocks apoptosis in growth-factor-restricted fibroblasts with physiologically expressed or deregulated Myc. Mol Cell Biol 16:6573–6581
49. Wendel HG, De Stanchina E, Fridman JS, Malina A, Ray S, Kogan S, Cordon-Cardo C, Pelletier J, Lowe SW (2004) Survival signalling by Akt and eIF4E in oncogenesis and cancer therapy. Nature 428:332–337
50. Wendel HG, Malina A, Zhao Z, Zender L, Kogan SC, Cordon-Cardo C, Pelletier J, Lowe SW (2006) Determinants of sensitivity and resistance to rapamycin-chemotherapy drug combinations in vivo. Cancer Res 66:7639–7646
51. De Benedetti A, Joshi-Barve S, Rinker-Schaeffer C, Rhoads RE (1991) Expression of antisense RNA against initiation factor eIF-4E mRNA in HeLa cells results in lengthened cell division times, diminished translation rates, and reduced levels of both eIF-4E and the p220 component of eIF-4F. Mol Cell Biol 11:5435–5445

52. Polunovsky VA, Gingras AC, Sonenberg N, Peterson M, Tan A, Rubins JB, Manivel JC, Bitterman PB (2000) Translational control of the antiapoptotic function of Ras. J Biol Chem 275:24776–24780
53. Herbert TP, Fahraeus R, Prescott A, Lane DP, Proud CG (2000) Rapid induction of apoptosis mediated by peptides that bind initiation factor eIF4E. Curr Biol 10:793–796
54. Moerke NJ, Aktas H, Chen H, Cantel S, Reibarkh MY, Fahmy A, Gross JD, Degterev A, Yuan J, Chorev M, Halperin JA, Wagner G (2007) Small-molecule inhibition of the interaction between the translation initiation factors eIF4E and eIF4G. Cell 128:257–267
55. Graff JR, Konicek BW, Vincent TM, Lynch RL, Monteith D, Weir SN, Schwier P, Capen A, Goode RL, Dowless MS, Chen Y, Zhang H, Sissons S, Cox K, McNulty AM, Parsons SH, Wang T, Sams L, Geeganage S, Douglass LE, Neubauer BL, Dean NM, Blanchard K, Shou J, Stancato LF, Carter JH, Marcusson EG (2007) Therapeutic suppression of translation initiation factor eIF4E expression reduces tumor growth without toxicity. J Clin Invest 117:2638–2648
56. Richter JD, Sonenberg N (2005) Regulation of cap-dependent translation by eIF4E inhibitory proteins. Nature 433:477–480
57. De Benedetti A, Graff JR (2004) eIF-4E expression and its role in malignancies and metastases. Oncogene 23:3189–3199
58. Rajasekhar VK, Viale A, Socci ND, Wiedmann M, Hu X, Holland EC (2003) Oncogenic Ras and Akt signaling contribute to glioblastoma formation by differential recruitment of existing mRNAs to polysomes. Mol Cell 12:889–901
59. Holcik M, Gordon BW, Korneluk RG (2003) The internal ribosome entry site-mediated translation of antiapoptotic protein XIAP is modulated by the heterogeneous nuclear ribonucleoproteins C1 and C2. Mol Cell Biol 23:280–288
60. Kim YK, Back SH, Rho J, Lee SH, Jang SK (2001) La autoantigen enhances translation of BiP mRNA. Nucleic Acids Res 29:5009–5016
61. Brenet F, Socci ND, Sonenberg N, Holland EC (2009) Akt phosphorylation of La regulates specific mRNA translation in glial progenitors. Oncogene 28:128–139
62. Evdokimova V, Ruzanov P, Anglesio MS, Sorokin AV, Ovchinnikov LP, Buckley J, Triche TJ, Sonenberg N, Sorensen PH (2006) Akt-mediated YB-1 phosphorylation activates translation of silent mRNA species. Mol Cell Biol 26:277–292
63. Palamarchuk A, Efanov A, Maximov V, Aqeilan RI, Croce CM, Pekarsky Y (2005) Akt phosphorylates and regulates Pdcd4 tumor suppressor protein. Cancer Res 65:11282–11286
64. LaRonde-LeBlanc N, Santhanam AN, Baker AR, Wlodawer A, Colburn NH (2007) Structural basis for inhibition of translation by the tumor suppressor Pdcd4. Mol Cell Biol 27:147–156
65. Benjamin D, Schmidlin M, Min L, Gross B, Moroni C (2006) BRF1 protein turnover and mRNA decay activity are regulated by protein kinase B at the same phosphorylation sites. Mol Cell Biol 26:9497–9507
66. Gherzi R, Trabucchi M, Ponassi M, Ruggiero T, Corte G, Moroni C, Chen CY, Khabar KS, Andersen JS, Briata P (2006) The RNA-binding protein KSRP promotes decay of beta-catenin mRNA and is inactivated by PI3K-AKT signaling. PLoS Biol 5:e5
67. Graham JR, Hendershott MC, Terragni J, Cooper GM (2010) mRNA degradation plays a significant role in the program of gene expression regulated by PI 3-kinase signaling. Mol Cell Biol 30(22):5295–5305
68. Auld GC, Campbell DG, Morrice N, Cohen P (2005) Identification of calcium-regulated heat-stable protein of 24 kDa (CRHSP24) as a physiological substrate for PKB and RSK using KESTREL. Biochem J 389:775–783
69. Mathews MB, Sonenberg N, Hershey JWB (2007) Translational control in biology and medicine. Cold Spring Harbor Laboratory Press, Cold Spring Harbor, New York, p 934
70. Sonenberg N, Hinnebusch AG (2009) Regulation of translation initiation in eukaryotes: mechanisms and biological targets. Cell 136:731–745
71. Harding HP, Zhang Y, Zeng H, Novoa I, Lu PD, Calfon M, Sadri N, Yun C, Popko B, Paules R, Stojdl DF, Bell JC, Hettmann T, Leiden JM, Ron D (2003) An integrated stress response regulates amino acid metabolism and resistance to oxidative stress. Mol Cell 11:619–633

72. Delepine M, Nicolino M, Barrett T, Golamaully M, Lathrop GM, Julier C (2000) EIF2AK3, encoding translation initiation factor 2-alpha kinase 3, is mutated in patients with Wolcott-Rallison syndrome. Nat Genet 25:406–409
73. Scheuner D, Song B, McEwen E, Liu C, Laybutt R, Gillespie P, Saunders T, Bonner-Weir S, Kaufman RJ (2001) Translational control is required for the unfolded protein response and in vivo glucose homeostasis. Mol Cell 7:1165–1176
74. Jefferson LS, Fabian JR, Kimball SR (1999) Glycogen synthase kinase-3 is the predominant insulin-regulated eukaryotic initiation factor 2B kinase in skeletal muscle. Int J Biochem Cell Biol 31:191–200
75. Welsh GI, Miller CM, Loughlin AJ, Price NT, Proud CG (1998) Regulation of eukaryotic initiation factor eIF2B: glycogen synthase kinase-3 phosphorylates a conserved serine which undergoes dephosphorylation in response to insulin. FEBS Lett 421:125–130
76. Cross DA, Alessi DR, Cohen P, Andjelkovich M, Hemmings BA (1995) Inhibition of glycogen synthase kinase-3 by insulin mediated by protein kinase B. Nature 378:785–789
77. Zhang HH, Lipovsky AI, Dibble CC, Sahin M, Manning BD (2006) S6K1 regulates GSK3 under conditions of mTOR-dependent feedback inhibition of Akt. Mol Cell 24:185–197
78. Wang X, Janmaat M, Beugnet A, Paulin FE, Proud CG (2002) Evidence that the dephosphorylation of Ser(535) in the epsilon-subunit of eukaryotic initiation factor (eIF) 2B is insufficient for the activation of eIF2B by insulin. Biochem J 367:475–481
79. Nairn AC, Matsushita M, Nastiuk K, Horiuchi A, Mitsui K, Shimizu Y, Palfrey HC (2001) Elongation factor-2 phosphorylation and the regulation of protein synthesis by calcium. Prog Mol Subcell Biol 27:91–129
80. Traugh JA (2001) Insulin, phorbol ester and serum regulate the elongation phase of protein synthesis. Prog Mol Subcell Biol 26:33–48

Chapter 9
AMP-Activated Protein Kinase and Cancer Cell Metabolism

Bin Zheng and Lewis C. Cantley

Introduction

Cancer cells undergo a number of almost stereotyped alterations in the course of neoplastic transformation. One such departure from normal cellular physiology is the difference in their metabolic profile, particularly as it relates to the utilization of glucose and the balance between energy production and anabolic processes necessary for cell division [1–3]. In contrast to the case for nonproliferating cells, most cancer cells prefer glycolysis instead of oxidative phosphorylation to utilize glucose even under oxygen-rich conditions. This is in spite of the fact that the latter is a more efficient pathway to generate ATP. This phenomenon is known as the "Warburg effect" [4]. As a result, cancer cells tend to exhibit less oxygen consumption and increased lactate production. Increased glycolytic flux through enhanced glucose uptake and upregulation of various key glycolytic enzymes may contribute to the Warburg effect. Significantly, the commonly used FDG-PET (^{18}fluorine labeled 2-deoxyglucose positron emission tomography) imaging technique takes advantage of this prominent metabolic feature of cancer cells for the detection of malignancy. In addition to glycolytic enzymes, the expression levels and activities of key metabolic enzymes involved in other metabolic pathways, including the TCA cycle, de novo fatty acid synthesis and other macromolecule synthesis, have also been shown to be regulated by various oncogenes and tumor suppressors [5, 6]. These metabolic

L.C. Cantley (✉)
Division of Signal Transduction, Beth Israel Deaconess Medical Center, Center for Life Sciences, Rm 417, 330 Brookline Avenue, Boston, MA 02115, USA

Department of Systems Biology, Harvard Medical School, Boston, MA 02115, USA
e-mail: lewis_cantley@hms.harvard.edu

I.G. Fantus (ed.), *Insulin Resistance and Cancer: Epidemiology, Cellular and Molecular Mechanisms and Clinical Implications*, Energy Balance and Cancer 1, DOI 10.1007/978-1-4419-9911-5_9,

alterations in cancer cells have been linked to their abilities to grow, proliferate, or survive. Understanding the molecular mechanisms underlying the metabolic reprogramming in cancer will be critical to develop better diagnostics tools and therapeutic strategies for cancer detection and treatment.

AMP-activated protein kinase (AMPK) is a critical evolutionarily conserved, energy sensor that regulates energy homeostasis by monitoring changes in the intracellular AMP and ATP concentrations [7] as its activity is regulated by the ratio of AMP to ATP (see below). Recent studies have suggested that AMPK is one of the major signaling players at the interface of metabolism and cancer. This suggestion is based not only on the fact that AMPK is well positioned to monitor metabolic changes in cancer cells but also on the observation that alteration of AMPK signaling activity has been shown to regulate growth, proliferation, survival, and metabolism of cancer cells.

AMPK: Structure and Regulation

Structure

AMPK exists as a heterotrimeric complex composed of a catalytic kinase subunit (α) and two regulatory subunits, β and γ (Fig. 9.1) [7]. There are two α, two β, and three γ isoforms in mammals. The α subunit contains an N-terminal Ser/Thr kinase domain, an autoinhibitory sequence (AIS), and a C-terminal region that binds to the β subunit. The β subunit serves as a scaffold that binds both α and γ subunits. In addition, the β subunit also contains a glycogen-binding domain that mediates glycogen-induced inhibition of the kinase activity [8]. The γ subunit contains a tandem repeat of four cystathionine-b-synthase (CBS) domains, each of which constitutes of a potential binding site for either AMP or ATP. A recent study on the crystal structure of mammalian AMPK $\gamma 1$ subunit revealed that only three of CBS domains bind to AMP and the other remains unoccupied [9]. Among the three AMP molecule bound, two of them are exchangeable with ATP. Full activation of AMPK requires both the allosteric regulation by AMP through binding to the γ subunit and phosphorylation of Thr172 in the activation loop of the α subunit by an upstream activating kinase (Fig. 9.1) [7]. It has been suggested that binding of AMP to the γ subunit may serve to protect Thr172 of the α subunit from dephosphorylation by protein phosphatases (Fig. 9.1), resulting in increased levels of phosphorylation at Thr172 and increased AMPK activity [10, 11]. However, a definitive understanding of how AMP binding affects the conformation and activity of AMPK holoenzyme remains a big challenge.

Activators of AMPK

In intact cells, the activation of AMPK can be triggered by stresses that cause increases in the AMP:ATP ratio, such as hypoxia, ischemia, or glucose deprivation.

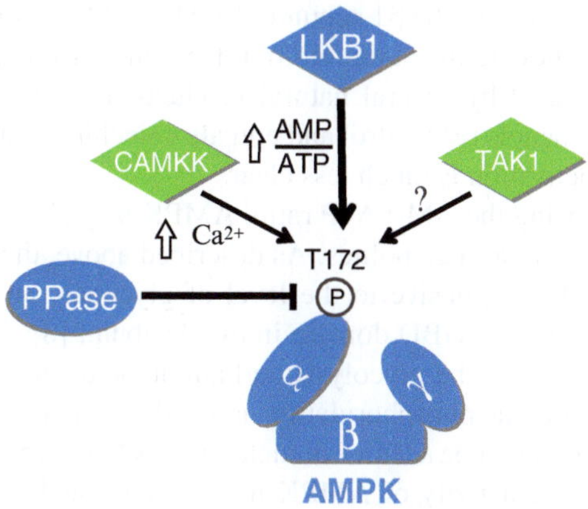

Fig. 9.1 Regulation of AMPK Activity. The heterotrimeric AMPK complex is composed of a catalytic alpha subunit, a scaffold beta subunit, and an AMP/ATP-binding γ subunit. Full activation of AMPK requires both the allosteric regulation by AMP through binding to the γ subunit and phosphorylation of Thr172 in the activation loop of α subunit by an upstream activating kinase. The tumor suppressor LKB1 is the primary upstream activating kinase under most conditions. In addition, CAMKK can phosphorylate and activate AMPK in response to an increase of intracellular calcium. Recent evidence suggests that TAK1 may also serve as another independent activating kinase of AMPK

In addition, AMPK can also be activated in response to physiological stimuli such as skeletal muscle contraction and various peptide hormones, including leptin and adiponectin [7, 12].

A number of pharmacological activators of AMPK have also been described. AICAR (5-Aminoimidazole-4-carboxamide-1-β-D-ribofuranoside) is one of the most common agents used to activate AMPK in cultured cells [13]. Once taken up into the cells, AICAR is converted to ZMP, which is the monophosphorylated derivative of AICAR and can mimic the effect of AMP on activating AMPK. However, it is worthy to note that AMPK-independent effects of AICAR have also been reported [13]. Interestingly, AMPK appears to be the major cellular target of two types of drugs commonly used to treat type II diabetes, biguanides (metformin and phenformin) and Thiazolidinediones (TZDs) (e.g., rosiglitazone) [14]. Metformin and phenformin may act indirectly on AMPK by inhibiting complex I of the mitochondrial respiratory chain, resulting in an increase in the intracellular AMP:ATP ratio and activation of AMPK indirectly [15]. Consistent with this idea, it has been shown that genetic inactivation of hepatic LKB1, a primary activating kinase of AMPK (see below), abolished the effect of metformin on lowering plasma glucose levels in mice [16]. TZDs have been shown to stimulate adiponectin production from adipocytes, which in turn activates AMPK. In addition, TZDs also have an adiponectin-independent effect on AMPK, probably through inhibiting complex I, similar to biguanides [14, 17, 18]. More recently, two direct and more specific AMPK activators, A-769662 [19] and PT-1 [20], have been reported. The effect of A-769662 is dependent on the presence of the β1 subunit of AMPK, whereas PT-1 may act at the α subunit through relieving the autoinhibition from the AIS domain. Furthermore, AMPK can be activated by several natural products, including the alkaloid berberine and the polyphenols resveratrol and epigallocatechin gallate (EGCG) [7], but the mechanism of activation is much less clear.

In addition to sensing the AMP:ATP ratio, AMPK may also be able to sense the levels of other intracellular metabolites. As described above, the activity of AMPK has been shown to be responsive to the level of glycogen, an important cellular energy reserve, through the GBD domain in the β subunit [8]. 3-phosphoglycerate (3-PG), an intermediate in the glycolysis and amino acid synthesis pathways, has been shown to promote the phosphorylation and activity of AMPK via an allosteric mechanism [21]. Nicotinamide adenine dinucleotide (NAD^+), a critical redox reagent, might also regulate the activity of AMPK indirectly through sirtuins, a family of NAD^+-dependent protein deacetylases [22, 23].

Upstream Activation Kinases of AMPK

Phosphorylation of Thr172 of the α subunit is critical for AMPK activation and several potential upstream kinases for this phosphorylation have been described, including LKB1, CAMKK (Ca^{2+}/Calmodulin-dependent protein kinase kinase), and TAK1 (TGF-β-activated kinase-1) (Fig. 9.1). Among them, LKB1 is considered the primary upstream kinase under most conditions.

LKB1

LKB1 (also known as Ser/Thr kinase 11 or STK11) is a tumor suppressor associated with the autosomal dominantly inherited Peutz-Jeghers syndrome (PJS), which is characterized by increased risk of benign and malignant tumors in multiple tissues, hamartomatous polyps in the gastrointestinal tract and mucocutaneous pigmentation [24, 25]. Somatic mutations in LKB1 have also been observed in a significant fraction (up to 30%) of sporadic lung adenocarcinoma and a lower percentage (5%) in pancreatic cancers and melanomas [26, 27]. In mice, targeted homozygous deletion of *Lkb1* results in mid-gestation embryonic lethality with multiple developmental defects and increased VEGF expression [28–30]. Heterozygous mice ($LKB1^{+/-}$) develop gastrointestinal polyps with similar histological features as those in PJS patients. Furthermore, multiple genetically engineered mouse models for inactivation of LKB1 have also supported LKB1's critical role as a tumor suppressor [27].

The LKB1 kinase contains an N-terminal nuclear localization signal (NLS), a catalytic kinase domain, and a C-terminal regulatory region [24, 25]. LKB1 forms a complex with two regulatory proteins, the pseudokinase STE20-related adaptor protein (STRAD), and an armadillo repeat-containing protein MO25 (mouse protein 25), which can induce the relocalization of LKB1 from the nucleus to the cytoplasm [31, 32]. This translocation has been shown to be required for the activation of the

LKB kinase activity. AMPK was the first physiological substrate of LKB1 identified [32–34]. Subsequently, LKB1 has been shown to serve as a master upstream kinase for 12 other AMPK-related kinases as well [35].

Before any of the LKB1 substrates was identified, earlier biochemical and genetic studies suggested that LKB1 might exert its role as a tumor suppressor through regulating cell proliferation and cell polarity [36]. For example, over-expression of LKB1 in HeLa cells, which do not express endogenous LKB1, resulted in the suppression of cell proliferation by imposing a kinase activity–dependent G1/S cell cycle arrest [37, 38]. Genetic studies in *Caenorhabditis elegans and Drosophila melanogaster* and mammalian cell culture studies have identified LKB1 as an important regulator in the establishment of early embryonic asymmetry, as well as epithelial and neuronal polarity [39–41]. With the identification of AMPK as a critical downstream kinase of LKB1, AMPK has become a focus of attention to understand how LKB1 may act as a tumor suppressor through regulating AMPK and its downstream effectors (see discussion below). However, it is equally important to investigate the contributions from 12 other AMPK-related kinases, which also require LKB1 for their activation.

Ca^{2+}/CaM-Dependent Kinase Kinase

CAMKKs (α and β) are members of the Ca^{2+}/CaM-dependent protein kinase family and function in the Ca^{2+}/CaM-dependent protein kinase cascade to phosphorylate and activate Ca^{2+}/CaM-dependent Kinases (CAMK) I and IV. Although earlier evidence suggested that CAMKK is capable of phosphorylating AMPK in vitro, only recently that the physiological roles of CAMKK in phosphorylation and activation of AMPK have been established [42–44]. Phosphorylation of AMPK by CAMKK is completely dependent on an increase of intracellular calcium level and independent of AMP. Moreover, unlike LKB1, the CAMKK is more restricted in its tissue expression, suggesting it may only contribute to AMPK activation in certain cell types, such as neurons and skeletal muscles [45, 46].

TGF-β–Activated Kinase-1

Mammalian TAK1, a cytokine-activated member of the mitogen-activated protein kinase kinase family, was recently identified in a yeast-based functional screen for activators of AMPK [47]. Recombinant TAK1, when fused with its binding partner TAK1-binding subunit 1 (TAB1), phosphorylates AMPK at Thr172 of the AMPK α subunit [47], just like LKB1 and CAMKKs. Based on siRNA knockdown analysis, TRAIL-induced AMPK activation and autophagy in epithelial cells was found to be dependent on TAK1, but not LKB1 or CAMKK β [48]. However, in a different study, LKB1 kinase activity was shown to be defective in TAK1-null mouse embryonic fibroblasts (MEFs), suggesting TAK1 might act upstream of LKB1 [49]. Further studies are still required to clarify whether TAK1 indeed serves as a third independent AMPK activating kinase.

Downstream Effects of AMPK

Traditionally, AMPK has been considered to be a critical player in metabolic regulation. In response to increased cellular AMP:ATP ratio, AMPK phosphorylates downstream regulatory proteins and enzymatic effectors to stimulate ATP-producing catabolic pathways and downregulate ATP-consuming anabolic pathways [7, 12]. A number of these AMPK targets involved in metabolism regulation have been described, including acetyl-CoA carboxylase (ACC), adipose triglyceride lipase, glutamine-fructose-6-phosphate transaminase, glycogen synthase, 3-hydroxy-3-methylglutaryl coenzyme A reductase, and 6-phosphofructo-2-kinase/fructose-2, 6-bisphosphatases [7, 12]. In addition, AMPK also plays an important role in energy homeostasis at the organismal level by regulating food intake behavior and whole-body energy expenditure in response to hormones and cytokines, such as gherlin, leptin, and adiponectin [7, 12]. These effects of AMPK on metabolism make it a promising target in treatment of type 2 diabetes, obesity, and other metabolic disorders. For recent reviews on the roles of AMPK in metabolism, please refer to [7, 12]. However, with the identification of the tumor suppressor LKB1 as a major upstream activating kinase of AMPK, a lot of progress has been made on understanding the role of AMPK in cancer, including its effects on cell growth and proliferation, epithelial cell polarity, and cancer cell metabolism (Fig. 9.2).

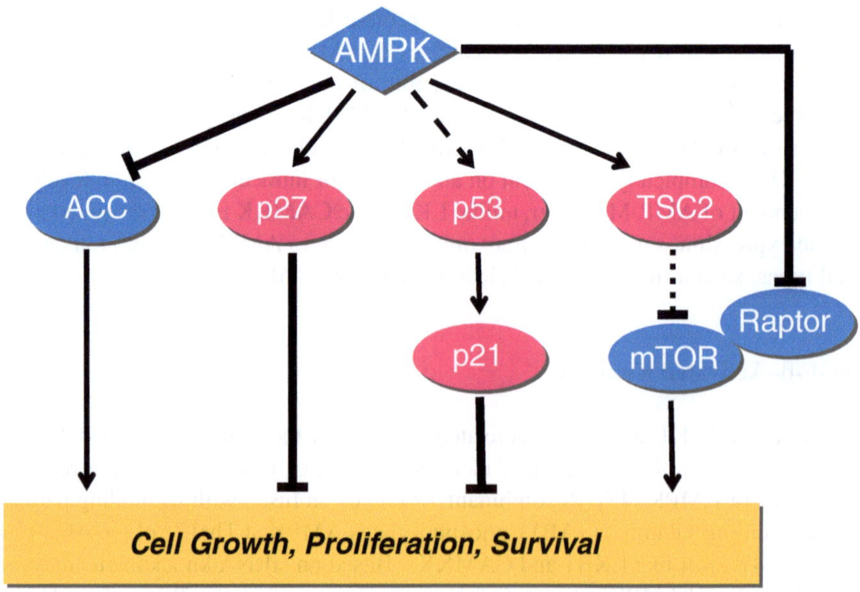

Fig. 9.2 Downstream effectors of AMPK involved in the regulation of cell growth, proliferation, and survival

AMPK and Cell Growth and Proliferation

mTOR Signaling

The mTOR (mammalian target of rapamycin) signaling network plays key roles in regulating cell growth, proliferation, and survival in response to growth factors and nutrients [50]. mTOR, a serine/threonine kinase in the phosphoinositide-3-kinase–related kinase family, can be found in two structurally and functionally distinct signaling complexes, mTORC1 and mTORC2. mTORC1 is sensitive to both nutrients and rapamycin, a macrolide antibiotic, and immunosuppressant, and is responsible for phosphorylating downstream targets such as S6K (ribosomal S6 kinase) and 4E-BP1 (eukaryotic initiation factor 4E bindingprotein-1), two regulators of mRNA translation. In contrast, the mTORC2 complex is insensitive to either nutrient or rapamycin, and it serves as an activating kinase for Akt and some other members of the AGC kinase family including PKC [51].

Under energy deprivation conditions, AMPK inhibits mTORC1 signaling by directly phosphorylating two different nodes in the pathway, TSC2 and Raptor, leading to suppression of protein synthesis and cell growth (Fig. 9.2) [52, 53]. TSC2 is a tumor suppressor and upstream negative regulator of mTORC1. Mutations in TSC2, or in its binding partner TSC1, are associated with the hamartomatous syndrome tuberous sclerosis complex (TSC) [50]. TSC2 possesses a GTPase activating protein (GAP) activity toward small GTPase Rheb, which, when in the GTP state, activates the mTORC1 complex [50]. Loss of TSC2 results in the accumulation of Rheb in the active GTP state and thus promotion of mTORC1 signaling. AMPK has been shown to phosphorylate TSC2 at Ser1387 in vitro and in vivo, thereby enhancing its ability to inhibit mTORC1 signaling [53]. Consistently, both MEFs lacking LKB1 and intestinal polyps from LKB1 heterozygous mice show hyperactivated mTORC1 signaling including increased phosphorylation of both S6K and 4EBP1 [54, 55]. However, phosphorylation of TSC2 does not appear to be the only mechanism by which AMPK suppresses mTORC1 because in cells lacking TSC2 mTORC1 signaling can still be further inhibited in response to AMPK activation [52]. AMPK also directly phosphorylates Raptor, a scaffold component and positive regulator of the mTORC1 complex [52]. Phosphorylation of Raptor by AMPK appears to inhibit mTOR kinase activity in the mTORC1 complex, probably through promoting the association between Raptor and 14-3-3 signaling adaptor proteins [52]. Furthermore, the phosphorylation of Raptor by AMPK is critical for cells to undergo cell cycle arrest and survive under energy stress conditions [52]. In the future, it would be interesting to dissect the relative contribution from TSC2 and Raptor in mediating the inhibition of mTOR signaling under energy stress conditions, and to further understand the biochemical mechanisms underlying the regulation of TSC2 and Raptor activities by AMPK phosphorylation.

p53

AMPK also regulates the tumor suppressor p53 as a metabolic cell cycle checkpoint regulatory mechanism (Fig. 9.2). It has been shown that in response to glucose restriction, MEFs undergo G1/S cell cycle arrest in a manner dependent on both AMPK and p53 [56]. Moreover, activation of AMPK by AICAR, glucose starvation, or expression of a constitutively active mutant of AMPK (CA-AMPK) induces p53 phosphorylation at Ser15 and expression of p53 downstream targets, including p21 CDK inhibitor [56]. Expression of CA-AMPK or glucose restriction also induces cell proliferation arrest in wild type, but not in p53 S15A mutant MEFs, suggesting that the regulation of p53 Ser15 phosphorylation is critical for growth arrest in response to metabolic stress [56]. These findings are consistent with earlier observations that ectopic expression of LKB1 in several LKB1-deficient cancer cells induces the expression of p21 CDK inhibitor in a p53-dependent manner [37]. However, it remains to be seen whether AMPK directly participate in the phosphorylation of p53 in vivo, because the flanking sequence of Ser15 in p53 does not conform well to the consensus AMPK phosphorylation motif. It is possible that AMPK may regulate the phosphorylation of Ser15 indirectly through a yet to be identified downstream kinase. Another possibility is that since Ser15 is tightly coupled to the stability of p53, AMPK may phosphorylate and regulate proteins involved in the control of p53 stability through such mechanisms.

Interestingly, recent evidence suggests that a reverse regulatory pathway from p53 back to AMPK may also exist. Two p53 target genes Sestrin1 and Sestrin2 have been shown to activate AMPK in response to genotoxic stresses, and promote its phosphorylation on TSC2, hence inhibiting mTOR signaling [57]. Moreover, activation of p53 by nutlin-3A, an inhibitor of the association between p53 and MDM2, has been shown to activate AMPK and downregulate mTOR signaling in mantle cell lymphoma cells [58].

p27

In addition to p53, the CDK inhibitor p27 (Kip1) represents another key cell cycle regulator that may be controlled by AMPK (Fig. 9.2). Activation of AMPK results in increased p27 expression in various cancer cells [59]. Recently, p27 was shown to be phosphorylated in response to AICAR and glucose starvation in an LKB1-dependent manner at Thr198 in the C-terminus Thr198 [60]. Expression of a phosphorylation-mimetic mutant of p27 (T198D), but not the phosphorylation-deficient mutant T198A, induces G1 cell cycle arrest as well as autophagy in the absence of external energy stress [60]. Likewise, the presence of p27 is required for cell survival and autophagy under glucose starvation conditions [60], but it is still unclear whether or not the phosphorylation of p27 at T198 is required. In addition to Thr198, AMPK has also been shown to phosphorylate p27 in vitro at Thr170 [61], which resides in sequence that is a less optimal fit to the AMPK phosphorylation motif, and the physiological relevance of this phosphorylation remains to be determined.

AMPK and Epithelial Polarity

Alterations in epithelial polarity play a critical role in the neoplastic transformation and progression of many carcinomas [62]. Loss of epithelial cell polarity has been linked to epithelial cell over-proliferation, epithelial mesenchymal transition (EMT), and metastasis [62]. LKB1 is a well-established and evolutionarily conserved regulator of cell polarity [63]. Par-4, the LKB1 ortholog in *C. elegans*, is one of six partitioning-defective genes identified in a genetic screen for anterior–posterior polarity during early embryo cell divisions [64]. *D. melanogaster* LKB1 (dLKB1) has also been shown to be required for proper follicular epithelium apical basolateral polarization [40]. Mammalian LKB1, when activated by association with its regulatory proteins STRAD and MO25, induces cell-autonomous polarization in intestinal epithelial cells [39]. In *C. elegans*, mutations in the microtubule affinity regulating kinases (MARKs) ortholog *par-1* were identified in the same screen that in which *par-4* (LKB1) was discovered [64]. This has led to the suggestion that the effects of LKB1 on polarity are probably mainly mediated by MARKs' family members [7].

However, accumulating evidence has revealed that AMPK also plays a critical role in regulation of epithelial polarity and serves as a link between energy stress and polarity regulation. Calcium depletion from the medium in a confluent monolayer of Madin-Darby Canine Kidney (MDCK) cells causes loss of cell–cell junctions; replenishment of calcium (calcium switch) triggers junction assembly and cell polarization. Using MDCK cells in this calcium switch model system, two groups independently reported that AMPK activity increases during epithelial tight junction formation and polarization [65, 66]. Both groups found that activation of AMPK by AICAR promotes tight junction assembly, whereas expression of a kinase-dead mutant of AMPK inhibits the process [65, 66]. More interestingly, one of the studies showed that treatment of AICAR partially prevents disassembly of tight junctions induced by calcium depletion from the media, suggesting that activation of AMPK could be beneficial to the maintenance of tight junction integrity under stress conditions [66]. Consistent with these findings, it was found in *D. melanogaster* that AMPKα mutant embryonic and follicular epithelial cells showed dramatic disorganization in the apical basolateral polarity [67, 68].

In the fly, MRLC (myosin regulatory light chain) has been shown to be a critical substrate of AMPK that mediates its effect on epithelial polarity regulation [67]. A previously known regulatory phosphorylation site of *Drosophila* MRLC (Ser19) turns out to be a direct target of AMPK both in vitro and in vivo [67]. Furthermore, forced transgene expression of a phospho-mimetic mutant of MRLC partially rescues some of the polarity phenotypes observed in AMPKα mutants [67]. However, whether mammalian MRLC also contributes significantly to AMPK-mediated epithelial polarity regulation remains to be clarified as targeted deletion of LKB1 in pancreatic epithelium failed to alter the phosphorylation of MRLC at Ser19, even though inactivation of AMPK and loss of acinar polarity and tight junctions were observed in these cells [69]. On the other hand, the incomplete rescue of the AMPKα mutant phenotype by over-expression of MRLC in fly suggests that additional downstream effectors must be involved. The contribution of mTORC1 was suggested in one study using the MDCK calcium switch model system [65], but was ruled out in another study examining the role of LKB1 in acinar structure formation using mammary epithelial cell 3D culture [70]. In the future, it would be interesting to further explore the molecular mechanism underlying the regulation of epithelial polarity by AMPK and to better understand its link to EMT and cancer metastasis.

Cancer Cell Metabolism

Regulation of cancer cell metabolism by AMPK also contributes to its suppression of cell growth and proliferation. AMPK inhibits the expression of two key enzymes in the fatty acid synthesis pathway, fatty acid synthase (FASN), and acetyl-CoA carboxylase-1 (ACC1) [7]. In addition, AMPK directly phosphorylates and inhibits ACC1 enzymatic activity. ACC1 is a rate-limiting enzyme that carboxylates acetyl-CoA to generate malonyl-CoA. FASN then uses malonyl-CoA and acetyl-CoA to make palmitate for long chain fatty acid synthesis. Upregulation of de novo fatty acid synthesis is a critical metabolic feature of cancer cells [1]. Not surprisingly, therefore, both ACC1 and FASN have been frequently found to be over-expressed in cancer cells [71] and knockdown of ACC1 or FASN in cancer cells has indicated that they are critical for cancer cell proliferation [72, 73]. More recently, ACC1 has been shown to interact with BRCA1, suggesting possible cooperation between these proteins in cellular homeostasis [74, 75]. The perturbation caused by oncogenic BRCA1 mutations may act, at least partially, through ACC1 in effecting neoplastic transformation. Specifically, the phospho-Ser/Thr binding BRCT domain in the C-terminus of BRCA1 interacts with a peptide containing phosphorylated Ser1263 from ACC1 [76, 77]. This phospho-Ser is distinct from the Ser residue phosphorylated by AMPK at Ser79, and the kinase responsible is still unknown. It would be interesting in the future to examine whether the phosphorylation of ACC1 at Ser79 by AMPK plays a role in regulating the association between ACC1 and BRCA1.

Members of the 6-phosphofructo-2-kinase/fructose-2, 6-bisphosphatase (PFK2/FBPase) family of enzymes can be regulated by AMPK, and these enzymes may play a critical role in cancer cell metabolism [78, 79]. This class of enzymes catalyzes the synthesis and turnover of fructose-2, 6-bisphosphate (F2,6BP), which is an allosteric activator of the first rate-limiting step in glycolysis catalyzed by 6-phosphofructo-1-kinase (PFK1) [78, 79]. There are four isoforms of PFK2/FBPase in mammalian cells and two of them, PFKFB2 and PFKFB3, have been shown to be substrates of AMPK [80–82]. However, the site at PFKFB3 (Ser461) appears to better conform to the AMPK consensus phosphorylation motif than the analogous site in PFKFB2 (Ser466), since the latter lacks a hydrophobic residue at the −5 position. PFKFB2 has been shown to be phosphorylated by AMPK in cardiomyocytes during ischemia and this phosphorylation leads to an increase of PFK2 activity, which may explain the increase in glycolytic flux in the heart under anaerobic conditions [81]. Consistent with a role for AMPK in this event, activation of

PFK2FB3 was found to correlate with increased AMPK activity in monocytes under hypoxia conditions [82]. Moreover, based on RNAi knockdown analysis, both AMPK and PFKFB3 were shown to be required for nitric oxide–dependent glycolysis activation and survival of astrocytes [80]. PFKFB3 has also been suggested to play a critical role in regulating glycolytic flux to lactate in cancer cells [83]. Interestingly, among all the isozymes, PFKFB3 has the highest ratio of PFK/FBPase activity and hence is believed to be the major regulator of intracellular F2,6BP level [78]. PFKFB3 is highly over-expressed in various cancer cell lines and tumor samples and can be upregulated by hypoxia [83–85]. Homozygous deletion of PFKFB3 results in embryonic lethality in mice. Heterozygous deletion of PFKFB3 in adult lung fibroblasts transformed with H-Ras suppresses anchorage-independent growth on soft agars and tumor growth in athymic mice, suggesting that PFKFB3 is critical for the transformation activity of H-Ras [86]. Moreover, knockdown of PFKFB3 by siRNA in HeLa and A549 cancer cells inhibited F2,6BP production and anchorage-independent growth [86, 87]. These findings support an important role of PFKFB3 in cancer. Further studies are needed to pinpoint the contribution of AMPK phosphorylation on PFKFB3 in regulating cell proliferation and tumor growth.

Regulation of AMPK Signaling in Cancer

As discussed earlier, activation of AMPK leads to suppression of cell growth and proliferation under conditions of energy stress conditions. It is conceivable that tumor cells must inactivate this signaling pathway in order to gain a growth advantage. There are at least four possible mechanisms to achieve this. First, cancer cells may maintain high level of cellular ATP through upregulation of HIF1 and subsequent transcriptional activation of genes involved in glucose-uptake and glycolysis-dependent ATP synthesis, hence relieving the energy stress [108–110]. Second, deletion or lost-of-function mutations in the components in the AMPK pathways would lead to inactivation of the pathway. Mutations in LKB1 have been found in PJS and several different types of cancers [24, 88], but mutations of AMPK subunits have not been reported in cancer yet. Third, epigenetic mechanisms for suppression of the expression of genes in this pathway might also be involved. Hypermethylation of the LKB1 promoter CpG island has been found in some cancer cells [89, 90]. LKB1 and AMPK genes might also be targeted for microRNA-mediated silencing in cancer. Finally, the activity of LKB1 and AMPK could be regulated at the posttranslational level. In this regard, we have recently found that AMPK is consistently suppressed in melanoma cells with the B-RAF V600E mutation and that downregulation of B-RAF signaling in turn activates AMPK (Fig. 9.3) [91]. It turns out that in these cells, LKB1 is constitutively phosphorylated at Ser325, an Ser428 by ERK and p90Rsk, two kinases downstream of B-RAF, respectively; and that this phosphorylation compromises the ability of LKB1 to bind and activate AMPK [91]. Furthermore, expression of a phosphorylation-deficient mutant of LKB1 allows activation of AMPK and results in inhibition

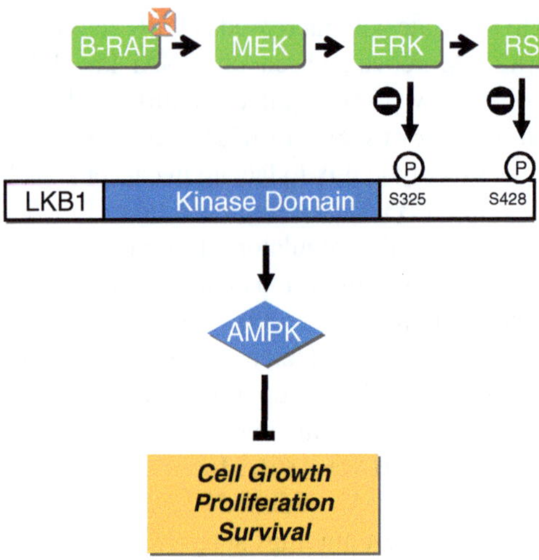

Fig. 9.3 Regulation of LKB1 and AMPK activity in BRAF V600E-driven melanoma. LKB1 is phosphorylated at Ser325 and Ser428, by ERK and p90RSK, two kinases activated downstream of oncogenic B-RAF V600E. Phosphorylation of LKB1 at these sites prevents its association with and activation on AMPK. Suppression of AMPK activity by oncogenic B-RAF V600E may be critical for B-RAF to release the inhibition of cell growth, proliferation, and survival imposed by AMPK under energy stress conditions

of melanoma cell proliferation and anchorage-independent cell growth, suggesting that suppression of LKB1 function by B-RAF V600E may contribute to B-RAF V600E-driven tumorigenesis [91]. An independent study also reported similar findings that B-RAF V600E induces the uncoupling of AMPK from LKB1 in melanoma cells [92].

It would be interesting to investigate whether similar posttranslational mechanisms of suppressing LKB1-AMPK signaling may also occur in cancer cells driven by other oncogenes or tumor suppressors. Treatment of GW-2974, an ErbB1/2 inhibitor, in ErbB2-driven breast cancer cells has been shown to activate AMPK and inhibit cell proliferation [93, 94]. Deletion of Fyn, Src family tyrosine kinases, leads to an increase in AMPK activity, which may contribute to the improved insulin sensitivity in the peripheral tissues in the knockout mice [95]. The molecular mechanism underlying the regulation of AMPK in these studies has not been characterized, but it would be interesting to find out whether tyrosine phosphorylation on components in the LKB1/AMPK pathway is involved. In addition to Ser325 and Ser428, residues discussed earlier, LKB1 has been shown to be phosphorylated at several other Ser/Thr residues [24]. Other types of posttranslational modification on LKB1 have also been reported, including farnesylation and acetylation [23, 24]. Ser/Thr phosphorylation of AMPK α and β subunits has also been described [7, 96]. Moreover, the stability of AMPKβ has also shown to be regulated through ubiquitination [97]. The biological significances of these modifications are largely unknown. It is conceivable that they could potentially serve as means for AMPK to crosstalk with other oncogenic or tumor-suppressing signaling pathways.

Implications in Cancer Therapeutic

The critical role of AMPK in suppressing cell growth and proliferation raises interesting possibilities that activation of this pathway would suppress tumor growth. This notion is especially appealing since AMPK activators, such as metformin/phenformin and TZDs, are already widely used for type 2 diabetes treatment and additional novel AMPK activators are being actively developed [15].

Indeed, in addition to numerous cell culture studies, increasing data from animal model studies and epidemiological studies support that metformin/phenformin and TZDs are promising effective cancer therapeutics. In a high-fat diet-induced pancreatic cancer hamster model, receiving metformin in drinking water for life prevents the formation of malignant lesions induced by N-nitrosobis-(2-oxopropyl)amine carcinogen [98]. Similar treatment with metformin has also been shown to delay the onset of tumor development, suppress tumor growth, and prolong lifespan in a mouse HER-2/neu mammary cancer model [99]. Moreover, administration of several AMPK activators metformin, phenformin, or A-769662 in the $PTEN^{+/-}$ mouse model has been shown to significantly delay the formation of various tumors, such as intestinal polyps, lymphoma, and prostate intraepithelial neoplasia [100]. More recently, metformin was found to suppress the formation of large intestinal polyps in Apc $Min^{+/-}$ mice, although the overall number of total polyps did not change [101]. Significantly, the plasma levels of glucose, insulin, and cholesterol did not change, suggesting that the effects of metformin are probably direct [101]. In addition to cancer prevention studies, the effect of metformin on the growth of pre-existing tumors has also been investigated. Introduction of metformin through IP injection or drinking water decreased the volume of xenograft tumors from LNCaP prostate cancer cells by ~35 and 55%, respectively [102]. Further studies using various genetic-modified mouse cancer models to investigate the effects on the tumor growth will further test the therapeutic value of AMPK activators.

In the $PTEN^{+/-}$ models, phenformin showed a more potent effect than metformin in delaying the tumor onset [100]. This probably is partly related to the observations that phenformin is less hydrophilic than metformin and that the uptake of metformin is dependent on organic cation transporters (OCT1 and OCT2) [103]. Phenformin was discontinued for the treatment of diabetes in the US due to its significant side effect in causing lactic acidosis, but it is still used in some European and Asian countries.

Two recent population-based cohort studies have shown that metformin treatment in patients with type 2 diabetes is associated with lower cancer risks. In one cohort study based in the UK, type 2 diabetes patients taking metformin were found to have a 23% reduced chance (in adjusted odds ratio) to be diagnosed with malignant cancer later on compared to those who never took metformin [104]. Interestingly, a potential dose–response relationship was also observed in this study [104]. Similarly, in another study based in Canada, patients with type 2 diabetes who were treated with sulfonylurea or insulin had a 30 and 90% higher risk (hazard risk 1.3 and 1.9), respectively, for cancer-related mortality, compared to those treated with metformin [105]. In addition to AMPK activators, metabolic stress conditions that lead to AMPK activation, such as exercise and calorie restriction, have been found to be associated with lower risk of cancer in human [106], although it would be difficult to tease out how much AMPK activation contributes to the overall beneficiary effect.

AMPK activators potentially could therefore be used in combination with other therapeutic agents to achieve better efficacy. For example, a recent study showed that metformin potentiated the cytotoxicity of cisplatin on OVCAR-3 ovarian cancer cells in cell viability assays [107]. Based on our recent findings on the molecular link between the LKB1/AMPK and B-RAF/MEK/ERK signaling pathways, we have proposed to use AMPK activators together with BRAF/MEK inhibitors for treating B-RAF V600E-driven cancers [91]. AMPK activators may also be used together with PI3K/Akt or mTOR inhibitors in the tumors driven by hyperactivation of the PI3K/Akt pathway.

Perspective

Recent studies have demonstrated that AMPK is a promising therapeutic target for cancer prevention and treatment. Based on results from preclinical studies, several clinical trials are currently ongoing to test metformin in various cancers, including breast, endometrial, kidney, lung, lymphoma, and prostate (http://clinicaltrials.gov). Further understanding of the structure of the AMPK complex, and additional knowledge about downstream effectors involved in cancer initiation and progression will provide new insight into developing more specific, effective, and personalized cancer therapeutics.

Acknowledgments We would like to thank Kenneth Swanson for critical reading the manuscript. This work is supported by National Institutes of Health Grant GM56203 and CA102694 to L.C.C., and K99CA133245 to B.Z.

References

1. Kroemer G, Pouyssegur J (2008) Tumor cell metabolism: cancer's Achilles' heel. Cancer Cell 13:472–482
2. Luo J, Solimini NL, Elledge SJ (2009) Principles of cancer therapy: oncogene and non-oncogene addiction. Cell 136:823–837
3. Vander Heiden MG, Cantley LC, Thompson CB (2009) Understanding the Warburg effect: the metabolic requirements of cell proliferation. Science 324(5930):1029–1033
4. Warburg O (1956) On the origin of cancer cells. Science 123:309–314
5. DeBerardinis RJ, Lum JJ, Hatzivassiliou G, Thompson CB (2008) The biology of cancer: metabolic reprogramming fuels cell growth and proliferation. Cell Metab 7:11–20
6. Hsu PP, Sabatini DM (2008) Cancer cell metabolism: warburg and beyond. Cell 134:703–707
7. Hardie DG (2007) AMP-activated/SNF1 protein kinases: conserved guardians of cellular energy. Nat Rev Mol Cell Biol 8:774–785
8. McBride A, Ghilagaber S, Nikolaev A, Hardie DG (2009) The glycogen-binding domain on the AMPK beta subunit allows the kinase to act as a glycogen sensor. Cell Metab 9:23–34
9. Xiao B, Heath R, Saiu P, Leiper FC, Leone P, Jing C, Walker PA, Haire L, Eccleston JF, Davis CT, Martin SR, Carling D, Gamblin SJ (2007) Structural basis for AMP binding to mammalian AMP-activated protein kinase. Nature 449:496–500

10. Sanders MJ, Grondin PO, Hegarty BD, Snowden MA, Carling D (2007) Investigating the mechanism for AMP activation of the AMP-activated protein kinase cascade. Biochem J 403:139–148
11. Steinberg GR, Michell BJ, van Denderen BJ, Watt MJ, Carey AL, Fam BC, Andrikopoulos S, Proietto J, Gorgun CZ, Carling D, Hotamisligil GS, Febbraio MA, Kay TW, Kemp BE (2006) Tumor necrosis factor alpha-induced skeletal muscle insulin resistance involves suppression of AMP-kinase signaling. Cell Metab 4:465–474
12. Kahn BB, Alquier T, Carling D, Hardie DG (2005) AMP-activated protein kinase: ancient energy gauge provides clues to modern understanding of metabolism. Cell Metab 1:15–25
13. Guigas B, Sakamoto K, Taleux N, Reyna SM, Musi N, Viollet B, Hue L (2009) Beyond AICA riboside: in search of new specific AMP-activated protein kinase activators. IUBMB Life 61:18–26
14. Hardie DG (2007) AMP-activated protein kinase as a drug target. Annu Rev Pharmacol Toxicol 47:185–210
15. Zhou G, Sebhat IK, Zhang BB (2009) AMPK activators – potential therapeutics for metabolic and other diseases. Acta Physiol (Oxf) 196(1):175–190
16. Shaw RJ, Lamia KA, Vasquez D, Koo SH, Bardeesy N, Depinho RA, Montminy M, Cantley LC (2005) The kinase LKB1 mediates glucose homeostasis in liver and therapeutic effects of metformin. Science 310:1642–1646
17. Hudson ER, Pan DA, James J, Lucocq JM, Hawley SA, Green KA, Baba O, Terashima T, Hardie DG (2003) A novel domain in AMP-activated protein kinase causes glycogen storage bodies similar to those seen in hereditary cardiac arrhythmias. Curr Biol 13:861–866
18. Polekhina G, Gupta A, Michell BJ, van Denderen B, Murthy S, Feil SC, Jennings IG, Campbell DJ, Witters LA, Parker MW, Kemp BE, Stapleton D (2003) AMPK beta subunit targets metabolic stress sensing to glycogen. Curr Biol 13:867–871
19. Cool B, Zinker B, Chiou W, Kifle L, Cao N, Perham M, Dickinson R, Adler A, Gagne G, Iyengar R, Zhao G, Marsh K, Kym P, Jung P, Camp HS, Frevert E (2006) Identification and characterization of a small molecule AMPK activator that treats key components of type 2 diabetes and the metabolic syndrome. Cell Metab 3:403–416
20. Pang T, Zhang ZS, Gu M, Qiu BY, Yu LF, Cao PR, Shao W, Su MB, Li JY, Nan FJ, Li J (2008) Small molecule antagonizes autoinhibition and activates AMP-activated protein kinase in cells. J Biol Chem 283:16051–16060
21. Ellingson WJ, Chesser DG, Winder WW (2007) Effects of 3-phosphoglycerate and other metabolites on the activation of AMP-activated protein kinase by LKB1-STRAD-MO25. Am J Physiol Endocrinol Metab 292:E400–E407
22. Hou X, Xu S, Maitland-Toolan KA, Sato K, Jiang B, Ido Y, Lan F, Walsh K, Wierzbicki M, Verbeuren TJ, Cohen RA, Zang M (2008) SIRT1 regulates hepatocyte lipid metabolism through activating AMP-activated protein kinase. J Biol Chem 283:20015–20026
23. Lan F, Cacicedo JM, Ruderman N, Ido Y (2008) SIRT1 modulation of the acetylation status, cytosolic localization, and activity of LKB1. Possible role in AMP-activated protein kinase activation. J Biol Chem 283:27628–27635
24. Alessi DR, Sakamoto K, Bayascas JR (2006) LKB1-dependent signaling pathways. Annu Rev Biochem 75:137–163
25. Katajisto P, Vallenius T, Vaahtomeri K, Ekman N, Udd L, Tiainen M, Makela TP (2007) The LKB1 tumor suppressor kinase in human disease. Biochim Biophys Acta 1775:63–75
26. Sanchez-Cespedes M, Parrella P, Esteller M, Nomoto S, Trink B, Engles JM, Westra WH, Herman JG, Sidransky D (2002) Inactivation of LKB1/STK11 is a common event in adenocarcinomas of the lung. Cancer Res 62:3659–3662
27. Hezel AF, Bardeesy N (2008) LKB1; linking cell structure and tumor suppression. Oncogene 27:6908–6919
28. Bardeesy N, Sinha M, Hezel AF, Signoretti S, Hathaway NA, Sharpless NE, Loda M, Carrasco DR, DePinho RA (2002) Loss of the Lkb1 tumour suppressor provokes intestinal polyposis but resistance to transformation. Nature 419:162–167
29. Jishage K, Nezu J, Kawase Y, Iwata T, Watanabe M, Miyoshi A, Ose A, Habu K, Kake T, Kamada N, Ueda O, Kinoshita M, Jenne DE, Shimane M, Suzuki H (2002) Role of Lkb1, the

causative gene of Peutz-Jegher's syndrome, in embryogenesis and polyposis. Proc Natl Acad Sci U S A 99:8903–8908

30. Ylikorkala A, Rossi DJ, Korsisaari N, Luukko K, Alitalo K, Henkemeyer M, Makela TP (2001) Vascular abnormalities and deregulation of VEGF in Lkb1-deficient mice. Science 293:1323–1326
31. Dorfman J, Macara IG (2008) STRADalpha regulates LKB1 localization by blocking access to importin-alpha, and by association with Crm1 and exportin-7. Mol Biol Cell 19:1614–1626
32. Hawley SA, Boudeau J, Reid JL, Mustard KJ, Udd L, Makela TP, Alessi DR, Hardie DG (2003) Complexes between the LKB1 tumor suppressor, STRAD alpha/beta and MO25 alpha/beta are upstream kinases in the AMP-activated protein kinase cascade. J Biol 2:28
33. Shaw RJ, Kosmatka M, Bardeesy N, Hurley RL, Witters LA, DePinho RA, Cantley LC (2004) The tumor suppressor LKB1 kinase directly activates AMP-activated kinase and regulates apoptosis in response to energy stress. Proc Natl Acad Sci U S A 101:3329–3335
34. Woods A, Johnstone SR, Dickerson K, Leiper FC, Fryer LG, Neumann D, Schlattner U, Wallimann T, Carlson M, Carling D (2003) LKB1 is the upstream kinase in the AMP-activated protein kinase cascade. Curr Biol 13:2004–2008
35. Lizcano JM, Goransson O, Toth R, Deak M, Morrice NA, Boudeau J, Hawley SA, Udd L, Makela TP, Hardie DG, Alessi DR (2004) LKB1 is a master kinase that activates 13 kinases of the AMPK subfamily, including MARK/PAR-1. EMBO J 23:833–843
36. Boudeau J, Sapkota G, Alessi DR (2003) LKB1, a protein kinase regulating cell proliferation and polarity. FEBS Lett 546:159–165
37. Tiainen M, Vaahtomeri K, Ylikorkala A, Makela TP (2002) Growth arrest by the LKB1 tumor suppressor: induction of p21(WAF1/CIP1). Hum Mol Genet 11:1497–1504
38. Tiainen M, Ylikorkala A, Makela TP (1999) Growth suppression by Lkb1 is mediated by a G(1) cell cycle arrest. Proc Natl Acad Sci U S A 96:9248–9251
39. Baas AF, Kuipers J, van der Wel NN, Batlle E, Koerten HK, Peters PJ, Clevers HC (2004) Complete polarization of single intestinal epithelial cells upon activation of LKB1 by STRAD. Cell 116:457–466
40. Martin SG, St Johnston D (2003) A role for Drosophila LKB1 in anterior-posterior axis formation and epithelial polarity. Nature 421:379–384
41. Watts JL, Morton DG, Bestman J, Kemphues KJ (2000) The *C. elegans* par-4 gene encodes a putative serine-threonine kinase required for establishing embryonic asymmetry. Development 127:1467–1475
42. Woods A, Dickerson K, Heath R, Hong SP, Momcilovic M, Johnstone SR, Carlson M, Carling D (2005) Ca2+/calmodulin-dependent protein kinase kinase-beta acts upstream of AMP-activated protein kinase in mammalian cells. Cell Metab 2:21–33
43. Hawley SA, Pan DA, Mustard KJ, Ross L, Bain J, Edelman AM, Frenguelli BG, Hardie DG (2005) Calmodulin-dependent protein kinase kinase-beta is an alternative upstream kinase for AMP-activated protein kinase. Cell Metab 2:9–19
44. Hurley RL, Anderson KA, Franzone JM, Kemp BE, Means AR, Witters LA (2005) The Ca2+/calmodulin-dependent protein kinase kinases are AMP-activated protein kinase kinases. J Biol Chem 280:29060–29066
45. Anderson KA, Ribar TJ, Lin F, Noeldner PK, Green MF, Muehlbauer MJ, Witters LA, Kemp BE, Means AR (2008) Hypothalamic CaMKK2 contributes to the regulation of energy balance. Cell Metab 7:377–388
46. Witczak CA, Sharoff CG, Goodyear LJ (2008) AMP-activated protein kinase in skeletal muscle: from structure and localization to its role as a master regulator of cellular metabolism. Cell Mol Life Sci 65:3737–3755
47. Momcilovic M, Hong SP, Carlson M (2006) Mammalian TAK1 activates Snf1 protein kinase in yeast and phosphorylates AMP-activated protein kinase in vitro. J Biol Chem 281:25336–25343
48. Herrero-Martin G, Hoyer-Hansen M, Garcia-Garcia C, Fumarola C, Farkas T, Lopez-Rivas A, Jaattela M (2009) TAK1 activates AMPK-dependent cytoprotective autophagy in TRAIL-treated epithelial cells. EMBO J 28:677–685

49. Xie M, Zhang D, Dyck JR, Li Y, Zhang H, Morishima M, Mann DL, Taffet GE, Baldini A, Khoury DS, Schneider MD (2006) A pivotal role for endogenous TGF-beta-activated kinase-1 in the LKB1/AMP-activated protein kinase energy-sensor pathway. Proc Natl Acad Sci U S A 103:17378–17383
50. Guertin DA, Sabatini DM (2007) Defining the role of mTOR in cancer. Cancer Cell 12:9–22
51. Jacinto E, Lorberg A (2008) TOR regulation of AGC kinases in yeast and mammals. Biochem J 410:19–37
52. Gwinn DM, Shackelford DB, Egan DF, Mihaylova MM, Mery A, Vasquez DS, Turk BE, Shaw RJ (2008) AMPK phosphorylation of raptor mediates a metabolic checkpoint. Mol Cell 30:214–226
53. Inoki K, Zhu T, Guan KL (2003) TSC2 mediates cellular energy response to control cell growth and survival. Cell 115:577–590
54. Corradetti MN, Inoki K, Bardeesy N, DePinho RA, Guan KL (2004) Regulation of the TSC pathway by LKB1: evidence of a molecular link between tuberous sclerosis complex and Peutz-Jeghers syndrome. Genes Dev 18:1533–1538
55. Shaw RJ, Bardeesy N, Manning BD, Lopez L, Kosmatka M, DePinho RA, Cantley LC (2004) The LKB1 tumor suppressor negatively regulates mTOR signaling. Cancer Cell 6:91–99
56. Jones RG, Plas DR, Kubek S, Buzzai M, Mu J, Xu Y, Birnbaum MJ, Thompson CB (2005) AMP-activated protein kinase induces a p53-dependent metabolic checkpoint. Mol Cell 18:283–293
57. Budanov AV, Karin M (2008) p53 target genes sestrin1 and sestrin2 connect genotoxic stress and mTOR signaling. Cell 134:451–460
58. Drakos E, Atsaves V, Li J, Leventaki V, Andreeff M, Medeiros LJ, Rassidakis GZ (2009) Stabilization and activation of p53 downregulates mTOR signaling through AMPK in mantle cell lymphoma. Leukemia 23(4):754–790
59. Rattan R, Giri S, Singh AK, Singh I (2005) 5-Aminoimidazole-4-carboxamide-1-beta-D-ribofuranoside inhibits cancer cell proliferation in vitro and in vivo via AMP-activated protein kinase. J Biol Chem 280:39582–39593
60. Liang J, Shao SH, Xu ZX, Hennessy B, Ding Z, Larrea M, Kondo S, Dumont DJ, Gutterman JU, Walker CL, Slingerland JM, Mills GB (2007) The energy sensing LKB1-AMPK pathway regulates p27(kip1) phosphorylation mediating the decision to enter autophagy or apoptosis. Nat Cell Biol 9:218–224
61. Short JD, Houston KD, Dere R, Cai SL, Kim J, Johnson CL, Broaddus RR, Shen J, Miyamoto S, Tamanoi F, Kwiatkowski D, Mills GB, Walker CL (2008) AMP-activated protein kinase signaling results in cytoplasmic sequestration of p27. Cancer Res 68:6496–6506
62. Lee M, Vasioukhin V (2008) Cell polarity and cancer–cell and tissue polarity as a non-canonical tumor suppressor. J Cell Sci 121:1141–1150
63. Baas AF, Smit L, Clevers H (2004) LKB1 tumor suppressor protein: PARtaker in cell polarity. Trends Cell Biol 14:312–319
64. Kemphues KJ, Priess JR, Morton DG, Cheng NS (1988) Identification of genes required for cytoplasmic localization in early *C. elegans* embryos. Cell 52:311–320
65. Zhang L, Li J, Young LH, Caplan MJ (2006) AMP-activated protein kinase regulates the assembly of epithelial tight junctions. Proc Natl Acad Sci U S A 103:17272–17277
66. Zheng B, Cantley LC (2007) Regulation of epithelial tight junction assembly and disassembly by AMP-activated protein kinase. Proc Natl Acad Sci U S A 104:819–822
67. Lee JH, Koh H, Kim M, Kim Y, Lee SY, Karess RE, Lee SH, Shong M, Kim JM, Kim J, Chung J (2007) Energy-dependent regulation of cell structure by AMP-activated protein kinase. Nature 447:1017–1020
68. Mirouse V, Swick LL, Kazgan N, St Johnston D, Brenman JE (2007) LKB1 and AMPK maintain epithelial cell polarity under energetic stress. J Cell Biol 177:387–392
69. Hezel AF, Gurumurthy S, Granot Z, Swisa A, Chu GC, Bailey G, Dor Y, Bardeesy N, Depinho RA (2008) Pancreatic LKB1 deletion leads to acinar polarity defects and cystic neoplasms. Mol Cell Biol 28:2414–2425
70. Partanen JI, Nieminen AI, Makela TP, Klefstrom J (2007) Suppression of oncogenic properties of c-Myc by LKB1-controlled epithelial organization. Proc Natl Acad Sci U S A 104:14694–14699

71. Baron A, Migita T, Tang D, Loda M (2004) Fatty acid synthase: a metabolic oncogene in prostate cancer? J Cell Biochem 91:47–53
72. Zhan Y, Ginanni N, Tota MR, Wu M, Bays NW, Richon VM, Kohl NE, Bachman ES, Strack PR, Krauss S (2008) Control of cell growth and survival by enzymes of the fatty acid synthesis pathway in HCT-116 colon cancer cells. Clin Cancer Res 14:5735–5742
73. Chajes V, Cambot M, Moreau K, Lenoir GM, Joulin V (2006) Acetyl-CoA carboxylase alpha is essential to breast cancer cell survival. Cancer Res 66:5287–5294
74. Brunet J, Vazquez-Martin A, Colomer R, Grana-Suarez B, Martin-Castillo B, Menendez JA (2008) BRCA1 and acetyl-CoA carboxylase: the metabolic syndrome of breast cancer. Mol Carcinog 47:157–163
75. Magnard C, Bachelier R, Vincent A, Jaquinod M, Kieffer S, Lenoir GM, Venezia ND (2002) BRCA1 interacts with acetyl-CoA carboxylase through its tandem of BRCT domains. Oncogene 21:6729–6739
76. Ray H, Moreau K, Dizin E, Callebaut I, Venezia ND (2006) ACCA phosphopeptide recognition by the BRCT repeats of BRCA1. J Mol Biol 359:973–982
77. Shen Y, Tong L (2008) Structural evidence for direct interactions between the BRCT domains of human BRCA1 and a phospho-peptide from human ACC1. Biochemistry 47:5767–5773
78. Chesney J (2006) 6-Phosphofructo-2-kinase/fructose-2,6-bisphosphatase and tumor cell glycolysis. Curr Opin Clin Nutr Metab Care 9:535–539
79. Rider MH, Bertrand L, Vertommen D, Michels PA, Rousseau GG, Hue L (2004) 6-phosphofructo-2-kinase/fructose-2,6-bisphosphatase: head-to-head with a bifunctional enzyme that controls glycolysis. Biochem J 381:561–579
80. Almeida A, Moncada S, Bolanos JP (2004) Nitric oxide switches on glycolysis through the AMP protein kinase and 6-phosphofructo-2-kinase pathway. Nat Cell Biol 6:45–51
81. Marsin AS, Bertrand L, Rider MH, Deprez J, Beauloye C, Vincent MF, Van den Berghe G, Carling D, Hue L (2000) Phosphorylation and activation of heart PFK-2 by AMPK has a role in the stimulation of glycolysis during ischaemia. Curr Biol 10:1247–1255
82. Marsin AS, Bouzin C, Bertrand L, Hue L (2002) The stimulation of glycolysis by hypoxia in activated monocytes is mediated by AMP-activated protein kinase and inducible 6-phosphofructo-2-kinase. J Biol Chem 277:30778–30783
83. Goren N, Manzano A, Riera L, Ambrosio S, Ventura F, Bartrons R (2000) 6-Phosphofructo-2-kinase/fructose-2,6-bisphosphatase expression in rat brain during development. Brain Res Mol Brain Res 75:138–142
84. Atsumi T, Chesney J, Metz C, Leng L, Donnelly S, Makita Z, Mitchell R, Bucala R (2002) High expression of inducible 6-phosphofructo-2-kinase/fructose-2,6-bisphosphatase (iPFK-2; PFKFB3) in human cancers. Cancer Res 62:5881–5887
85. Minchenko A, Leshchinsky I, Opentanova I, Sang N, Srinivas V, Armstead V, Caro J (2002) Hypoxia-inducible factor-1-mediated expression of the 6-phosphofructo-2-kinase/fructose-2,6-bisphosphatase-3 (PFKFB3) gene. Its possible role in the Warburg effect. J Biol Chem 277:6183–6187
86. Telang S, Yalcin A, Clem AL, Bucala R, Lane AN, Eaton JW, Chesney J (2006) Ras transformation requires metabolic control by 6-phosphofructo-2-kinase. Oncogene 25:7225–7234
87. Calvo MN, Bartrons R, Castano E, Perales JC, Navarro-Sabate A, Manzano A (2006) PFKFB3 gene silencing decreases glycolysis, induces cell-cycle delay and inhibits anchorage-independent growth in HeLa cells. FEBS Lett 580:3308–3314
88. Launonen V (2005) Mutations in the human LKB1/STK11 gene. Hum Mutat 26:291–297
89. Esteller M, Avizienyte E, Corn PG, Lothe RA, Baylin SB, Aaltonen LA, Herman JG (2000) Epigenetic inactivation of LKB1 in primary tumors associated with the Peutz-Jeghers syndrome. Oncogene 19:164–168
90. Trojan J, Brieger A, Raedle J, Esteller M, Zeuzem S (2000) 5′-CpG island methylation of the LKB1/STK11 promoter and allelic loss at chromosome 19p13.3 in sporadic colorectal cancer. Gut 47:272–276

91. Zheng B, Jeong JH, Asara JM, Yuan YY, Granter SR (2009) Oncogenic B-RAF negatively regulates the tumor suppressor LKB1 to promote melanoma cell. Mol Cell 33(2):237–247
92. Esteve-Puig R, Canals F, Colome N, Merlino G, Recio JA (2009) Uncoupling of the LKB1-AMPKalpha energy sensor pathway by growth factors and oncogenic BRAF. PLoS ONE 4:e4771
93. Shell SA, Lyass L, Trusk PB, Pry KJ, Wappel RL, Bacus SS (2008) Activation of AMPK is necessary for killing cancer cells and sparing cardiac cells. Cell Cycle 7:1769–1775
94. Spector NL, Yarden Y, Smith B, Lyass L, Trusk P, Pry K, Hill JE, Xia W, Seger R, Bacus SS (2007) Activation of AMP-activated protein kinase by human EGF receptor 2/EGF receptor tyrosine kinase inhibitor protects cardiac cells. Proc Natl Acad Sci U S A 104:10607–10612
95. Bastie CC, Zong H, Xu J, Busa B, Judex S, Kurland IJ, Pessin JE (2007) Integrative metabolic regulation of peripheral tissue fatty acid oxidation by the SRC kinase family member Fyn. Cell Metab 5:371–381
96. Hurley RL, Barre LK, Wood SD, Anderson KA, Kemp BE, Means AR, Witters LA (2006) Regulation of AMP-activated protein kinase by multisite phosphorylation in response to agents that elevate cellular cAMP. J Biol Chem 281:36662–36672
97. Qi J, Gong J, Zhao T, Zhao J, Lam P, Ye J, Li JZ, Wu J, Zhou HM, Li P (2008) Downregulation of AMP-activated protein kinase by Cidea-mediated ubiquitination and degradation in brown adipose tissue. EMBO J 27:1537–1548
98. Schneider MB, Matsuzaki H, Haorah J, Ulrich A, Standop J, Ding XZ, Adrian TE, Pour PM (2001) Prevention of pancreatic cancer induction in hamsters by metformin. Gastroenterology 120:1263–1270
99. Anisimov VN, Egormin PA, Bershtein LM, Zabezhinskii MA, Piskunova TS, Popovich IG, Semenchenko AV (2005) Metformin decelerates aging and development of mammary tumors in HER-2/neu transgenic mice. Bull Exp Biol Med 139:721–723
100. Huang X, Wullschleger S, Shpiro N, McGuire VA, Sakamoto K, Woods YL, McBurnie W, Fleming S, Alessi DR (2008) Important role of the LKB1-AMPK pathway in suppressing tumorigenesis in PTEN-deficient mice. Biochem J 412:211–221
101. Tomimoto A, Endo H, Sugiyama M, Fujisawa T, Hosono K, Takahashi H, Nakajima N, Nagashima Y, Wada K, Nakagama H, Nakajima A (2008) Metformin suppresses intestinal polyp growth in ApcMin/+ mice. Cancer Sci 99:2136–2141
102. Ben Sahra I, Laurent K, Loubat A, Giorgetti-Peraldi S, Colosetti P, Auberger P, Tanti JF, Le Marchand-Brustel Y, Bost F (2008) The antidiabetic drug metformin exerts an antitumoral effect in vitro and in vivo through a decrease of cyclin D1 level. Oncogene 27:3576–3586
103. Shu Y, Sheardown SA, Brown C, Owen RP, Zhang S, Castro RA, Ianculescu AG, Yue L, Lo JC, Burchard EG, Brett CM, Giacomini KM (2007) Effect of genetic variation in the organic cation transporter 1 (OCT1) on metformin action. J Clin Invest 117:1422–1431
104. Evans JM, Donnelly LA, Emslie-Smith AM, Alessi DR, Morris AD (2005) Metformin and reduced risk of cancer in diabetic patients. BMJ 330:1304–1305
105. Bowker SL, Majumdar SR, Veugelers P, Johnson JA (2006) Increased cancer-related mortality for patients with type 2 diabetes who use sulfonylureas or insulin. Diabetes Care 29:254–258
106. Hursting SD, Lashinger LM, Colbert LH, Rogers CJ, Wheatley KW, Nunez NP, Mahabir S, Barrett JC, Forman MR, Perkins SN (2007) Energy balance and carcinogenesis: underlying pathways and targets for intervention. Curr Cancer Drug Targets 7:484–491
107. Gotlieb WH, Saumet J, Beauchamp MC, Gu J, Lau S, Pollak MN, Bruchim I (2008) In vitro metformin anti-neoplastic activity in epithelial ovarian cancer. Gynecol Oncol 110:246–250
108. Ashrafian H (2006) Cancer's sweet tooth: the Janus effect of glucose metabolism in tumorigenesis. Lancet 367:618–621
109. Gatenby RA, Gillies RJ (2004) Why do cancers have high aerobic glycolysis? Nat Rev Cancer 11:891–899
110. Shaw RJ. (2006) Glucose metabolism and cancer. Curr Opin Cell Biol 6:598–608

Chapter 10
The Role of the IGF Axis in Human Malignancy: Evidence from Epidemiological Studies and Tissue Analysis

Julia V. Burnier, Shun Li, and Pnina Brodt

Abbreviations

ALS	Acid-labile subunit
CRC	Colorectal carcinoma
ECM	Extracellular matrix
ELISA	Enzyme-linked immunosorbent assay
GH	Growth hormone
GI	Gastrointestinal
HCC	Hepatocellular carcinoma
HGF	Hepatocyte growth factor
HNSCC	Head and neck squamous cell carcinoma
HPV	Human papilloma virus
IGF	Insulin-like growth factor
IGFBP	Insulin-like growth factor binding protein
IGFIR	Insulin-like growth factor-I receptor
IHC	Immunohistochemistry
IR	Insulin receptor
IRMA	Immunoradiometric assay
MCF	Human breast adenocarcinoma cell line
MMP	Matrix metalloproteinase
MT1-MMP	Membrane type 1 matrix metalloproteinase
NSCLC	Non–small-cell lung cancer

P. Brodt (✉)
Department of Medicine, McGill University, Montreal, QC, Canada H3A 1A1

Department of Oncology, McGill University, Montreal, QC, Canada H3A 1A1

Department of Surgery, McGill University, Surgical Labs, Royal Victoria Hospital, Room H6.25 687 Pine Avenue, Montreal, QC, Canada H3A 1A1
e-mail: pnina.brodt@muhc.mcgill.ca

I.G. Fantus (ed.), *Insulin Resistance and Cancer: Epidemiology, Cellular and Molecular Mechanisms and Clinical Implications*, Energy Balance and Cancer 1,
DOI 10.1007/978-1-4419-9911-5_10,

PDGF	Platelet-derived growth factor
PIN	Prostatic intraepithelial neoplasia
PSA	Prostate specific antigen
RIA	Radioimmunoassay
SCLC	Small-cell lung cancer
SIL	Squamous intraepithelial lesion
uPA	Urokinase plasminogen activator
uPAR	uPA receptor

Role of the IGF Axis in Normal Development

The insulin-like growth factor (IGF) axis consists of the two highly homologous IGF ligands, IGF-I and IGF-II, three receptors that mediate the biological effects of the IGFs, namely, the insulin-like growth factor-I receptor (IGF-IR), the IGF-II receptor (IGF-IIR) and one of the two insulin receptor isoforms (IR-A), and six high affinity IGF binding proteins, IGFBP1–6.

IGF-I and IGF-II are the products of two independently regulated genes. Hepatocytes are the major source of IGF-I, producing 70% of IGF-I in the body. Liver IGF-I is regulated mainly by growth hormone (GH), although nutrition and insulin also play a role [1, 2]. In turn, IGF-I regulates GH production through a tightly controlled feedback loop [3]. In extra-hepatic tissues, *IGF-I* gene expression is regulated by tissue-specific factors, as well as by GH [4]. *IGF-II* gene expression is GH independent and regulated by hormones and tissue-specific growth factors [5]. In humans, IGF-I and IGF-II play a major role during embryogenesis and in growth and development. Circulating IGF-I levels decrease after puberty, while IGF-II levels remain high and are higher than those of IGF-I throughout adulthood. In rodents, however, IGF-II is functional during fetal growth and development but IGF-I is the major circulating ligand in postnatal and adult animals (reviewed in [5]). The endocrine, as well as the autocrine/paracrine growth promoting effects of IGF-I and IGF-II are mediated mainly through binding to, and activation of the IGF-IR that conveys survival and growth signals to the cell through a complex network of signaling mechanisms (reviewed in [6]).

IGF-I levels can be affected by altered catabolic states (e.g., sepsis and trauma) [7]. Lifestyle parameters such as nutrition, obesity, exercise, and smoking are associated with changes in IGF-I levels that can be transient or long lasting. In certain pathological conditions associated with malnutrition, such as cachexia, anorexia, and inflammatory bowel disease, serum IGF-I levels are reduced [8], whereas obesity is associated with increased circulating levels of free IGF-I due, in part, to reduced IGFBP levels [9].

The IGF-IR is expressed in most cell types, but not in hepatocytes and T lymphocytes. During development, it plays a crucial role in cell survival and growth. Mice lacking the IGF-IR are 45% smaller in size at birth as compared to wild type littermates due to organ hypoplasia [10], develop lung, skin, bone, and neurological defects, and invariably die due to respiratory failure [10, 11].

In the circulation, the IGFs are found mostly in a complex with IGFBPs. The six high affinity binding proteins can modulate IGF action in complex ways that involve both inhibiting IGF action by blocking its binding to the receptor (e.g., IGFBP-1 and -2) or promoting its activity by stabilizing and increasing IGF half-life (e.g., IGFP-3). In the circulation, IGF-I and IGF-II are normally found in a ternary complex with IGFBP-3 and an acid-labile subunit (ALS) [12]. Once this complex dissociates, the binary IGFBP–IGF complex is removed from the circulation and can cross the vascular endothelium to interact with cell surface receptors in the target tissue. In the microenvironment of a target tissue, IGFBPs can serve as a reservoir, releasing the ligands slowly in response to signals that activate IGFBP-degrading proteases [5, 13]. In addition to their IGF-dependent effects, IGFBPs can also have direct, growth-modulating effects and stimulate cell growth (e.g., IGFBP-5) or induce apoptosis (e.g., IGFBP-3) in a ligand-independent manner [13].

The IGF System in Human Malignancy-Epidemiological Studies

Early Epidemiological Studies Implicate the GH-IGF Axis in Malignancy

IGF levels are tightly regulated and an imbalance in their production or function can lead to uncontrolled cell growth and malignant transformation. Early indications for a possible association between serum IGF levels and cancer risk came from epidemiological studies that examined the correlation between body height (regulated by IGF) and cancer risk and found that taller individuals had a 20–60% increased risk for several cancers, with leg length most significantly correlated with risk (reviewed in [14]). Increased birth weight, height, and caloric intake have been linked to circulating IGF-I levels and cancer risk in other studies [15, 16]. In addition, a higher cancer incidence, particularly for colon cancer, has been observed in acromegaly, a condition characterized by chronically elevated GH levels resulting from a pituitary adenoma and a sustained increase in circulating GH levels and IGF-I production suggesting that circulating IGF levels were relevant to cancer development (reviewed in [17]).

Increased IGF-I levels could result in increased cancer risk due to several potential mechanisms, including increased protection of damaged cells from apoptosis, stimulation of cellular proliferation, and in the case of hormone-dependent malignancies such as breast and prostate carcinoma, increased sex hormone production. However, when interpreting epidemiological data based on measurements of circulating IGF-I levels, several factors should be considered. There is a wide person-to-person variation in circulating IGF levels and even in the same individual, serum IGF-I concentrations can fluctuate significantly over time [18]. Among the many factors affecting IGF-I levels are genetic determinants, diet, lifestyle, time of measurement, hormone levels, ligand bioavailability, as well as the method of measurements and confounding factors such as the levels of other growth factors and blood markers. These factors are discussed at greater length in Sect. 2.6 and should be borne in mind when assessing the data reviewed below. A selection of large studies performed in the past 10 years (since 1999) for breast, prostate, and gastrointestinal (GI) cancer patients is summarized in Table 10.1.

The IGF Axis in Breast Cancer

More than half a century ago, Ray practiced hypophysectomy as a treatment for metastatic breast cancer and showed an effect in some patients, thereby providing early evidence for a link between pituitary hormones and the progression of this disease [19]. This effect was initially attributed to the depletion of prolactin, but it has since become clear that serum IGF-I, under the control of pituitary GH, may be a major factor in breast cancer growth and progression [20, 21].

In 1995, Bruning et al. [22] reported the results of a case–control study involving 150 women presenting with stage I or II breast cancer whose circulating IGF-I and IGFBP-3 levels were investigated prior to, or after, surgery. They showed that in premenopausal women, serum IGF-I concentrations were elevated and IGFBP-3 levels were decreased, resulting in increased IGF-I/IGFBP-3 ratios and concluded that the serum IGF-I/IGFBP-3 ratio is a significant breast cancer risk factor. These findings were confirmed by a subsequent large prospective study involving more than a thousand nurses that identified serum IGF-I levels as a risk factor for breast cancer in premenopausal women regardless of age, although the association was stronger in women younger than 50 years of age [23]. A third study by Vadgama et al. showed that serum IGF-I and IGFBP-3 levels correlated with tumor histopathology, recurrence rates and probability of survival in premenopausal African American women, leading the authors to conclude that lowering plasma IGF-I levels may reduce the risk of developing breast cancer, slow the progression of the disease, lower the risk of recurrence and increase survival [24]. This was further supported by two meta-analyses of epidemiologic and clinical studies that concluded that a positive association existed between high IGF-I and IGFBP-3 levels and breast cancer risk in pre- but not in postmenopausal women [25, 26], while a large prospective, nested case–control study confirmed this association, but only in patients diagnosed after the age of 50 years [27]. However, the authors of the latter study found a significant heterogeneity in the relationship of breast cancer with serum IGF-I and IGFBP-3 levels depending on the time interval between blood donation and tumor diagnosis, with the best correlation found in women whose breast cancer diagnosis was made more the 2 years after blood collection. Pansanisi et al. found that IGF-I may increase the risk of breast cancer recurrence in postmenopausal women but only in the presence of high platelet-derived growth factor (PDGF) levels [28]. Furthermore, a study by Bryne et al. later showed that mammographic breast density – a strong predictor of breast cancer – correlated with increased plasma IGF-I:IGFBP-3 ratios in premenopausal women and proposed that premenopausal levels of IGF-I and IGFBP-3 may be etiological factors that

Table 10.1 Results of representative large clinical studies performed for breast, prostate and GI cancer patients between 1999 and 2009

Type of cancer	Year	Experimental design	Patients/ controls	Sample and method of analysis	Parameters analyzed	Findings and conclusions	References
Breast cancer	2009	Prospective Case-Cohort, nested		Serum (ELISA)	Total and free **IGF-I and IGFBP-3**[a] Insulin, glucose, estradiol	Increase in breast cancer risk most associated with free IGF-I levels	[136]
	2008	Nested case-control	325/647	Serum (RIA)	**IGF-I, IGFBP-3**	Modest positive association between IGF-I levels and risk of cancer	[34]
	2008	Prospective study	110 post meno-pausal women	Serum (RIA)	**IGF-I** PDGF, fructosamine, C-reactive protein	High IGF-I and PDGF together (but not separately) are associated with increased relapse	[28]
	2008	Tissue Collection	348 fresh tissues	mRNA and peptide levels measured by RT-PCR and ELISA, respectively	**IGF-I, IGF-II, IGFBP-3**	High mRNA associated with small tumors, early TMN stage or low grade; high expression of IGFI associated with lower risk of disease recurrence	[137]
	2008	Case-control	43/38	Serum (IRMA, ELISA, RIA)	Total and free **IGF-I and II**, **Pro-IGFII**, **IGFBP-1**, **IGFBP-2**, **IGFBP-3**, **IGFBP-4**, **IGFBP-6**	Patients showed elevated free IGF-I and IGF-II, reduced total IGF-II and altered IGFBPs levels as compared to healthy controls	[36]
	2008	Cross-sectional	737	Plasma (ELISA)	**IGFBP3 and IGF-1**	Total (intact and fragmented) and intact IGFBP-3 forms correlated differently with other breast cancer risk factors	[138]

(continued)

Table 10.1 (continued)

Type of cancer	Year	Experimental design	Patients/ controls	Sample and method of analysis	Parameters analyzed	Findings and conclusions	References
	2007	Tissue Collection	508/206	mRNA levels	**IGF-I, IGF-IR**	IGF-I mRNA expression was higher in benign breast disease than in breast cancer tissue (in both tumor and adjacent tissue). In breast cancer patients, IGF-I expression was higher in the tumor-adjacent than in tumor tissue. Higher IGF-I gene expression in these patients was associated with a more favorable outcome	[139]
	2007	Cross-sectional	977	Plasma (ELISA)	**IGF-I, IGFBP-3** mammographic density	IGF-I and the IGF-I/IGFBP-3 ratio were positively associated with mammographic density in postmenopausal women	[30]
	2006	Nested case-control	317/317	Plasma (ELISA)	**IGF-I, IGFBP-1, IGFBP-3, GH**	No association was found between IGF-I, IGFBP1, IGFBP-3, or GH levels and risk	[35]
	2006	Population-based nested case-control study	15,192 in 1974 and 18,724 in 1989	Serum and plasma (ELISA)	**IGF-I and IGFBP-3**	An association between IGF-I:IGFBP-3 ratio and risk was found in the oldest postmenopausal and youngest premenopausal groups, only after age stratification	[140]
	2005	Large, nested case-control study	800/1,129	Plasma (ELISA)	**IGF-I, free IGF, IGFBP-3, and IGFBP-1**	Among postmenopausal women, IGFBP-3, IGFBP-1, and IGF-1 were not associated with breast cancer risk. Among premenopausal women, higher IGF-I levels were associated with a modestly increased risk	[23]
	2004	Meta-analysis	N/A	N/A	**IGF-I, IGFBP-3**	The data support an association between high IGF-I and IGFBP-3 levels and increased risk of cancer in premenopausal women	[26]
	2000	Cross-sectional study	250+	Plasma (ELISA)	**IGF-I, IGFBP-3** breast density	Mammographic density is positively associated with plasma IGF-I levels and inversely associated with plasma IGFBP-3 levels among premenopausal women	[29]
	1999	Retrospective study	130	Plasma and serum (RIA)	**IGF-I, IGFBP-3**	Increased plasma IGF-I and serum IGFBP-3 correlate with tumor histopathology, recurrence,	[24]

Prostate[b]	2009	Tissue staining study	644 TMA cores	Tissue	**IGF-IR**, **IR**	Immunoreactivity was seen with anti-IGF-IR and anti IR antibodies suggesting that hybrid receptors may also be present. Insulin receptor staining was higher on malignant than on benign prostate epithelial cells	[64]
	2007	Nested case-control study	630/630	Serum (ELISA)	**IGF-I**, **IGFBP-3**	The results were compatible with a small increase in risk in patients with high IGF-I concentrations, particularly for advanced-stage disease. There was no association with IGFBP-3 levels	[57]
	2007	Retrospective	281/305	Serum (ELISA)	**IGF-I**, **IGFBP-3** Free PSA (fPSA)	IGF-I/fPSA ratios enhanced detection	[141]
	2007	Prospective nested case-control	727/887	Serum (ELISA)	**IGF-I**, **IGFBP-3**	There was no clear overall association between IGF-I, IGFBP-3 and IGF-1:IGFBP-3 molar ratio and risk	[142]
	2006	Case-cohort	524/2,167	Plasma (ELISA)	**IGF-I**, **IGFBP-3**	High levels of IGFBP-3 but not IGF-I were associated with an increased risk of prostate cancer	[143]
	2005		462/462	Plasma (ELISA)	**IGF-I**, **IGFBP-3**	Men with higher concentrations of IGF-1 and IGFBP-3 had a higher risk of prostate cancer	[144]
	2005	Nested case-control	100/400	Plasma (several methods)	**IGF-1**, **IGF-II**, **IGFBP-2**, **IGFBP-3**	The results suggested that IGF axis variables are not long-term predictors of the occurrence of prostate cancer	[145]
	2005	Nested case-control	174/174	Plasma (IRMA, RIA)	**IGF-I**, **IGFBP-3**	IGF-I levels were not positively associated with the risk of prostate carcinoma; however, an increase in the IGFBP-3 level was associated with a modest decrease in risk	[146]

(continued)

Table 10.1 (continued)

Type of cancer	Year	Experimental design	Patients/ controls	Sample and method of analysis	Parameters analyzed	Findings and conclusions	References
	2004	Prospective study in a population-based non-screened cohort	281/560	Plasma (IRMA)	**IGF-I**, **IGFBP-3**	There was an increase in risk with increasing plasma IGF-I levels which was attenuated after adjustment for IGFBP-3. The risk for men younger was significantly stronger than for men older than 59	[51]
	2003	Retrospective	408/437	Serum (ELISA)	**IGF-I**, **IGFBP-3**	A high IGF-I:IGFBP-3 molar ratio was associated with increased risk. High IGF-I was associated with increased risk among men with less advanced disease at diagnosis	[147]
	2003	Prospective nested case-control	100/400	Plasma (ELISA)	**IGF-I**, **IGFBP-3**	There was no significant association between either IGF-I or IGFBP-3 levels and prostate cancer risk	[148]
	2002		120/44	Plasma (ELISA, RIA)	**IGF-I**, **IGFBP-2**, **IGFBP-3**	Plasma IGFBP-3 levels were lowest in patients with bone metastases. IGFBP-2 levels were inversely correlated with prostatic tumor volume	[149]
	2001	Case-control	128/306	Plasma (ELISA)	**IGF-I**, **IGF-II**, **IGFBP-1**, **IGFBP-3**	There was a positive association between IGF-I levels and risk, and inverse association with IGFBP-3 levels and no significant association with IGF-II levels	[150]
	2000	Prospective case-control	171/67	Serum (chemiluminescence method, RIA)	**IGF-I**	There was no significant association between IGF-I serum levels and prostate cancer	[151]
	2000		179/486	Serum (ELISA, IFMA)	**IGF-I**, **IGFBP-3**, PSA	In men with elevated serum PSA, serum IGF-I is not a useful diagnostic test for prostate cancer, but it may be associated with benign prostatic hyperplasia	[56]

	2000	Prospective, cohort, case-control	72/127	Serum (RIA)	**IGF-I**, **IGF-II**, **IGFBP-3**, PSA	High IGF-I and low IGF-II are independently associated with increased risk, but PSA level is a much stronger predictor	[52]
	1999	Prospective	71/174	Serum (IRMA)	**IGF-1**, **IGFD**, **and IGF-1**/PSA ratio	IGF-1, IGF density, IGF-1/PSA ratio, and PSA were significantly higher in patients with PC than in those with benign disease. IGF-1 levels did not enhance the performance of PSA but the IGF-1/PSA ratio significantly improved PC detection over PSA alone	[54]
	1999	Prospective	37/57	Serum (IRMA)	**IGF-I**, PSA	Serum IGF-1 does not help to predict patients with prostate cancer. PSA level and even age were better predictors of the presence of cancer than serum IGF-1 levels	[55]
G.I. malignancies							
CRC[c]	2008	Prospective case-cohort	438/816	Serum (ELISA)	**IGF-I**, **free IGF-I**, **IGFBP3** Insulin, glucose, total estradiol, waist circumference	Insulin, waist circumference and free IGF-I were each associated with colorectal cancer incidence in multivariate models. However, these associations became nonsignificant when adjusted for one another	[71]
	2008		527	Plasma (ELISA)	**IGF-I**, **IGF-II**, **IGFBP-3**, C-peptide[d]	Higher baseline plasma IGFBP-3 levels were associated with a significantly greater chemotherapy response rate after adjusting for other prognostic factors, whereas neither IGF-I nor IGF-II levels significantly predicted tumor response	[82]
	2008	Case-control	52/52	??????	**IGF-I**, **GH**, Insulin, C-peptide[d]	A positive correlation was found between increased blood IGF-I levels and colon cancer incidence.	[82]
	2007	Nested case-control study	375/750	Plasma (IRMA)	**IGF-I**, **IGFBP-1**, **IGFBP-3**, C-peptide	IGF peptides were not associated with colon cancer risk in either men or women. Only plasma C-peptide levels were associated with colorectal cancer risk (in men)	[79]

(continued)

Table 10.1 (continued)

Type of cancer	Year	Experimental design	Patients/ controls	Sample and method of analysis	Parameters analyzed	Findings and conclusions	References
	2007	Nested case-control study	1,078/1,078	Serum (RIA, IRMA)	**IGFBP-1**, **IGFBP-2**, C-peptide	No clear colon or rectal cancer risk associations were observed for IGFBP-1 or -2 An association was found with C-peptide levels	[152]
	2006	Prospective, cohort study	526	Plasma (ELISA)	**IGF-I**, **IGFBP-3** level of physical activity	For the physically active, increased IGFBP-3 levels were associated with reduced colorectal cancer-associated deaths. No association was seen for IGF-1. The authors concluded that the beneficial effects of physical activity in reducing colorectal cancer mortality may involve IGFBP-3	[153]
	2003	Nested case-control	282/282	Serum (ELISA)	**IGF-I**, **IGFBP-3**	No significant association between IGF-I, IGFBP-3 and CRC risk	[70]
	2003	Nested case-control	168/336	Plasma (IRMA, RIA)	**IGFBP-1**, **IGFBP-2**, **insulin**	IGFBP-1 and IGFBP-2 showed no association but chronic hyperinsulinemia was moderately associated with CRC risk	[154]
	2002	Nested case-control	102/200	Serum (IRMA)	**IGF-II**	High IGF-II increases risk of CRC	[155]
	2001	Cohort	135/661	Serum (RIA)	**IGF-I**, **IGF-II**, **IGFBP-3**	Serum IGF-I was not associated with risk but increased circulating IGF-II and IGFBP-3 may indicate impending CRC	[156]
	2001	Prospective	53/47	Serum (RIA, IRMA)	**IGF-I**, **IGFBP-3**	IGF-I and IGFBP-3 levels are associated with risk of CRC and adenoma progression	[76]
	2000	Nested case-control	276/236	Plasma (ELISA)	**IGF-I**, **IGFBP-3**	Increased IGF-I and decreased IGFBP-3 are associated with increased risk of colorectal adenoma and cancer	[72]

	2000	Nested case-control study in women	102/200	Serum (RIA, IRMA)	**IGF-I**, **IGFBP-1**, **-2**, **-3**, C-peptide,	A statistically significant decrease in colorectal cancer risk was observed for increasing levels of IGFBP-1 or IGFBP-2 and an increased risk for IGFBP-3, but the association with IGF-I levels was not statistically significant	[157]
	2000	Nested case-control	193/318	Plasma (ELISA)	**IGF-I**, **IGF-II IGFBP-3**	Circulating IGF-I and IGFBP-3, but not IGF-II levels, are associated with development of CRC	[73]
	2000	Comparative	52/293	Serum (RIA, IRMA)	**IGF-I**, **IGF-II**, **IGFBP-2**, **IGFBP-3**	There was a significant association between IGF-II and IGFBP-2 levels and the occurrence of adenomas (detected by colonoscopies) but no association with IGF-I and/or IGFBP-3 levels. Serum IGF-II may be a marker for adenomas	[83]
	2000	Prospective colonoscopic evaluation	66	Serum (RIA)	**IGF-I**	The development of additional adenomas in previously diagnosed acromegaly patients was associated with elevated serum IGF-I	[158]
	2000	Case-control	92/57	Serum (RIA, IRMA)	**IGF-I**, **IGF-II**, **IGFBP-2 and -3**	There was a Significant association between increased IGF-II and IGFBP-2 levels and the occurrence of adenomas	[159]
	1999	Case-control	41/50	Serum(IRMA)	**IGF-I**, **IGF-II and IGFBP-3**	High circulating IGF-I and -II levels may be associated with colorectal cancer	[160]
Multiple malignancies							
Breast, prostate, colon, lung	2004	Systematic review and meta-regression analysis of case-control studies, including studies nested in cohorts	3,609/7,137	N/A	**IGF-I**, **IGFBP3**	In men, high concentrations of IGF-I were associated with increased risk for prostate cancer and in premenopausal women, for breast cancer. High concentrations of IGFBP-3 were associated with increased risk for breast cancer premenopausal women Associations were stronger when assessing plasma than serum samples and in case-control studies vs. nested studies	[25]

(continued)

Table 10.1 (continued)

Type of cancer	Year	Experimental design	Patients/ controls	Sample and method of analysis	Parameters analyzed	Findings and conclusions	References
						Conclusion: Circulating IGF-I and IGFBP-3 levels are associated with increased risk for common cancers, but the associations are modest and vary among different tumor types. Laboratory methods need to be standardized	
Fourteen different cancers including prostate, colorectal and lung carcinoma	2006	Nested case-control study in men with meta analysis for CRC, prostate and lung cancer.	1,051/3,142	Serum	**IGF-I, IGF-II, IGFBP-3**	The odds ratio between the highest and lowest quartile IGF-1 groups were 1.31 for prostate, 1.37 for colorectal and 1.02 for lung cancer Conclusion: IGF-I, IGF-II, and IGFBP-3 measurements have no value in cancer screening but IGF-I and IGF-II may be of aetiological significance in relation to colorectal and prostate cancer (modestly increased risk when comparing highest to lowest IGF-I quartiles)	[161]

[a] IGF axis proteins are in bold letters
[b] The information in this section is based, in part, on ref. [59]
[c] The information in this section is based, in part, on ref. [162]
[d] C-peptide is a marker for insulin secretion

link breast density and breast cancer risk [29]. A positive but weak association between plasma IGF-I concentrations and mammographic density was also recently found in a Norwegian study of postmenopausal women [30]. In several studies, IGF-I levels were found to be significantly higher [31, 32], while IGFBP-3 levels were lower [33] in breast cancer patients as compared to healthy controls, and a recent nested, case–control study among more than 35,000 Norwegian women found IGF-I to be modestly correlated with risk of breast cancer development in women younger than 50 years of age [34], while IGFBP-3 levels correlated inversely with risk. Taken together these studies suggest that IGF-I:IGFBP-3 ratios rather than total serum IGF-I levels may be the more relevant risk factor in premenopausal women, suggesting that IGF-I bioavailability is the critical factor and indirectly implicating IGF-IR receptor activation in breast cancer initiation and progression. This issue remains highly controversial however, and a recent study, reported by some of the same authors that initially documented the circulating IGF-I/breast cancer link [23], has in fact concluded that circulating IGF-I, IGFBP-1, IGFBP-3, and GH levels have no important association with breast cancer risk in premenopausal women [35].

The significance of IGF-II levels in breast cancer development has also been investigated. For example, Espelund et al. recently reported that breast cancer patients had elevated circulating free IGF-I and IGF-II, reduced total IGF-II, and altered IGFBPs levels as compared to healthy controls [36].

In several studies that analyzed IGF-I receptor levels in breast cancers, receptor expression has been documented in the majority of breast tumor samples and found to be elevated in primary breast malignancies relative to benign hyperplasia and normal breast tissue [37–39]. In one of these studies, Pezzino et al. [38] used a sensitive radioimmunoassay (RIA) to measure IGF-IR content in over 200 breast cancer specimens and found that IGF-IR was detectable in >80% of breast cancer tissues but in only 31% of normal breast specimens, with the mean IGF-IR content value tenfold higher in the malignant specimens. When the IGF-IR content in the cancer tissues was then correlated with various host and tumor variables, no correlation with age, menopausal status, body weight, histological type, tumor size, tumor grade, and axillary node involvement was found, but a significant correlation was observed with insulin receptor (IR) levels, and to a lesser extent, with the estrogen receptor content of the tumors. Interestingly, Voskuil et al. measuring IGF-IR, IGF-I, and IGF-II mRNA levels in surgical specimens found that they were higher in normal than in malignant breast tissue, suggesting that post-translational mechanisms may be important [40] and highlighting the fact that results of such analyses and the conclusions derived may vary considerably, depending on the assay used.

Several studies suggest that increased expression and/or function of IGF-IR in primary breast carcinomas may be relevant to disease progression and outcome in several ways. For example, Peyrat and Bonneterre [37] and Railo et al. [41] reported that in ER-negative cancers, IGF-IR positivity correlated with a poorer outcome. This may also be due to the rescue effect of IGF-IR because it has been shown that increased IGF-IR expression levels correlated with resistance to radiation, increased tumor recurrence, and a shorter disease-free survival time [42].

In more recent studies, low levels of activated IGF-IR were shown to be associated with local recurrence in lymph node negative breast cancers [43], and an IGF-I–activated gene transcription program that was first identified in cultured breast carcinoma MCF-7 cells was found to be manifest in the majority of ER-negative and a subset of ER-positive breast tumors analyzed and correlated with poor prognosis [44]. Taken together, these studies have collectively identified the IGF-IR as a target for breast cancer therapy and provided a rationale for the inclusion of breast carcinoma among several primary malignancies being targeted with IGF-IR inhibitors in ongoing phase I and II clinical trials [45–47].

The IGF Axis in Prostate Cancer

Similar to breast cancer, an association between circulating IGF-I levels and cancer risk was also documented for prostate cancer, first by Mantzoros et al. in 1997 and later, in larger population-based case–control studies reported by other groups [48–50]. In one such study, high serum IGF-I measured as early as 9–10 years before diagnosis were found to be associated with increased prostate cancer risk [51]. Interestingly, in some studies, an inverse correlation was found between serum IGF-II levels and prostate cancer risk leading the authors to conclude that IGF-II may actually inhibit the development of prostate cancer [52], possibly by inducing a differentiation program in prostate epithelial cells. Shaneyfelt et al. in a meta-analysis of all studies on hormonal predictors of risk for prostate cancer performed up to the year 2000 concluded that serum testosterone or IGF-I levels were risk factors for developing prostate cancer [53]. Importantly, a prospective study examining the importance of IGF-I and prostate specific antigen (PSA) levels, together or separately, as markers for prostate cancer found that IGF-I/PSA ratios were a superior indicator of the presence of prostate cancer than either measurement alone [54], leading the authors of this study to conclude that increased IGF-1/PSA ratios may be a useful tool for early detection of prostate cancer.

However, the importance of circulating IGF-I levels as predictors of increased prostate cancer risk remains a controversial issue, as contradicting evidence has also been documented. In several reported studies, IGF-I was not found to be a useful marker for prostate cancer [55–57] and in one study, a significant association between low circulating IGF-I levels and prostate cancer was actually observed, when IGF-I levels were measured at the time of prostatectomy [58].

Rowlands et al. performed a meta-analysis of all published studies linking prostate cancer to IGF levels and concluded that while increased circulating IGF-I levels were positively associated with prostate cancer risk, there was no consistent association with IGFBP-3 levels and there was little evidence for an association of risk with IGF-II, IGFBP-1 or IGFBP-2 levels [59]. Similarly, analysis of 12 prospective studies led to the conclusion that elevated circulating IGF-I, but not IGF-II or IGFBP-2 concentrations were associated with a moderately increased risk for prostate cancer [60].

In reviewing these seemingly conflicting data, LeRoith and Roberts have noted that while no association between IGF-I levels, and prostatic cancer was evident in cross-sectional studies, there was, nevertheless, a consistent correlation in all prospective studies [4]. Based on the data, the authors concluded that although IGF-I levels at the time of diagnosis may not be highly informative, there is a predictive value to serum IGF-I levels when measured in younger men, prior to onset of the disease. This suggests that the prolonged exposure of the prostate to high circulating IGF-I levels may increase the risk of hyperplasia and cancer later in life. Serum IGF-I levels may therefore be a better prostate cancer predictor early in life than a tumor marker or a prognostic indicator in prostate cancer patients. The studies thus identify serum IGF-I as a potential target in preventative prostate cancer care [4].

The role of the IGF-I receptor in prostate cancer progression has also been a subject of conflicting results. Findings of decreased IGF-IR expression levels in malignant vs. benign prostatic epithelium [61], of no measurable differences in expression [62] and of significantly upregulated IGF-IR expression, at both the protein and mRNA levels in primary prostate cancer relative to benign prostatic epithelium have all been reported [63]. Expression of IGF-IR in bone metastases was reported to be either similar to or downregulated in comparison to the primary tumors [62, 63] (reviewed in [6]). In a recent study, immunoreactivity with antibodies to both IGF-IR and IR was observed in prostate carcinoma specimens, and IR staining intensity was significantly higher in malignant than in benign prostate epithelial cells. This raises the possibility that prostate cancer cells express hybrid IR/IGF-IR receptors that can also contribute to cell survival and proliferation. The authors of this study also suggested that the IR isoform A expressed in prostate carcinoma cells may be functionally significant to disease progression [64]. Taken together, the data suggest that the IGF-IR is only one of several prostate epithelial cell receptors that can be activated by IGF ligands and that further examination of all of these receptors in cancer cells, both in the primary tumors and in bone metastases may be warranted and could be more informative with regard to the role of the IGF axis in tumor progression in this disease than analysis of IGF-IR alone.

The IGF Axis in Gastrointestinal (GI) Malignancies

Early evidence for an association between the IGF axis and GI malignancies came from epidemiological data on acromegaly patients who have abnormally high circulating levels of GH and IGF-I. These studies revealed a significant association between acromegaly and increased incidence of colorectal cancer [65–67]. Later evidence implicated insulin and IGF-I, as well as other growth factors, such as EGF, TGF-α, and PDGF in the development of colon cancer [68, 69].

In the last decade, the link between colon cancer and IGF has been examined in several studies including large-scale correlation studies between serum IGF levels and cancer risk. While only a weak correlation was found in one study of Japanese–American men [70], the data overall showed a positive correlation between colon cancer risk and serum IGF-I levels [71–73], an inverse correlation with serum IGFBP-3 levels [72], and no correlation with circulating IGF-II levels [72, 74]. A recent case–control study involving 52 colon cancer patients revealed significantly higher levels of IGF-I in the blood of these patients than in the control group [75]. Prospective studies revealed an increased risk of developing colon cancer in individuals with increased serum/plasma IGF-I levels [74, 76] and found that patients with adenomas who had a higher risk of developing colon cancer also had increased IGF-I levels and lower IGFBP-3 levels than controls [76]. Similarly, low expression of IGFBP-3 mRNA in normal colonic mucosa was found to predict increased risk of adenomas [77]. In addition, studies on healthy individuals revealed an association between IGF-I levels and colorectal carcinoma (CRC) risk. A meta-analysis based on five case–control studies also concluded that there was a positive association between elevated IGF-I levels and CRC risk [25] (and reviewed in [78]). These results were not, however, supported by a nested, case–control study in Japanese men [79], suggesting that IGF-related risk may be affected by other factors that vary among different cohorts.

Several studies have examined IGF-IR expression in colon cancer specimens. In a retrospective study using immunohistochemistry (IHC), positive IGF-IR staining was found to correlate with the stage of the disease and was strong in metastatic CRC [80]. These results were essentially confirmed by another study that measured IGF-IR mRNA and protein levels in 40 paired samples of CRC and adjacent normal mucosa and documented an overexpression in the tumor tissue [81]. Furthermore, an association between circulating IGF axis proteins and a therapeutic response was also demonstrated. In a first-line chemotherapy trial for metastatic colorectal cancer, Fuchs et al. showed that higher baseline plasma IGFBP-3 levels correlated with a better response rate to chemotherapy, although no such correlation was observed with total circulating IGF-I and IGF-II levels, suggesting that similarly to data obtained for breast cancer patients, free IGF levels and IGF:IGFBP-3 ratios may be a more pertinent measure of the impact of IGF on disease progression and response to therapy [82] than the ligand levels alone.

In this context, it should also be noted that loss of imprinting for IGF-II was documented in CRC and therefore autocrine, IGF-II–mediated effects may be as important in this disease as the endocrine effects of circulating IGF. Moreover, Renehan et al. found that IGF-II levels increased in Dukes A and B but not in metastatic CRC disease, while serum IGFBP-2 levels correlated with the stage of the disease and decreased following curative surgery, suggesting that circulating IGFBP-2 levels more accurately reflected tumor load and could potentially serve as a marker for disease progression [83].

The IGF Axis in Other Malignancies

While IGF proteins as potential risk factors were analyzed most extensively in prostate, breast, and colon cancer, their association with other malignancies has also been investigated. For example, in a study of metastatic uveal melanoma, a significant association was found between high IGF-IR expression levels and death due to metastasis [84]. This was later confirmed in a study that found high levels of IGF-IR immunoreactivity in uveal melanoma tumors with liver metastasis [85]. Recent data also implicated the IGF axis in the development of ovarian tumors. In a study of 215 ovarian carcinoma patients, high levels of free, but not total, IGF-I were associated with elevated risk for disease progression [86]. This finding was supported by other studies where similar correlations were found but only in women who developed ovarian cancer at the age of 55 or younger [87, 88]. However, a case–control study by Dal Maso et al. found an inverse association between serum IGF-I and IGFBP-3 levels and ovarian cancer risk but identified IGFBP-1 levels as a potential risk factor, concluding that IGFBP-3 may play a protective role in ovarian cancer [89]. IGF-II expression levels in tumor specimens have also been studied in ovarian cancer patients. One study found elevated IGF-II and decreased IGFBP-3 mRNA expression levels to be associated with poor prognosis and concluded that patients with high IGF-II expression had increased risk for disease progression and death [90]. However an IHC-based analysis by another group failed to reveal an increase in IGF-II levels in ovarian carcinoma as compared to benign tissue and only a slight increase was seen in endometrial cancers. This may have been due to the small sample size used in this analysis (five ovarian cancer specimens), but may also indicate variations between mRNA and protein expression levels in this malignancy [91].

There are contradictory data on the link between IGF and the incidence or progression of cervical cancer. In a case–control study, patients with either high or low-grade squamous intraepithelial lesions (SILs) of the cervix had significantly higher serum IGF-I and IGFBP-3 levels and IGF-I:IGFBP-3 ratios than control subjects [92]. In contrast, however, another study reported an association between reduced risk for high-grade cervical intraepithelial neoplasia and human papilloma virus (HPV) infection and increased IGF-I levels, suggesting that IGF-I may actually play a protective role in the development of this disease [93]. IGF-II levels were found to be higher in cervical cancers than in matched control tissue. Interestingly, in this study, small nests of lymph node metastases could be identified by IHC using IGF-II as a marker [91].

Finally, the relationship between IGF proteins and lung cancer was also studied. In one such study, serum IGF-I and IGF-II levels were found to be higher in non–small-cell (NSCLC) and small-cell lung cancer (SCLC) patients than in healthy controls [94]. In another, hospital-based case–control study, IGF-I levels in the highest quartile were associated with a twofold increase in lung cancer and with distant vs. localized disease, while IGFBP-3 levels, once adjusted for IGF-I levels, were associated with a greater than 50% reduced risk for lung cancer [95]. However, in a subsequent study by the same authors, the data did not support the same conclusions [96] and other studies also failed to identify an association between serum IGFs or IGFBPs and lung cancer risk [97, 98]. The role of IGF-IR has also been analyzed in lung cancer. In a study of stage I NSCLC using IHC, no significant relationship was found between clinical/histopathological parameters and IGF-IR expression levels [99].

Factors Contributing to the Disparity in Results Obtained from Different Epidemiological Studies

When evaluating the data reviewed above, and in an effort to reconcile the disparate data and conclusions from different studies, several factors should be considered. Circulating IGF levels vary widely among individuals and can be affected by multiple factors such as nutrition, weight, and age (reviewed in [100]). Hormonal status may also affect individual IGF levels [101] and both IGF-I and IGFBP levels are altered during pregnancy [102, 103]. Finally, genetic factors have also been identified that can contribute to person-to-person variations in IGF levels. Hong et al., studying 97 pairs of monozygotic twins showed that genetic factors played a role in determining IGF levels, although several nongenetic, metabolic factors have been identified in this study such as circulating insulin, glucose, and IGFBP-1 levels that contributed to individual variations between twins [104]. Several studies have shown that gene polymorphisms also contribute to differences in serum IGF-I and IGFBP-3 levels. For example, Vaessen et al. [105] examined the role of IGF-I promoter region polymorphism in the variation in circulating IGF-I levels as related to height and the incidence of type II diabetes and found that carriers of a 192-bp allele had higher IGF-I levels and increased body height. In studies by Jernstrom et al., circulating IGF-I levels were found to be positively associated with the absence of an IGF-I 19-repeat allele and the presence of the CYP3A4 variant and the AIB1 26-repeat alleles, while a single base pair polymorphism in the promoter region of the IGFBP-3 gene was found to be related to the level of IGFBP-3 in the circulation [106] (reviewed in [107]). Collectively, the results show that the regulation of circulating IGF-I and IGFBP-3 levels is multifactorial and influenced by a number of interacting genetic and nongenetic factors.

Even in the same individual, IGF levels may fluctuate daily [18]. For example, in a study reported by Milani et al., IGF-I levels were measured repeatedly in the same individuals over a 2-week period and found to fluctuate considerably in some of the subjects, resulting in a shift in the quartile position for over 40% of the subjects during this interval [108]. Similarly, Shalet et al. have shown that daily fluctuations can change the circulating IGF levels from the normal to abnormal range within days [109].

In the studies reviewed above, there is a marked variation in the overall reported levels of circulating IGFs and IGFBP. In addition to the factors already noted above, other variables such as the sampling method (e.g., plasma or serum), the type of epidemiological study performed (e.g., prospective or case–control studies), the method used to quantify serum/plasma levels, and the variability in population cohorts (e.g., age, ethnicity, hormonal status) could all have contributed to these differences (see Table 10.1). Sampling and quantification methods can have a significant impact on the results. IGF-I levels were found to be 10% higher overall in serum when compared to plasma levels [110] and an analysis of blood samples from 173 individuals that compared the Nichols Advantage IGF-I Assay and four other, commercially available IGF-I test kits, revealed differences in the readings obtained from different assays [111]. This suggests that a standardization of the sampling and quantification methods and a tighter control of the subjects' health background and pretest conditions such as nutritional intake may be required in order to obtain more consistent data on the clinical significance of circulating IGF as a predictor of cancer risk or a marker for cancer detection.

Gene and Protein Expression Profiling Identify IGF Axis Proteins As Tumor Progression Factors and Potential Biomarkers

Circulating IGF levels can impact cancer development and progression through multiple pathways including the promotion of hyperplasia and increased survival of transformed cells. In addition, the IGF axis has been implicated in the induction of an invasive/metastatic phenotype, among others, by promoting the expression/production of extracellular matrix (ECM) degrading enzymes such as the matrix metalloproteinases (MMPs) [112, 113]. A comprehensive review of the evidence in support of a causative/mechanistic link between human malignant disease progression and the activation of the IGF axis is beyond the scope of this chapter and the reader is referred to previous reviews by our group [6, 114] and other chapters in this collection for critical discussions of this subject matter. Here, we review recent evidence from gene and protein profiling of clinical specimens that have collectively identified IGF axis proteins as potential tumor biomarkers and that show that these proteins are often coordinately upregulated with molecular mediators of invasion and metastasis, providing indirect evidence for a functional link between these molecules. One such study is a protein microarray analysis performed on 30 paired head and neck squamous cell carcinomas (HNSCCs) and benign epithelial cells that revealed a significant upregulation of IGF-II and MMP-7 [115] in the cancer specimens. MMP-7 and IGF ligands were also identified as biomarkers for other tumor types including ovarian carcinoma and gastric cancer [115–117]. In addition, a protein microarray analysis that compared 210 hepatocellular carcinoma (HCC) specimens and corresponding normal liver found that IGF-II expression in the tumor cells was upregulated together with ADAM (a disintegrin and metalloprotease) levels [118]. Recent studies provide a functional basis for the link between MMP-7 and the IGF axis. Namely, Nakamura et al. have shown that tumor cell–derived MMP-7 can cleave all six IGF binding proteins and thereby increase IGF-I and IGF-II bioavailability in the tumor microenvironment and as a result enhance tumor cell survival and growth [119]. This group has also shown that MMP-7–mediated proteolysis of IGFBP-3 increased IGF-I bioavailability and thereby IGF-IR activation in two human colon cancer cell lines [120] and could generate bioactive IGF-II by degrading an ECM-bound IGF-II/IGFBP-2 complex, triggering IGF-II–induced signal transduction in human colon cancer cells [121]. Interestingly, in a recent study by Oshima et al. that analyzed 205 CRC specimens and adjacent normal mucosa by qRT-PCR, increased *mmp-7* and *igf-ir* gene expression were found in the cancerous tissue and IGF-IR levels correlated with the incidence of liver metastasis [122].

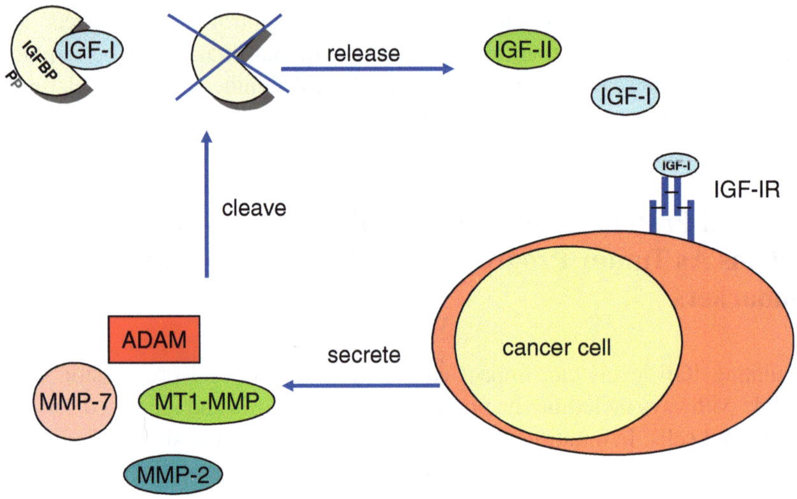

Fig. 10.1 The matrix metalloproteinases regulate IGF bioavailability and enhance IGF-IR signaling. Depicted is a diagrammatic representation of the reciprocal crosstalk between the IGF axis and the matrix metalloproteinases (MMPs)

Moreover, a recent study revealed that in colon cancer patients undergoing chemotherapy, serum IGFBP-3 levels increased during or after treatment, in the absence of progressive disease, but significantly decreased during disease progression, as MMP-7 levels increased. This suggests that tumor-derived circulating MMP-7 may contribute to an acquired resistance to chemotherapy (and tumor cell survival) by degrading IGFBP-3 and increasing IGF bioavailability [123] (see diagrammatic representation in Fig. 10.1).

Membrane type 1 matrix metalloproteinase (MT1-MMP) is another IGF-regulated metalloproteinase that was implicated in tumor invasion and metastasis [113, 114]. When MT1-MMP and IGF-IR expression and localization were examined in human prostate cancer and benign epithelium using IHC, high MT1-MMP expression was observed in prostatic intraepithelial neoplasia (PIN) and prostate cancer cells but not in the benign tissues. IGF-IR was also highly expressed in prostate carcinoma tissue. Using human prostate cancer cell lines, the authors of this study also found that treatment of the cells with a synthetic androgen together with IGF-I increased MT1-MMP expression, suggesting a potential regulatory link in prostate cancer cells in vivo [124].

The urokinase plasminogen activator (uPA) is another ECM-degrading enzyme that can be regulated by IGF [6]. Studies using several different human malignant cell lines including pancreatic [125] and CRC [126] cells have shown that IGF-I can induce tumor cell migration and invasion by activating the uPA/uPA receptor (uPAR) system in coordination with other factors such as hepatocyte growth factor (HGF) [125]. The potential relevance of this association to tumor progression in vivo was demonstrated in a breast cancer tissue microarray analysis that identified IGF-IR and uPA upregulation in over 50% of breast cancer cases and found that increased expression of either IGF-IR or uPA or both was associated with a worse disease outcome [127].

While increased expression of IGF-IR and/or IGF ligands has frequently been noted in microarray analysis of malignant specimens and metastases from different tumor types including colorectal, gallbladder, prostate, hepatocellular, renal cell, and ovarian carcinoma and meningioma [118, 128–133], a recent study based on tissue microarray analysis suggests that IGFBPs may also be important biomarkers of progression and possibly targets for therapy. In this study, over 4,000 primary invasive breast cancers and 120 benign breast tissue samples were analyzed, revealing a significant increase in IGFBP-2 in the breast cancer as compared to benign tissue [134]. A significantly increased expression of IGFBP-2 and IGFBP-3 was also found in pediatric medulloblastoma and this correlated with poor prognosis [135]. However, the role of these binding proteins in tumor progression in these malignancies remains unclear. Taken together, these studies suggest that IGF axis proteins may be effective biomarkers of progression, at least in some malignancies. Moreover, they indicate that IGF axis proteins may be most useful as biomarkers when measured in combination with other indicators of acquired tumor aggressiveness such as the MMPs and uPA/uPAR axis proteins.

Summary and Conclusions

IGF axis proteins have been linked to increased cancer risk in various malignancies. First indications of this link came from early studies that implicated GH in tumor development and this has led to identification of circulating IGF-I levels as a potential risk factor for some of the most common human malignancies including prostate, breast, and CRC. A careful review of the literature reveals, however, that the data linking circulating IGFs to cancer risk should be subjected to careful scrutiny and interpreted with caution as it varied significantly from study to study and could not always be reproducibly observed even in different studies reported by the same groups. The factors that may be contributing to this disparity have been summarized above. In addition, the data suggest that results of different studies may be most consistent when adjusted to the variability in other parameters such as the levels of circulating IGFBPs, particularly IGFBP-3, that determine IGF bioavailability, other circulating markers such as PSA (for prostate cancer), estrogen levels, and the estrogen receptor status (for breast cancer), as well as variables such as IR status of the tumors and host parameters such as age, weight, and nutritional status. Circulating IGF levels may therefore be most valuable as a clinical indicator when considered in combination with, and in the context of other host factors and tumor markers. This may also apply to the utility of IGF axis proteins as tumor biomarkers. Namely, the data suggest that when the expression of any one of the axis proteins (i.e., IGF-IR, IGF ligands, or IGFBPs) is examined in isolation, the correlation with tumor progression is likely to be highly variable, even for the same tumor type. However, a combined analysis of several axis proteins within the same tumor specimens may reveal significant perturbations in IGF-IR signaling and function that correlate with tumor stage and this may be further refined by assessing the expression of other IGF-IR–regulated proteins with known pro-malignant functions such as the MMPs. In summary, therefore, the studies suggest that while IGF axis proteins (in the circulation or expressed in malignant cells) are functionally relevant to disease progression, their value as clinical indicators may be more limited and best assessed in the context of additional host and tumor-specific factors.

References

1. Le Roith D, Bondy C, Yakar S, Liu J-L, Butler A (2001) The somatomedin hypothesis: 2001. Endocr Rev 22:53–74
2. Sell C (2003) Caloric restriction and insulin-like growth factors in aging and cancer. Horm Metab Res 35:705–711
3. Tannenbaum GS, Guyda HJ, Posner BI (1983) Insulin-like growth factors: a role in growth hormone negative feedback and body weight regulation via brain. Science 220:77–79
4. LeRoith D, Roberts CT (2003) The insulin-like growth factor system and cancer. Cancer Lett 195:127–137
5. Yakar S, LeRoith D, Brodt P (2005) The role of the growth hormone/insulin-like growth factor axis in tumor growth and progression: lessons from animal models. Cytokine Growth Factor Rev 16:407–420
6. Samani AA, Yakar S, LeRoith D, Brodt P (2007) The role of the IGF system in cancer growth and metastasis: overview and recent insights. Endocr Rev 28:20–47
7. Yu H, Rohan T (2000) Role of the insulin-like growth factor family in cancer development and progression. J Natl Cancer Inst 92:1472–1489
8. Thissen JP, Ketelslegers JM, Underwood LE (1994) Nutritional regulation of the insulin-like growth factors. Endocr Rev 15:80–101
9. Nam SY, Lee EJ, Kim KR et al (1997) Effect of obesity on total and free insulin-like growth factor (IGF)-1, and their relationship to IGF-binding protein (BP)-1, IGFBP-2, IGFBP-3, insulin, and growth hormone. Int J Obes Relat Metab Disord 21:355–359
10. Liu JP, Baker J, Perkins AS, Robertson EJ, Efstratiadis A (1993) Mice carrying null mutations of the genes encoding insulin-like growth factor I (Igf-1) and type 1 IGF receptor (Igf1r). Cell 75:59–72
11. Powell-Braxton L, Hollingshead P, Warburton C et al (1993) IGF-I is required for normal embryonic growth in mice. Genes Dev 7:2609–2617
12. Jones JI, Clemmons DR (1995) Insulin-like growth factors and their binding proteins: biological actions. Endocr Rev 16:3–34
13. Mohan S, Baylink DJ (2002) IGF-binding proteins are multifunctional and act via IGF-dependent and -independent mechanisms. J Endocrinol 175:19–31
14. Gunnell D (2001) Height, leg length, and cancer risk: a systematic review. Epidemiol Rev 23(2):313–342
15. Gunnell DJ, Smith GD, Holly JM, Frankel S (1998) Leg length and risk of cancer in the Boyd Orr cohort. BMJ 317:1350–1351
16. Frankel S, Gunnell DJ, Peters TJ, Maynard M, Davey Smith G (1998) Childhood energy intake and adult mortality from cancer: the Boyd Orr Cohort Study. BMJ 316:499–504
17. Loeper S, Ezzat S (2008) Acromegaly: re-thinking the cancer risk. Rev Endocr Metab Disord 9:41–58
18. Borofsky ND, Vogelman JH, Krajcik RA, Orentreich N (2002) Utility of insulin-like growth factor-1 as a biomarker in epidemiologic studies. Clin Chem 48:2248–2251

19. Ray BS (1967) Current cancer concepts. Hypophysectomy as palliative treatment. JAMA 200:974–975
20. Hankinson SE, Willett WC, Colditz GA et al (1998) Circulating concentrations of insulin-like growth factor-I and risk of breast cancer. Lancet 351:1393–1396
21. Yee D, Rosen N, Favoni RE, Cullen KJ (1991) The insulin-like growth factors, their receptors, and their binding proteins in human breast cancer. Cancer Treat Res 53:93–106
22. Bruning PF, Van Doorn J, Bonfrer JM et al (1995) Insulin-like growth-factor-binding protein 3 is decreased in early-stage operable pre-menopausal breast cancer. Int J Cancer 62:266–270
23. Schernhammer ES, Holly JM, Pollak MN, Hankinson SE (2005) Circulating levels of insulin-like growth factors, their binding proteins, and breast cancer risk. Cancer Epidemiol Biomarkers Prev 14:699–704
24. Vadgama JV, Wu Y, Datta G, Khan H, Chillar R (1999) Plasma insulin-like growth factor-I and serum IGF-binding protein 3 can be associated with the progression of breast cancer, and predict the risk of recurrence and the probability of survival in African-American and Hispanic women. Oncology 57:330–340
25. Renehan AG, Zwahlen M, Minder C, O'Dwyer ST, Shalet SM, Egger M (2004) Insulin-like growth factor (IGF)-I, IGF binding protein-3, and cancer risk: systematic review and meta-regression analysis. Lancet 363:1346–1353
26. Shi R, Yu H, McLarty J, Glass J (2004) IGF-I and breast cancer: a meta-analysis. Int J Cancer 111:418–423
27. Rinaldi S, Peeters PH, Berrino F et al (2006) IGF-I, IGFBP-3 and breast cancer risk in women: the European Prospective Investigation into Cancer and Nutrition (EPIC). Endocr Relat Cancer 13:593–605
28. Pasanisi P, Venturelli E, Morelli D, Fontana L, Secreto G, Berrino F (2008) Serum insulin-like growth factor-I and platelet-derived growth factor as biomarkers of breast cancer prognosis. Cancer Epidemiol Biomarkers Prev 17:1719–1722
29. Byrne C, Colditz GA, Willett WC, Speizer FE, Pollak M, Hankinson SE (2000) Plasma insulin-like growth factor (IGF) I, IGF-binding protein 3, and mammographic density. Cancer Res 60:3744–3748
30. Bremnes Y, Ursin G, Bjurstam N, Rinaldi S, Kaaks R, Gram IT (2007) Insulin-like growth factor and mammographic density in postmenopausal Norwegian women. Cancer Epidemiol Biomarkers Prev 16:57–62
31. Peyrat JP, Bonneterre J, Hecquet B et al (1993) Plasma insulin-like growth factor-1 (IGF-1) concentrations in human breast cancer. Eur J Cancer 29A:492–497
32. Barni S, Lissoni P, Brivio F et al (1994) Serum levels of insulin-like growth factor-I in operable breast cancer in relation to the main prognostic variables and their perioperative changes in relation to those of prolactin. Tumori 80:212–215
33. Ng EH, Ji CY, Tan PH, Lin V, Soo KC, Lee KO (1998) Altered serum levels of insulin-like growth-factor binding proteins in breast cancer patients. Ann Surg Oncol 5:194–201
34. Vatten LJ, Holly JM, Gunnell D, Tretli S (2008) Nested case-control study of the association of circulating levels of serum insulin-like growth factor I and insulin-like growth factor binding protein 3 with breast cancer in young women in Norway. Cancer Epidemiol Biomarkers Prev 17:2097–2100
35. Schernhammer ES, Holly JM, Hunter DJ, Pollak MN, Hankinson SE (2006) Insulin-like growth factor-I, its binding proteins (IGFBP-1 and IGFBP-3), and growth hormone and breast cancer risk in The Nurses Health Study II. Endocr Relat Cancer 13:583–592
36. Espelund U, Cold S, Frystyk J, Orskov H, Flyvbjerg A (2008) Elevated free IGF2 levels in localized, early-stage breast cancer in women. Eur J Endocrinol 159:595–601
37. Peyrat JP, Bonneterre J (1992) Type 1 IGF receptor in human breast diseases. Breast Cancer Res Treat 22:59–67
38. Pezzino V, Papa V, Milazzo G, Gliozzo B, Russo P, Scalia PL (1996) Insulin-like growth factor-I (IGF-I) receptors in breast cancer. Ann N Y Acad Sci 784:189–201
39. Ando S, Panno ML, Salerno M et al (1998) Role of IRS-1 signaling in insulin-induced modulation of estrogen receptors in breast cancer cells. Biochem Biophys Res Commun 253:315–319

40. Voskuil DW, Bosma A, Vrieling A, Rookus MA, van't Veer LJ (2004) Insulin-like growth factor (IGF)-system mRNA quantities in normal and tumor breast tissue of women with sporadic and familial breast cancer risk. Breast Cancer Res Treat 84:225–233
41. Railo MJ, von Smitten K, Pekonen F (1994) The prognostic value of insulin-like growth factor-I in breast cancer patients. Results of a follow-up study on 126 patients. Eur J Cancer 30A:307–311
42. Turner BC, Haffty BG, Narayanan L et al (1997) Insulin-like growth factor-I receptor overexpression mediates cellular radioresistance and local breast cancer recurrence after lumpectomy and radiation. Cancer Res 57:3079–3083
43. Peiro G, Benlloch S, Sanchez-Tejada L et al (2009) Low activation of Insulin-like Growth Factor 1-Receptor (IGF1R) is associated with local recurrence in early breast carcinoma. Breast Cancer Res Treat 117(2):433–441
44. Creighton CJ, Casa A, Lazard Z et al (2008) Insulin-like growth factor-I activates gene transcription programs strongly associated with poor breast cancer prognosis. J Clin Oncol 26:4078–4085
45. Yee D (2002) The insulin-like growth factor system as a treatment target in breast cancer. Semin Oncol 29:86–95
46. Sachdev D, Yee D (2006) Inhibitors of insulin-like growth factor signaling: a therapeutic approach for breast cancer. J Mammary Gland Biol Neoplasia 11:27–39
47. Yee D (2007) Targeting insulin-like growth factor pathways. Br J Cancer 96(Suppl):R7–R10
48. Wolk A, Mantzoros CS, Andersson SO et al (1998) Insulin-like growth factor 1 and prostate cancer risk: a population-based, case-control study. J Natl Cancer Inst 90:911–915
49. Mantzoros CS, Tzonou A, Signorello LB, Stampfer M, Trichopoulos D, Adami HO (1997) Insulin-like growth factor 1 in relation to prostate cancer and benign prostatic hyperplasia. Br J Cancer 76:1115–1118
50. Stattin P, Bylund A, Rinaldi S et al (2000) Plasma insulin-like growth factor-I, insulin-like growth factor-binding proteins, and prostate cancer risk: a prospective study. J Natl Cancer Inst 92:1910–1917
51. Stattin P, Rinaldi S, Biessy C, Stenman UH, Hallmans G, Kaaks R (2004) High levels of circulating insulin-like growth factor-I increase prostate cancer risk: a prospective study in a population-based nonscreened cohort. J Clin Oncol 22:3104–3112
52. Harman SM, Metter EJ, Blackman MR, Landis PK, Carter HB (2000) Serum levels of insulin-like growth factor I (IGF-I), IGF-II, IGF-binding protein-3, and prostate-specific antigen as predictors of clinical prostate cancer. J Clin Endocrinol Metab 85:4258–4265
53. Shaneyfelt T, Husein R, Bubley G, Mantzoros CS (2000) Hormonal predictors of prostate cancer: a meta-analysis. J Clin Oncol 18:847–853
54. Djavan B, Bursa B, Seitz C et al (1999) Insulin-like growth factor 1 (IGF-1), IGF-1 density, and IGF-1/PSA ratio for prostate cancer detection. Urology 54:603–606
55. Cutting CW, Hunt C, Nisbet JA, Bland JM, Dalgleish AG, Kirby RS (1999) Serum insulin-like growth factor-1 is not a useful marker of prostate cancer. BJU Int 83:996–999
56. Finne P, Auvinen A, Koistinen H et al (2000) Insulin-like growth factor I is not a useful marker of prostate cancer in men with elevated levels of prostate-specific antigen. J Clin Endocrinol Metab 85:2744–2747
57. Allen NE, Key TJ, Appleby PN et al (2007) Serum insulin-like growth factor (IGF)-I and IGF-binding protein-3 concentrations and prostate cancer risk: results from the European Prospective Investigation into Cancer and Nutrition. Cancer Epidemiol Biomarkers Prev 16:1121–1127
58. Baffa R, Reiss K, El-Gabry EA et al (2000) Low serum insulin-like growth factor 1 (IGF-1): a significant association with prostate cancer. Tech Urol 6:236–239
59. Rowlands MA, Gunnell D, Harris R, Vatten LJ, Holly JM, Martin RM (2009) Circulating insulin-like growth factor peptides and prostate cancer risk: a systematic review and meta-analysis. Int J Cancer 124(10):2416–2429
60. Roddam AW, Allen NE, Appleby P et al (2008) Insulin-like growth factors, their binding proteins, and prostate cancer risk: analysis of individual patient data from 12 prospective studies. Ann Intern Med 149(461–71):W83–W88

61. Tennant M, Thrasher J, Twomey P, Drivdahl R, Birnbaum R, Plymate S (1996) Protein and messenger ribonucleic acid (mRNA) for the type 1 insulin- like growth factor (IGF) receptor is decreased and IGF-II mRNA is increased in human prostate carcinoma compared to benign prostate epithelium. J Clin Endocrinol Metab 81:3774–3782
62. Chott A, Sun Z, Morganstern D et al (1999) Tyrosine kinases expressed in vivo by human prostate cancer bone marrow metastases and loss of the type 1 insulin-like growth factor receptor. Am J Pathol 155:1271–1279
63. Hellawell GO, Turner GD, Davies DR, Poulsom R, Brewster SF, Macaulay VM (2002) Expression of the type 1 insulin-like growth factor receptor is up-regulated in primary prostate cancer and commonly persists in metastatic disease. Cancer Res 62:2942–2950
64. Cox ME, Gleave ME, Zakikhani M et al (2009) Insulin receptor expression by human prostate cancers. Prostate 69:33–40
65. Orme SM, McNally RJ, Cartwright RA, Belchetz PE (1998) Mortality and cancer incidence in acromegaly: a retrospective cohort study. United Kingdom Acromegaly Study Group. J Clin Endocrinol Metab 83:2730–2734
66. Pines A, Rozen P, Ron E, Gilat T (1985) Gastrointestinal tumors in acromegalic patients. Am J Gastroenterol 80:266–269
67. Ron E, Gridley G, Hrubec Z, Page W, Arora S, Fraumeni JF Jr (1991) Acromegaly and gastrointestinal cancer. Cancer 68:1673–1677
68. Richter M, Jurek D, Wrba F et al (2002) Cells obtained from colorectal microadenomas mirror early premalignant growth patterns in vitro. Eur J Cancer 38:1937–1945
69. Singer CF, Hudelist G, Lamm W, Mueller R, Czerwenka K, Kubista E (2004) Expression of tyrosine kinases in human malignancies as potential targets for kinase-specific inhibitors. Endocr Relat Cancer 11:861–869
70. Nomura AM, Stemmermann GN, Lee J, Pollak MN (2003) Serum insulin-like growth factor I and subsequent risk of colorectal cancer among Japanese-American men. Am J Epidemiol 158:424–431
71. Gunter MJ, Hoover DR, Yu H et al (2008) Insulin, insulin-like growth factor-I, endogenous estradiol, and risk of colorectal cancer in postmenopausal women. Cancer Res 68:329–337
72. Giovannucci E, Pollak MN, Platz EA et al (2000) A prospective study of plasma insulin-like growth factor-1 and binding protein-3 and risk of colorectal neoplasia in women. Cancer Epidemiol Biomarkers Prev 9:345–349
73. Ma J, Pollak M, Giovannucci E et al (2000) A prospective study of plasma levels of insulin-like growth factor I (IGF-I) and IGF-binding protein-3, and colorectal cancer risk among men. Growth Horm IGF Res 10(Suppl A):S28–S29
74. Ma J, Pollak MN, Giovannucci E et al (1999) Prospective study of colorectal cancer risk in men and plasma levels of insulin-like growth factor (IGF)-I and IGF-binding protein-3. J Natl Cancer Inst 91:620–625
75. Tripkovic I, Tripkovic A, Strnad M, Capkun V, Zekan L (2007) Role of insulin-like growth factor-1 in colon cancerogenesis: a case-control study. Arch Med Res 38:519–525
76. Renehan AG, Painter JE, Atkin WS, Potten CS, Shalet SM, O'Dwyer ST (2001) High-risk colorectal adenomas and serum insulin-like growth factors. Br J Surg 88:107–113
77. Keku TO, Sandler RS, Simmons JG et al (2008) Local IGFBP-3 mRNA expression, apoptosis and risk of colorectal adenomas. BMC Cancer 8:143
78. Donovan EA, Kummar S (2008) Role of insulin-like growth factor-1R system in colorectal carcinogenesis. Crit Rev Oncol Hematol 66:91–98
79. Otani T, Iwasaki M, Sasazuki S, Inoue M, Tsugane S (2007) Plasma C-peptide, insulin-like growth factor-I, insulin-like growth factor binding proteins and risk of colorectal cancer in a nested case-control study: the Japan public health center-based prospective study. Int J Cancer 120:2007–2012
80. Hakam A, Yeatman TJ, Lu L et al (1999) Expression of insulin-like growth factor-1 receptor in human colorectal cancer. Hum Pathol 30:1128–1133
81. Weber MM, Fottner C, Liu SB, Jung MC, Engelhardt D, Baretton GB (2002) Overexpression of the insulin-like growth factor I receptor in human colon carcinomas. Cancer 95:2086–2095

82. Fuchs CS, Goldberg RM, Sargent DJ et al (2008) Plasma insulin-like growth factors, insulin-like binding protein-3, and outcome in metastatic colorectal cancer: results from intergroup trial N9741. Clin Cancer Res 14:8263–8269
83. Renehan AG, Jones J, Potten CS, Shalet SM, O'Dwyer ST (2000) Elevated serum insulin-like growth factor (IGF)-II and IGF binding protein-2 in patients with colorectal cancer. Br J Cancer 83:1344–1350
84. All-Ericsson C, Girnita L, Seregard S, Bartolazzi A, Jager MJ, Larsson O (2002) Insulin-like growth factor-1 receptor in uveal melanoma: a predictor for metastatic disease and a potential therapeutic target. Invest Ophthalmol Vis Sci 43:1–8
85. Mallikarjuna K, Pushparaj V, Biswas J, Krishnakumar S (2006) Expression of insulin-like growth factor receptor (IGF-1R), c-Fos, and c-Jun in uveal melanoma: an immunohistochemical study. Curr Eye Res 31:875–883
86. Brokaw J, Katsaros D, Wiley A et al (2007) IGF-I in epithelial ovarian cancer and its role in disease progression. Growth Factors 25:346–354
87. Lukanova A, Lundin E, Toniolo P et al (2002) Circulating levels of insulin-like growth factor-I and risk of ovarian cancer. Int J Cancer 101:549–554
88. Peeters PH, Lukanova A, Allen N et al (2007) Serum IGF-I, its major binding protein (IGFBP-3) and epithelial ovarian cancer risk: the European Prospective Investigation into Cancer and Nutrition (EPIC). Endocr Relat Cancer 14:81–90
89. Dal Maso L, Augustin LS, Franceschi S et al (2004) Association between components of the insulin-like growth factor system and epithelial ovarian cancer risk. Oncology 67:225–230
90. Lu L, Katsaros D, Wiley A et al (2006) The relationship of insulin-like growth factor-II, insulin-like growth factor binding protein-3, and estrogen receptor-alpha expression to disease progression in epithelial ovarian cancer. Clin Cancer Res 12:1208–1214
91. Mathur SP, Landen CP, Datta SM, Hoffman MC, Mathur RS, Young RC (2003) Insulin-like growth factor II in gynecological cancers: a preliminary study. Am J Reprod Immunol 49:113–119
92. Wu X, Tortolero-Luna G, Zhao H, Phatak D, Spitz MR, Follen M (2003) Serum levels of insulin-like growth factor I and risk of squamous intraepithelial lesions of the cervix. Clin Cancer Res 9:3356–3361
93. Schaffer A, Koushik A, Trottier H et al (2007) Insulin-like growth factor-I and risk of high-grade cervical intraepithelial neoplasia. Cancer Epidemiol Biomarkers Prev 16:716–722
94. Izycki T, Chyczewska E, Naumnik W, Talalaj J, Panek B, Ossolinska M (2004) Serum levels of IGF-I and IGF-II in patients with lung cancer during chemotherapy. Exp Oncol 26:316–319
95. Yu H, Spitz MR, Mistry J, Gu J, Hong WK, Wu X (1999) Plasma levels of insulin-like growth factor-I and lung cancer risk: a case-control analysis. J Natl Cancer Inst 91:151–156
96. Spitz MR, Barnett MJ, Goodman GE, Thornquist MD, Wu X, Pollak M (2002) Serum insulin-like growth factor (IGF) and IGF-binding protein levels and risk of lung cancer: a case-control study nested in the beta-Carotene and Retinol Efficacy Trial Cohort. Cancer Epidemiol Biomarkers Prev 11:1413–1418
97. Ahn J, Weinstein SJ, Snyder K, Pollak MN, Virtamo J, Albanes D (2006) No association between serum insulin-like growth factor (IGF)-I, IGF-binding protein-3, and lung cancer risk. Cancer Epidemiol Biomarkers Prev 15:2010–2012
98. Lukanova A, Toniolo P, Akhmedkhanov A et al (2001) A prospective study of insulin-like growth factor-I, IGF-binding proteins-1, -2 and -3 and lung cancer risk in women. Int J Cancer 92:888–892
99. Lee CY, Jeon JH, Kim HJ et al (2008) Clinical significance of insulin-like growth factor-1 receptor expression in stage I non-small-cell lung cancer: immunohistochemical analysis. Korean J Intern Med 23:116–120
100. Brabant G, Wallaschofski H (2007) Normal levels of serum IGF-I: determinants and validity of current reference ranges. Pituitary 10:129–133
101. Ho KK, Gibney J, Johannsson G, Wolthers T (2006) Regulating of growth hormone sensitivity by sex steroids: implications for therapy. Front Horm Res 35:115–128

102. Caufriez A, Frankenne F, Hennen G, Copinschi G (1993) Regulation of maternal IGF-I by placental GH in normal and abnormal human pregnancies. Am J Physiol 265:E572–E577
103. Monaghan JM, Godber IM, Lawson N et al (2004) Longitudinal changes of insulin-like growth factors and their binding proteins throughout normal pregnancy. Ann Clin Biochem 41:220–226
104. Hong Y, Brismar K, Hall K, Pedersen NL, de Faire U (1997) Associations between insulin-like growth factor-I (IGF-I), IGF-binding protein-1, insulin and other metabolic measures after controlling for genetic influences: results from middle-aged and elderly monozygotic twins. J Endocrinol 153:251–257
105. Vaessen N, Heutink P, Janssen JA et al (2001) A polymorphism in the gene for IGF-I: functional properties and risk for type 2 diabetes and myocardial infarction. Diabetes 50:637–642
106. Jernstrom H, Deal C, Wilkin F et al (2001) Genetic and nongenetic factors associated with variation of plasma levels of insulin-like growth factor-I and insulin-like growth factor-binding protein-3 in healthy premenopausal women. Cancer Epidemiol Biomarkers Prev 10:377–384
107. Fletcher O, Gibson L, Johnson N et al (2005) Polymorphisms and circulating levels in the insulin-like growth factor system and risk of breast cancer: a systematic review. Cancer Epidemiol Biomarkers Prev 14:2–19
108. Milani D, Carmichael JD, Welkowitz J et al (2004) Variability and reliability of single serum IGF-I measurements: impact on determining predictability of risk ratios in disease development. J Clin Endocrinol Metab 89:2271–2274
109. Shalet SM, Toogood A, Rahim A, Brennan BM (1998) The diagnosis of growth hormone deficiency in children and adults. Endocr Rev 19:203–223
110. Renehan AG, Jones J, O'Dwyer ST, Shalet SM (2003) Determination of IGF-I, IGF-II, IGFBP-2, and IGFBP-3 levels in serum and plasma: comparisons using the Bland-Altman method. Growth Horm IGF Res 13:341–346
111. Krebs A, Wallaschofski H, Spilcke-Liss E et al (2008) Five commercially available insulin-like growth factor I (IGF-I) assays in comparison to the former Nichols advantage IGF-I in a growth hormone treated population. Clin Chem Lab Med 46:1776–1783
112. Zhang D, Bar-Eli M, Meloche S, Brodt P (2004) Dual regulation of MMP-2 expression by the type 1 insulin-like growth factor receptor: the phosphatidylinositol 3-kinase/Akt and Raf/ERK pathways transmit opposing signals. J Biol Chem 279:19683–19690
113. Zhang D, Brodt P (2003) Type 1 insulin-like growth factor regulates MT1-MMP synthesis and tumor invasion via PI 3-kinase/Akt signaling. Oncogene 22:974–982
114. Zhang D, Samani AA, Brodt P (2003) The role of the IGF-I receptor in the regulation of matrix metalloproteinases, tumor invasion and metastasis. Horm Metab Res 35:802–808
115. Weber A, Hengge UR, Stricker I et al (2007) Protein microarrays for the detection of biomarkers in head and neck squamous cell carcinomas. Hum Pathol 38:228–238
116. Davidson B, Zhang Z, Kleinberg L et al (2006) Gene expression signatures differentiate ovarian/peritoneal serous carcinoma from diffuse malignant peritoneal mesothelioma. Clin Cancer Res 12:5944–5950
117. Ajisaka H, Fushida S, Yonemura Y, Miwa K (2001) Expression of insulin-like growth factor-2, c-MET, matrix metalloproteinase-7 and MUC-1 in primary lesions and lymph node metastatic lesions of gastric cancer. Hepatogastroenterology 48:1788–1792
118. Tannapfel A, Anhalt K, Hausermann P et al (2003) Identification of novel proteins associated with hepatocellular carcinomas using protein microarrays. J Pathol 201:238–249
119. Nakamura M, Miyamoto S, Maeda H et al (2005) Matrix metalloproteinase-7 degrades all insulin-like growth factor binding proteins and facilitates insulin-like growth factor bioavailability. Biochem Biophys Res Commun 333:1011–1016
120. Miyamoto S, Yano K, Sugimoto S et al (2004) Matrix metalloproteinase-7 facilitates insulin-like growth factor bioavailability through its proteinase activity on insulin-like growth factor binding protein 3. Cancer Res 64:665–671
121. Miyamoto S, Nakamura M, Yano K et al (2007) Matrix metalloproteinase-7 triggers the matricrine action of insulin-like growth factor-II via proteinase activity on insulin-like growth factor binding protein 2 in the extracellular matrix. Cancer Sci 98:685–691

122. Oshima T, Akaike M, Yoshihara K et al (2008) Clinicopathological significance of the gene expression of matrix metalloproteinase-7, insulin-like growth factor-1, insulin-like growth factor-2 and insulin-like growth factor-1 receptor in patients with colorectal cancer: insulin-like growth factor-1 receptor gene expression is a useful predictor of liver metastasis from colorectal cancer. Oncol Rep 20:359–364
123. Gallego R, Codony-Servat J, Garcia-Albeniz X et al (2009) Serum IGF-I, IGFBP-3, and matrix metalloproteinase-7 levels and acquired chemo-resistance in advanced colorectal cancer. Endocr Relat Cancer 16:311–317
124. Sroka IC, McDaniel K, Nagle RB, Bowden GT (2008) Differential localization of MT1-MMP in human prostate cancer tissue: role of IGF-1R in MT1-MMP expression. Prostate 68:463–476
125. Bauer TW, Liu W, Fan F et al (2005) Targeting of urokinase plasminogen activator receptor in human pancreatic carcinoma cells inhibits c-Met- and insulin-like growth factor-I receptor-mediated migration and invasion and orthotopic tumor growth in mice. Cancer Res 65:7775–7781
126. Bauer TW, Fan F, Liu W et al (2005) Insulinlike growth factor-I-mediated migration and invasion of human colon carcinoma cells requires activation of c-Met and urokinase plasminogen activator receptor. Ann Surg 241:748–756; discussion 56–58
127. Nielsen TO, Andrews HN, Cheang M et al (2004) Expression of the insulin-like growth factor I receptor and urokinase plasminogen activator in breast cancer is associated with poor survival: potential for intervention with 17-allylamino geldanamycin. Cancer Res 64:286–291
128. Kornprat P, Rehak P, Ruschoff J, Langner C (2006) Expression of IGF-I, IGF-II, and IGF-IR in gallbladder carcinoma. A systematic analysis including primary and corresponding metastatic tumours. J Clin Pathol 59:202–206
129. Schips L, Zigeuner R, Ratschek M, Rehak P, Ruschoff J, Langner C (2004) Analysis of insulin-like growth factors and insulin-like growth factor I receptor expression in renal cell carcinoma. Am J Clin Pathol 122:931–937
130. Varghese S, Burness M, Xu H, Beresnev T, Pingpank J, Alexander HR (2007) Site-specific gene expression profiles and novel molecular prognostic factors in patients with lower gastrointestinal adenocarcinoma diffusely metastatic to liver or peritoneum. Ann Surg Oncol 14:3460–3471
131. Savli H, Szendroi A, Romics I, Nagy B (2008) Gene network and canonical pathway analysis in prostate cancer: a microarray study. Exp Mol Med 40:176–185
132. Wrobel G, Roerig P, Kokocinski F et al (2005) Microarray-based gene expression profiling of benign, atypical and anaplastic meningiomas identifies novel genes associated with meningioma progression. Int J Cancer 114:249–256
133. Sayer RA, Lancaster JM, Pittman J et al (2005) High insulin-like growth factor-2 (IGF-2) gene expression is an independent predictor of poor survival for patients with advanced stage serous epithelial ovarian cancer. Gynecol Oncol 96:355–361
134 So AI, Levitt RJ, Eigl B et al (2008) Insulin-like growth factor binding protein-2 is a novel therapeutic target associated with breast cancer. Clin Cancer Res 14:6944–6954
135. de Bont JM, van Doorn J, Reddingius RE et al (2008) Various components of the insulin-like growth factor system in tumor tissue, cerebrospinal fluid and peripheral blood of pediatric medulloblastoma and ependymoma patients. Int J Cancer 123:594–600
136. Gunter MJ, Hoover DR, Yu H et al (2009) Insulin, insulin-like growth factor-I, and risk of breast cancer in postmenopausal women. J Natl Cancer Inst 101:48–60
137. Mu L, Katsaros D, Wiley A et al (2008) Peptide concentrations and mRNA expression of IGF-I, IGF-II and IGFBP-3 in breast cancer and their associations with disease characteristics. Breast Cancer Res Treat 115(1):151–162
138. Diorio C, Brisson J, Berube S, Pollak M (2008) Intact and total insulin-like growth factor-binding protein-3 (IGFBP-3) levels in relation to breast cancer risk factors: a cross-sectional study. Breast Cancer Res 10:R42

139. Shin A, Ren Z, Shu XO, Cai Q, Gao YT, Zheng W (2007) Expression patterns of insulin-like growth factor 1 (IGF-I) and its receptor in mammary tissues and their associations with breast cancer survival. Breast Cancer Res Treat 105:55–61
140. Rollison DE, Newschaffer CJ, Tao Y, Pollak M, Helzlsouer KJ (2006) Premenopausal levels of circulating insulin-like growth factor I and the risk of postmenopausal breast cancer. Int J Cancer 118:1279–1284
141. Zhigang Z, Jieming L, Su L, Wenlu S (2007) Serum insulin-like growth factor I/free prostate specific antigen (IGF-I/fPSA) ratio enhances prostate cancer detection in men with total PSA 4.0–10.0 ng/ml. J Surg Oncol 96:54–61
142. Weiss JM, Huang WY, Rinaldi S et al (2007) IGF-1 and IGFBP-3: risk of prostate cancer among men in the Prostate, Lung, Colorectal and Ovarian Cancer Screening Trial. Int J Cancer 121:2267–2273
143. Severi G, Morris HA, MacInnis RJ et al (2006) Circulating insulin-like growth factor-I and binding protein-3 and risk of prostate cancer. Cancer Epidemiol Biomarkers Prev 15:1137–1141
144. Platz EA, Pollak MN, Leitzmann MF, Stampfer MJ, Willett WC, Giovannucci E (2005) Plasma insulin-like growth factor-1 and binding protein-3 and subsequent risk of prostate cancer in the PSA era. Cancer Causes Control 16:255–262
145. Meyer F, Galan P, Douville P et al (2005) A prospective study of the insulin-like growth factor axis in relation with prostate cancer in the SU.VI.MAX trial. Cancer Epidemiol Biomarkers Prev 14:2269–2272
146. Chen C, Lewis SK, Voigt L, Fitzpatrick A, Plymate SR, Weiss NS (2005) Prostate carcinoma incidence in relation to prediagnostic circulating levels of insulin-like growth factor I, insulin-like growth factor binding protein 3, and insulin. Cancer 103:76–84
147. Li L, Yu H, Schumacher F, Casey G, Witte JS (2003) Relation of serum insulin-like growth factor-I (IGF-I) and IGF binding protein-3 to risk of prostate cancer (United States). Cancer Causes Control 14:721–726
148. Woodson K, Tangrea JA, Pollak M et al (2003) Serum insulin-like growth factor I: tumor marker or etiologic factor? A prospective study of prostate cancer among Finnish men. Cancer Res 63:3991–3994
149. Shariat SF, Lamb DJ, Kattan MW et al (2002) Association of preoperative plasma levels of insulin-like growth factor I and insulin-like growth factor binding proteins-2 and -3 with prostate cancer invasion, progression, and metastasis. J Clin Oncol 20:833–841
150. Chokkalingam AP, Pollak M, Fillmore CM et al (2001) Insulin-like growth factors and prostate cancer: a population-based case-control study in China. Cancer Epidemiol Biomarkers Prev 10:421–427
151. Kurek R, Tunn UW, Eckart O, Aumuller G, Wong J, Renneberg H (2000) The significance of serum levels of insulin-like growth factor-1 in patients with prostate cancer. BJU Int 85:125–129
152. Jenab M, Riboli E, Cleveland RJ et al (2007) Serum C-peptide, IGFBP-1 and IGFBP-2 and risk of colon and rectal cancers in the European Prospective Investigation into Cancer and Nutrition. Int J Cancer 121:368–376
153. Haydon AM, Macinnis RJ, English DR, Morris H, Giles GG (2006) Physical activity, insulin-like growth factor 1, insulin-like growth factor binding protein 3, and survival from colorectal cancer. Gut 55:689–694
154. Palmqvist R, Stattin P, Rinaldi S et al (2003) Plasma insulin, IGF-binding proteins-1 and -2 and risk of colorectal cancer: a prospective study in northern Sweden. Int J Cancer 107:89–93
155. Hunt KJ, Toniolo P, Akhmedkhanov A et al (2002) Insulin-like growth factor II and colorectal cancer risk in women. Cancer Epidemiol Biomarkers Prev 11:901–905
156. Probst-Hensch NM, Yuan JM, Stanczyk FZ, Gao YT, Ross RK, Yu MC (2001) IGF-1, IGF-2 and IGFBP-3 in prediagnostic serum: association with colorectal cancer in a cohort of Chinese men in Shanghai. Br J Cancer 85:1695–1699

157. Kaaks R, Toniolo P, Akhmedkhanov A et al (2000) Serum C-peptide, insulin-like growth factor (IGF)-I, IGF-binding proteins, and colorectal cancer risk in women. J Natl Cancer Inst 92:1592–1600
158. Jenkins PJ, Frajese V, Jones AM et al (2000) Insulin-like growth factor I and the development of colorectal neoplasia in acromegaly. J Clin Endocrinol Metab 85:3218–3221
159. Renehan AG, Painter JE, O'Halloran D et al (2000) Circulating insulin-like growth factor II and colorectal adenomas. J Clin Endocrinol Metab 85:3402–3408
160. Manousos O, Souglakos J, Bosetti C et al (1999) IGF-I and IGF-II in relation to colorectal cancer. Int J Cancer 83:15–17
161. Morris JK, George LM, Wu T, Wald NJ (2006) Insulin-like growth factors and cancer: no role in screening. Evidence from the BUPA study and meta-analysis of prospective epidemiological studies. Br J Cancer 95:112–117
162. Durai R, Yang W, Gupta S, Seifalian AM, Winslet MC (2005) The role of the insulin-like growth factor system in colorectal cancer: review of current knowledge. Int J Colorectal Dis 20:203–220

Chapter 11
IGF-I and Insulin Receptor Families in Cancer

Antonino Belfiore, Ira D. Goldfine, and Roberta Malaguarnera

Introduction

It has been the general opinion that the IGF-IR and its ligands (IGF-I and IGF-II) are mediators of mitogenic effects, whereas insulin and its receptor (IR) are mediators of metabolic effects. However, the actions and interactions of these two systems are complex. Moreover, in recent years, several lines of evidence indicate that components of the IGF system are involved in cancer pathogenesis along with the insulin and the IR. The role of insulin and its receptor in tumorigenesis is supported by several epidemiological studies indicating that diseases characterized by hyperinsulinemia (type 2 diabetes and obesity) are associated with an increased risk for cancer [1]. Furthermore, recent studies have partially elucidated the molecular basis of IR involvement in cancer. These studies include the aberrant expression of the IR in malignant cells, in particular IR isoform A (IR-A), which is a second receptor for IGF-II, and the formation of IR/IGF-IR hybrids. These new receptors expand the pool of functional binding sites for IGF-I and IGF-II and trigger various biological effects. Moreover, atypical IRs and IGF-IRs may also be expressed in cancer cells, thus further increasing the complexity of these systems. This "IGF network" is also complicated by its cross-talk with other molecular systems, such as oncogenes/anti-oncogenes, other growth factor receptors, and sex steroid hormones. In this chapter, we will focus on the role of IGF-IR and IR systems and their cognate ligands in tumorigenesis. These systems have important implications for both the prevention and the treatment of common human malignancies that are characterized by dysregulation of the IGF system.

A. Belfiore (✉)
Department of Clinical and Experimental Medicine, University of Catanzaro,
Campus Universitario, loc. Germaneto, 88100 Catanzaro, Italy
e-mail: belfiore@unicz.it

I.G. Fantus (ed.), *Insulin Resistance and Cancer: Epidemiology, Cellular and Molecular Mechanisms and Clinical Implications*, Energy Balance and Cancer 1,
DOI 10.1007/978-1-4419-9911-5_11,

Receptors of the IGF and IR Systems and Downstream Signaling

The IGF-I Receptor (IGF-IR) and the Insulin Receptor (IR)

The IR and IGF-IR are related transmembrane receptors with intrinsic tyrosine kinase activity. They are encoded by distinct genes and are expressed on the cell surface as heterotetrameric receptors. Each receptor is formed by two dimers containing two $\alpha\beta$ chains joined by disulfide bridges (Fig. 11.1). The genes encoding the IR and IGF-IR have evolved by a common ancestral gene and belong to a highly conserved system, which plays a crucial role in the regulation of metabolism, growth, and differentiation in multicellular organisms in response to nutrient availability [2]. Indeed, the two receptors share a high degree of sequence homology, which at the level of cDNA, ranges from 45 to 65% in the ligand binding domains to 60–85% in the tyrosine kinase and substrate recruitment domains [3,4].

The IR has a high affinity for insulin with an approximately 100-fold lower affinity for IGF-I. Conversely, the IGF-IR has high affinity for both IGF-I and IGF-II, but an approximately 100-fold lower affinity for insulin. Unlike the IGF-IR, the human IR exists in two isoforms characterized by the inclusion (IR-B) or the exclusion (IR-A) of exon 11, which encodes a 12 amino acid residue located at the carboxyl terminus of the IR α-subunit [5]. The IR-B is predominantly expressed in classical targets of insulin's metabolic effects (liver, muscle, and fat); IR-A is mostly expressed in tissues that are nonclassical targets of insulin (spleen, lymphocytes, and brain) [6].

Upon ligand binding, these receptors activate their tyrosine kinase activity and become phosphorylated on multiple tyrosine residues [7]. These tyrosine residues occur in three clusters: in the juxtamembrane region; in the catalytic domain; and in the carboxyl terminus [8]. These phosphotyrosine residues are docking sites for Src homology 2 (SH2)-containing domain substrates. The primary substrates that bind to both IR and IGF-IR include the four insulin receptor substrate proteins [9], Shc, GAB-1, Cbl, APS, and the signal regulatory protein family (SIRP) [10,11]. The primary site of binding of the IRS and Shc proteins is the juxtamembrane domain of both the IR and the IGF-IR. The interaction of the IRS and Shc molecules with the IR and the IGF-IR allows the kinase domains of the receptors to phosphorylate these proteins on tyrosine residues. These phosphotyrosine residues, in turn, are docking sites for other kinases or adaptors, such as the phosphatidyl-inositol-3-kinase (PI3K) [12], Grb2 [13], and others.

The Insulin-Like Growth Factor-II (IGF-II) Receptor (M6P/IGF-IIR)

In addition to the binding to IGF-IR, and IR-A, IGF-II but not IGF-I also binds to the cation-independent mannose 6-phosphate (M6P) receptor (M6P/IGF-IIR). This

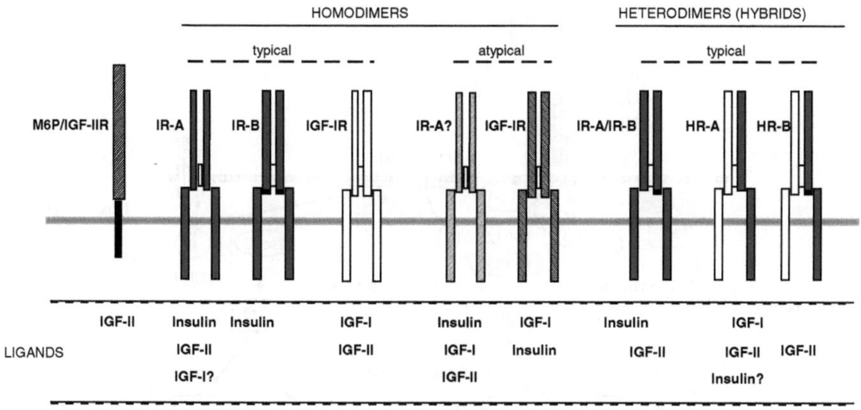

Fig. 11.1 Schematic representation of receptors of the IGF system. The M6P/IGF-IIR and typical homodimers and heterodimers derived from assembly of IR isoforms and IGF-IR hemidimers have been characterized concerning their ligand binding affinity. Their ligands are also indicated, although some uncertainty still remains. Unlike IR and IGF-IR and their hybrid heterodimers, the M6P/IGF-IIR has no enzymatic activity and targets IGF-II to degradation. Atypical receptors are less well characterized and most likely derive from differential post-translational processing of typical counterparts. Whether they are able to form hybrids with typical receptors is unknown

multifunctional transmembrane glycoprotein has a large extracellular domain and a small cytoplasmic domain [14] (Fig. 11.1). M6P/IGF-IIR has no enzymatic activity and targets IGF-II to lysosomes for degradation. Therefore, the strength of the IGF-II signaling is inversely related to the abundance of the M6P/IGF-IIR.

The IR and IGF-IR Signaling Pathways

Upon ligand binding, both the IR and the IGF-IR lead to the activation of two main signaling pathways: (1) the mitogen activated protein kinases cascade (MAPKs), which is mainly implicated in mitogenic effects and; (2) the PI3K signaling pathway that is mainly responsible for metabolic actions, although this pathway is also implicated in the mitogenic and survival effects. Furthermore, components of both signaling pathways, MAPK and PI3K, are interconnected and converge on the common mTOR/p70S6k axis that is involved in cell growth, survival, and metabolism (Fig. 11.2). It is worth noting that different cell types can use different pathways for proliferation and apoptosis and, during the different stages of the development, some pathways are more significant than others.

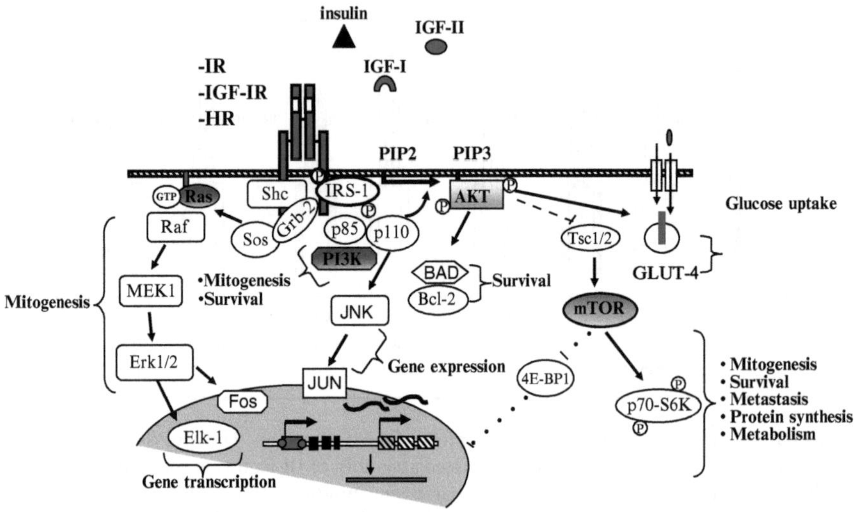

Fig. 11.2 The IGF signaling transduction pathway. Schematic representation of the major signaling cascades that can be stimulated by autophosphorylated insulin receptor (IR) or IGF-I receptor (IGF-IR) or hybrids receptors (HR). After the binding of the ligands (IGFs, insulin) to their specific receptors, adaptor proteins belonging to the IRS family or Shc are phosphorylated. Activation of IRS and SHC leads to stimulation of extracellular signal regulated kinase Erk1/2 of the MAPK cascade through the growth factor receptor binding protein 2 (Grb2)/Sos/Ras/Raf/Mek. Erk1/2, in the nucleus, stimulates gene transcription via activation of the transcription factor Elk-1 and Fos. MAPK signaling pathway is mainly involved in mediating the mitogenic effects of insulin and IGFs. IRS proteins also bind to the p110 subunit of phosphatidylinositol 3-kinase (PI3K) leading to the generation of phosphatidylinositol 3,4,5-triphopshate (PIP3) and AKT phosphorylation. Activated AKT, in turn, activates the antiapoptotic factors Bad and Bcl2 and inhibits tuberous sclerosis complex 1/2 (Tsc1/2). The inhibition of Tsc1/2 induces mammalian target of rapamycin (mTOR) that activates p70S6K and inhibits 4EBP1. Both mTOR downstream substrates, p70S6K and 4EBP1, regulate protein synthesis and enhance proliferation, survival and cell migration. AKT pathway is responsible not only for mediating insulin and IGFs mitogenic and pro-survival functions but it is also involved in the insulin-dependent regulation of glucose uptake

The MAPK Signaling Pathway

The Ras/Raf/MEK/Erk cascade is activated by either insulin or IGFs following the phosphorylation of Shc and the recruitment of Grb/Sos complex. This complex, in turn, triggers the activation of GTPase Ras, and subsequently the RAF isoforms (MAPKKKs) and their downstream signaling effectors MEK1/2 (MAPKKs) and ERK1/2 (MAPKs). Activated ERK1/2 phosphorylates cytosolic proteins then translocate to the nucleus, where they regulate gene expression [15] (Fig. 11.2). The Ras-Raf-MEK-ERK pathway is hyperactivated in ~30% of human cancers [16] where it provides growth and survival signals. Dysregulation of the IGF system occurs through (1) IGF-IR overexpression; (2) autocrine/paracrine production of IGF-I and IGF-II; or (3) autocrine IGF-II/IR-A loop activation. All can induce constitutive stimulation of the MAPK signaling cascade.

The PI3K Signaling Pathway

The second pathway stimulated by the IR and the IGF-IR involves the PI3K system (Fig. 11.2). The binding of insulin and IGFs to either the IR or the IGF-IR results in the recruitment of PI3K to the plasma membrane. PI3K is then phosphorylated and activated by the IRS adaptor proteins and leads to increased production of phosphatidylinositol-3,4,5-triphosphate (PIP3), which, in turn, activates the 3-phosphoinositide–dependent protein kinase 1 (PDK1) and AKT. The PI3K/AKT pathway is negatively regulated by the lipid phosphatase PTEN (phosphatase and tensin homolog deleted on chromosome 10 gene) which dephosphorylates PIP3.

AKT phosphorylates and activates other targets involved in several processes including cell survival (BCL-X_L/BCL-2 associated death, BAD), glycogen synthesis (glycogen synthetase kinase 3, GSK3), glucose uptake (Rab-GTPase activating protein, AS160, and translocation of the glucose transporter GLUT4 to the plasma membrane), gene transcription (Forkhead box O transcription factors, FoxO), and ribosome biogenesis (tuberous sclerosis complex, TSC1/TSC2 and mammalian target of rapamycin, mTOR) [17]. The mTOR axis plays also an important role in signaling pathways that respond to growth factors and nutrients [18]. mTOR exists in two distinct multiprotein complexes: mTORC1 (mTOR-raptor) and mTORC2 (mTOR-rictor). Extracellular signals, such as growth factors and hormones, modulate mTORC1 complex activity primarily through the activation of MAPK and PI3K. Upon activation, mTORC1 enhances protein synthesis by the phosphorylation of two major targets: ribosomal S6 kinase (p70S6K) and eukaryotic initiation factor 4E binding protein (4EBP1), both of which may be involved in cancer [19]. The IGF-I system coordinates with the mTOR axis through the phosphorylation and inhibition of the TSC1/2 complex by AKT, which in turn activates Rheb and mTOR. mTOR is also involved in a negative feedback regulation of the insulin/IGFs signal by inducing IRS-1 serine phosphorylation and degradation [20]. Moreover, when mTOR is assembled into the mTORC2 complex, it directly phosphorylates and activates AKT, thus placing AKT upstream and downstream of the mTOR signaling network. AKT activation is crucial for the regulation of glucose homeostasis, but exerts also an important role in regulation of cell size, cell division, and survival. The putative role of the AKT signaling pathway in cancer biology derives from the evidence that the deregulation of this signaling is seen in up to 30% of all human cancers [21], and occurs through different mechanisms: (1) constitutive activation of RTKs, such as the IR or the IGF-IR; (2) Ras oncogene overexpression and activating mutations; (3) amplification or mutations of genes encoding the p110α PI3K catalytic subunit (PIK3CA); and (4) inactivation of PTEN [22].

Insulin vs. IGF Signaling: Molecular Bases of Signal Specificity and Diversification

The IGF system plays a crucial role in development, growth, and metabolism. The mechanisms of signal diversification required to accomplish these various functions have been the subject of numerous studies; yet they are not fully clarified. The different cellular distribution of the IR and the IGF-IR only partially explains how insulin, IGF-I, and IGF-II induce different cellular and physiological responses despite activating similar signaling pathways. Other mechanisms may include: (a) differences in internalization and subcellular distribution of the ligand–receptor complexes [23]; (b) different abundance of signaling substrates among various cells with different receptor expression; (c) differential activation of intracellular substrates by the IR and the IGF-IR; (d) tissue-specific abundance of specific substrates for each receptor; (e) signaling differences between IR isoforms; (f) the presence of IR/IGF-IR hybrid receptors (HRs); and (g) the possible presence of atypical receptors.

Differences in Intracellular Substrate Activation Between the IR and the IGF-IR

Studies carried out in 3T3 fibroblasts overexpressing either the IR or the IGF-IR have shown that global gene expression profiling is partially different in response to each ligand [24]. The differential activation of intracellular pathways has been studied by expressing, in 3T3-L1 adipocytes, chimaeras consisting of the extracellular portion of the neurotrophin receptor TrkC (tyrosine kinase C receptor) fused to the intracellular portions of either the IR or the IGF-IR [25]. These data indicate that stimulation of the TrkC-IR chimaera predominantly activates the IRS-1/PI3K pathway and glucose uptake, while stimulation of the TrkC-IGF-IR chimaera predominantly activates the Shc/Grb2/MAPK pathway and mitogenesis [25].

We have found a mechanism that partially accounts for these differences in biological effects between insulin and IGFs that involves c-Abl. Insulin, but not IGF-I, stimulates c-Abl tyrosine phosphorylation, with consequent de-phosphorylation of focal adhesion kinase (FAK) and increased metabolic effects of insulin [26]. In contrast, in cells with a functionally impaired c-Abl, insulin stimulates FAK phosphorylation in a manner similar to IGF-I, promoting cell proliferation and migration [26].

Other substrates differentially activated by the IR and the IGF-IR have been described. Ceacam2 is a substrate specific for the IR [27] and is involved in IR internalization and termination of the mitogenic response to insulin. The mitotic arrest deficient 2 (MAD2), a cell cycle checkpoint regulator, binds to the IR carboxyl terminus, but not to the homologous region of the IGF-IR [28]. Crk-II, a SH2-SH3 adapter protein, is directly phosphorylated by the IGF-IR tyrosine kinase, but not by the IR tyrosine kinase [29]. Other proteins specifically interacting with the IGF-IR, but not the IR, include 14-3-3, a scaffolding protein, and Twist, a transcription factor, both with an antiapoptotic role [30].

The Role of Insulin Receptor Isoforms

IR isoform switching greatly contributes to the regulation of ligand affinity and specificity in the IGF system. IR-A shows an approximately twofold higher affinity for insulin [31] and a faster internalization and recycling time than IR-B [32]. In contrast, IR-B may have stronger tyrosine kinase activity than IR-A [33]. However, the greatest functional difference between the two isoforms is their binding affinities for IGFs. IR-A is a second receptor for the IGF-II [34,35]. IR-A binds IGF-II with an affinity that is only threefold lower than that for insulin. Moreover, the affinity of IGF-II for the IR-A is similar to its affinity for the IGF-IR. In contrast, IR-B only binds insulin with high affinity and not IGF-II [34]. IGF-I binds to the IR-A with a low affinity than IGF-II, but IGF-I binding to IR-B is 5–10 times higher than IGF-I binding to IR-B [35,36].

When both IR-A and IR-B isoforms are coexpressed, heterodimerization may occur by the assembly of one IR-A hemireceptor with one IR-B hemireceptor, leading to the formation of hybrid IR-A/IR-B receptors (HIR-AB) [35,37]. Preliminary evidence now indicates that HIR-AB receptors behave functionally like IR-A rather than IR-B [37]. If confirmed, these studies indicate that even a small excess of IR-A may greatly affect IR ligand specificity.

The two IR isoforms may also mediate different intracellular signaling and biological effects. Possible differential effects of the two IR isoforms are seen in both apoptosis protection and cell differentiation. Neonatal hepatocytes expressing only IR-B are more prone to apoptosis than those expressing only IR-A, although only the coexistence of both isoforms effectively protects these cells from apoptosis [38]. Moreover, isoform switching to obtain a predominant IR-B expression is characteristically associated with cell differentiation in various model systems [39–41].

In pancreatic β cells, it has been reported that IR-A and IR-B are located in different membrane compartments and may activate differential intracellular signaling and gene transcription [42]. Another possible mechanism of signal diversification concerns the intracellular signaling of IGF-II through the IR-A. Available evidence indicates that IGF-II may differ in a subtle way from that of insulin [34,43,44] both in the differential phosphorylation of intracellular substrates and in the modulation of gene transcription [45].

Cross-Talk Between the IGF-IR and the IR Pathways: Role of Hybrid and Atypical Receptors

Hybrid Receptors

Because of the high degree of homology between the IR and the IGF-IR [3,46], an IR hemireceptor may assemble with an IGF-IR hemireceptor, forming IR/IGF-IR hybrids (Fig. 11.1). As IR hemireceptors may exclude or include exon 11, IR/IGF-IR hybrids may contain either IR-A (HR-A) or IR-B hemireceptors (HR-B), respectively. The existence of IR/IGF-IR HRs was first identified in the human placenta [47], but then confirmed in both normal and neoplastic tissues [48]. Functional studies indicate that a consequence of HR formation is the expansion of IGF-I and IGF-II binding sites [49,50]. The possibility also exists that HR activation results in the activation of a unique signaling pathway, distinct from those activated by the homodimeric IRs and IGF-IR, but this area has not been studied in detail.

Early studies carried out with purified HRs indicated that these receptors bound IGF-I with high affinity, while they bound insulin with a much lower affinity [51]. Indeed, several studies have found that both IR and IGF-IR β-subunits of HRs are autophosphorylated in response to both ligands, although IGF-I is more efficient than insulin [52–54]. Binding displacement studies in HRs have shown that the binding of labeled IGF-I is displaced by low concentrations of IGF-I, but only by high concentrations of insulin, whereas the binding of labeled insulin is displaced by low concentrations of both insulin and IGF-I [51], suggesting that IGF-I binding allosterically inhibits HR insulin binding.

However, functional studies have yielded discrepant results. In one study, IGF-I, IGF-II, and insulin were all able to bind and phosphorylate HR-A with the following hierarchy: IGF-I>IGF-II>>insulin. In contrast, only IGF-I and IGF-II, but not insulin, were able to phosphorylate HR-B with the following hierarchy: IGF-I>>IGF-II (Fig. 11.1). These data were interpreted as HR-A being a promiscuous receptor that may be activated by both IGFs and insulin (although to a lesser extent than the IGFs) while IR-B behaves very much similarly to the homodimeric IGF-IR [55]. In this study, insulin was able to phosphorylate the IGF-IR β-subunit and IGF-IR–specific intracellular substrates [55].

However, two other studies were unable to confirm this different affinity of the two HR subtypes for insulin [35,56] while showing that IGF-I could stimulate transphosphorylation of the IR β-subunit [35,56]. In chick neuroretina, it was found that while IGF-I bound mostly to IGF-IR homodimers, insulin bound preferentially to HR-A, which had similar binding affinity for insulin and IGF-I [57].

Atypical IGF-IRs and IRs

Atypical IGF-IRs and IRs refer to receptors immunologically similar to typical IRs or IGF-IRs but with unusual binding characteristics (Fig. 11.1). Although poorly characterized, these atypical receptors have mostly been described in fetal and cancer tissues and probably derive from differential posttranslational processing. They often have the characteristics of promiscuous receptors for both insulin and IGFs and may contribute to signal diversification in certain tissues. Atypical IGF-IRs that are phosphorylated by both insulin and IGF-I have been found in fetal muscle [58]. A subclone of a mouse myoblast cell line expresses an IGF-IR that binds IGF-II with a higher affinity than IGF-I or insulin [59]. An atypical IGF-IR with high affinity for both IGF-I and insulin was also found in human breast cancer cells MCF-7 [60]. Conversely, atypical IRs with high affinity binding for IGFs have been described both in human placenta [61] and in human lymphoblastoid cells IM-9 [62].

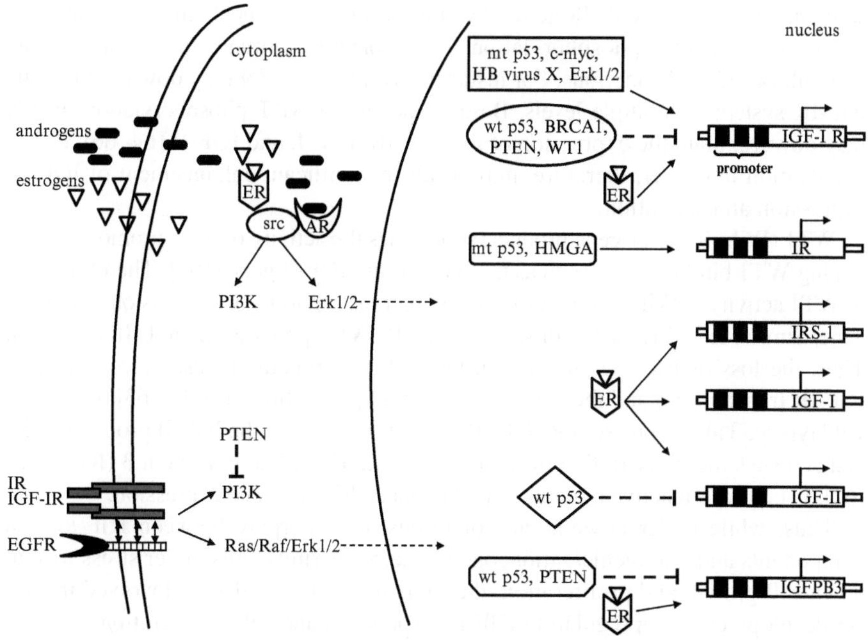

Fig. 11.3 Interplay between tumor suppressors, oncogenes, steroid hormones, tyrosine kinase receptors and the IGF system components. In the cytoplasm, ER and AR markedly upregulate the IGF-IR, but not the IR, by a nongenotropic mechanism. This steroid hormones mediated nongenotropic event consists in the activation of tyrosine kinase Src and in the subsequent induction of extracellular signal regulated kinase (Erk1/2) and, to a lesser extent, phosphatidylinositol 3-kinase (PI3K). Erk1/2, translocated into the nucleus, increases IGF-IR gene transcription. MAPK and PI3K survival pathways, can be also activated by the autophosphorylation of IR and IGF-IR as well as by the direct interaction between IGF-IR and other tyrosine kinase receptors as EGFR/HER2. In the nucleus tumor suppressors, oncogenes, estrogens and PI3K /MAPK effectors interact with the IGF system components stimulating (*solid arrows*) or suppressing (*dashed lines*) the IGF system genes transcription. *mt* mutant; *wt* wild type; *ER* estrogen receptor; *AR* androgen receptor

Cross-Talk of the IGF-IR System with Other Signaling Systems

Interactions with Oncogenes and Tumor Suppressors

A role for the IGF-IR signaling system in cancer is also based on the finding that certain components of the IGF-IR system interact with onco-suppressors as well as with activated proto-oncogenes (Fig. 11.3). The IGF-IR promoter is a downstream target for oncogenes such as c-myc, Src, and hepatitis B virus X. This interaction occurs both at transcriptional and at nontranscriptional levels. Constitutive overexpression of the proto-oncogene c-myc in Balb/c-3T3 cells as well as oncogene hepatitis B virus X in hepatic cells induces overexpression of both IGF-I and the IGF-IR through increased transcriptional activity [63]. Yet, the Src oncogene of the Rous sarcoma virus affects IGF-IR action by nontranscriptional mechanisms, resulting in constitutive receptor phosphorylation [63]. Conversely, many tumor suppressors may inhibit IGF-IR functions. For instance, wild type PTEN may downregulate the IGF-IR system at multiple levels. Besides increasing AKT phosphorylation, PTEN may downregulate the expression of the IGF-IR, IGF-I, and IGF-II [64–66]. PTEN inactivation in cancer, therefore, may result in significant enhancement of IGF-IR expression and activation.

WT1 (Wilm's tumor gene product) suppresses the activity of gene promoters, containing WT1 binding sites, such as the IGF-IR and IGF-II genes [63]. Therefore, loss of WT1 activity in Wilm's tumor may result in transcriptional de-repression of IGF-IR gene. Similar to WT1, the tumor suppressor BRCA1 suppresses the IGF-IR promoter. Thus, the loss of BRCA1 function in familial and sporadic breast cancers induces IGF-IR transcription and the autocrine/paracrine production of IGFs [63]. Likewise, wild type p53 also represses the IGF-IR promoter as well as the IGF-II promoter [63], and activates the transcription of the proapoptotic IGF binding protein 3 (IGFBP-3) [67]. In contrast, inactive mutants of p53 enhance IGF-IR gene expression.

Thus, while under physiologic conditions, the interplay between IGF system components and oncogenic/antioncogenic factors permits cells under stress to shut down cell growth and proliferation; the same network can also be involved in cancer development by upregulating IGF-IR expression and cell proliferation.

Interactions with Other Tyrosine Kinase Receptors

Whereas there are little data demonstrating an interplay between the IR (in particular IR-A isoform) and the EGFR/HER2 signaling system, several studies provide evidence interactions between the IGF-IR and the EGFR/HER2 (Fig. 11.3). In normal human mammary epithelial cells, the IGF-IR physically interacts with the EGFR inducing the activation of ERK pathway and cell proliferation [68]. A direct interaction between the IGF-IR and HER2 has also been reported [69], providing evidence that IGF-IR is necessary for the activation of HER2 by the heregulin family ligands. IGF-IR heterodimerization with HER2 may contribute to the development of resistance to the anti-HER2 monoclonal antibody, trastuzumab, in breast cancer cells [70]. Moreover, in Cos 7 cells overexpressing the IGF-IR, an EGFR inhibitor was able to reduce ERK activation mediated by IGF-I [71]. These data suggest that IGF-I requires the EGFR both to induce ERK activation and to exert mitogenic effects. These studies are important not only for developing targeted therapies for tumors showing IGF-IR/EGFR/HER2 deregulation but also to overcome resistance to these anticancer therapies.

Interactions with Steroid Hormones

The interactions between IGF system and steroid hormones have been extensively studied in breast and prostate cancers, and have been recently reviewed [72].

Breast cancer cells express the IGF-IR, the IR, and the HRs. They also produce both IGF-I, and IGF-II, and IGF binding proteins (IGFBP2-3-4-5) in greater amounts than in normal breast cells. A reciprocal potentiation between the ER and IGF-IR signaling pathways has been reported in several studies [72–74]. Estrogens induce increased gene transcription and upregulation of IGF-IR, IGF-II, and IRS-1 [72], although they do not affect IR expression (Fig. 11.3). This synergy between IGF and estrogens can explain the resistance to antiestrogen therapies. Both estrogens and androgens induce IGF-IR (but not IR) upregulation in prostate cancer cells [75,76] and sensitize cells to the biological effects of IGF-I. Androgens do not affect IGF-IR expression in androgen receptor negative prostate cancer cells. These observations suggest that the cross-talk between sex steroids and IGF-IR may play an important role in prostate cancer progression.

Involvement of the IGF-IR and IR in Cancer: Experimental Evidence and Clinical Aspects

A Possible Role in Cell Transformation and Tumorigenesis

In addition to its well-established role in mediating cell growth and resistance to apoptosis, the IGF-IR has also been hypothesized to have a permissive role in cell transformation. This concept has evolved from the observation that fibroblasts derived from mice with a targeted disruption of the IGF-IR gene (R-cells) are unable to undergo transformation after transfection with several viral and cellular oncogenes [77]. The reintroduction of the IGF-IR restores their ability to undergo transformation [78]. Although the IGF-IR does not need to be overexpressed in order to permit cell transformation by oncogenes, IGF-IR overexpression in R-cells as well as in NIH-3T3 cells was sufficient to activate ligand-dependent transformation [79,80], which was directly related to the degree of IGF-IR expression.

Whether the IR may recapitulate the effects of the IGF-IR transformation is unclear. In contrast to results obtained with the IGF-IR, R-cells transfected with the IR were unable to form colonies in soft agar when treated with insulin [78,80]. This observation led to the hypothesis that the transforming effect of IGF-IR is not shared by the IR because transformation is linked to the IGF-IR carboxyl terminus, which is not homologous to the carboxyl terminus of the IR [78,80]. However, NIH-3T3 cells transfected with the IR showed ligand-dependent colony formation [81]. At variance with R-cells, these cells express the endogenous IGF-IR.

Studies obtained with insulin analogs have provided further evidence of a possible direct involvement of IR in cancer [82]. Some of these analogs bind to the IR with a low dissociation rate and form receptor–ligand complexes with an increased half-life that results in enhanced mitogenic potency [82]. Prolonged treatment with one of these analogs (AspB10) caused both benign and malignant mammary tumors in female rats [83]. AspB10 also induced foci formation in the immortalized human breast cells MCF-10 [84]. Whether and to what extent these effects of AspB10 could be affected by cross-talk with the IGF-IR is unclear.

Transgenic models have provided further support to the possible role of the IGF-IR in transformation. Transgenic mice expressing a constitutively active form of the IGF-IR developed salivary and mammary adenocarcinomas [85]. Moreover, mice engineered to express the human IGF-IR in mammary cells under an inducible promoter revealed that IGF-IR overexpression induces mammary epithelial hyperplasia and tumor formation [86].

When endogenous IGF-IR activation in transgenic animals has been obtained by IGF-I overexpression, the transforming effect is less than that obtained with IGF-IR overexpression. Transgenic mice overexpressing the ligand IGF-I did not develop cancer in most tissues but did develop selective organomegaly [87]. However, transgenic mice expressing human IGF-I in basal epithelial cells of prostate caused IGF-IR activation and led to stepwise development of neoplasia [88]. Targeted IGF-I expression to the mammary gland in transgenic mice was associated with the development of mammary adenocarcinomas but only in animals undergone multiple lactations [89]. The frequency of mammary tumors was increased by the coexistence of a mutant p53 [90].

IGF-II overexpression in transgenic mice seems to have a stronger effect than IGF-I overexpression. In transgenic mice, where IGF-II was overexpressed in the mammary gland, the animals developed both benign and malignant mammary tumors [91] and a delay in mammary gland involution [92].

Since IGF-II binds to and activates not only the IGF-IR but also the IR-A and HRs, the stronger transforming effect of IGF-II overexpression in transgenic models, as compared with the effect of IGF-I, may be via the additional contribution of both IR-A and HR activation. However, direct evidence for the transforming potential of IR isoforms using transgenic models is lacking.

Deregulated Receptor Expression in Human Cancer

Both the IGF-IR and the IR are ubiquitously expressed in adult tissues. While IGF-IR is believed to mediate trophic effects in terminally differentiated cells, the biological role of IR expression in nonclassical insulin target tissues is mostly unclear. In the last two decades, a wealth of evidence has shown that both the IGF-IR and the IR are expressed, and often overexpressed, in a variety of human malignancies and, as a consequence, HRs often are also overexpressed in these malignancies (Table 11.1). In many of these malignancies, these receptors may be activated by locally produced IGF-I and/or IGF-II, which may be secreted either in autocrine or in paracrine manner depending on the tumor histotype (Table 11.1).

Table 11.1 Expression of the IGF-IR and IR systems in common malignancies

Receptor and/or IGFs expression	Breast cancer	Thyroid cancer	Colon cancer	Ovary cancer	Prostate cancer	Sarcomas
IR	Papa et al. [105]; Kalli et al. [108]	Frasca et al. [34]; Vella et al. [99]	Frasca et al. [34]	Kalli et al. [108]		
IR-A	Sciacca et al. [107]	Frasca et al. [34]; Vella et al. [99]	Frasca et al. [34]	Kalli et al. [108]		Sciacca et al. [44]; Avnet et al. [114]
Increased IRA:IRB ratio	Frasca et al. [34]	Frasca et al. [34]		Kalli et al. [108]		
IGF-IR	Peyrat et al. [93]; Cullen et al. [94]; Papa et al. [95]; Pandini et al. [48]; Koda et al. [96]; Ouban et al. [150]	Frasca et al. [34]	Guo et al. [151]; Ouban et al. [150]	Ouban et al. [150]	Iwamura et al. [152]; Nickerson et al. [153]; Hellawell et al. [133]; Ouban et al. [150]	Avnet et al. [114]
HRs	Pandini et al. [48]	Vella et al. [99]				Avnet et al. [114]
IGF-I	Huff et al. [154]; Yee et al. [155]	Maiorano et al. [156]	Michell et al. [157]		Pietrzkowski et al. [158]; DiGiovanni et al. [88]; Nickerson et al. [153]	
IGF-II	Paik [159]; Sciacca et al. [107]	Vella et al. [99]	Singh et al. [160]; Jehle et al. [161]	Kalli et al. [108]	Tennant et al. [132]; Li et al. [162]	Sciacca et al. [44]

IGF-IR Overexpression

IGF-IR is expressed or overexpressed in a variety of human malignancies (Table 11.1). IGF-IR has been extensively characterized in breast cancer and found widely expressed in human breast cancer specimens [93,94]. In a study on a large series of breast cancer specimens, it was found that the IGF-IR content is approximately tenfold higher in cancer when compared to normal breast tissue [95]. The IGF-IR may be overexpressed not only in primary breast cancers but also in nodal metastases [96], and may have constitutive tyrosine kinase activity [97]. It should be noted that IGF-II and not IGF-I is the predominant IGF ligand in breast cancer, as it is widely expressed in breast cancer either in stromal cells adjacent to epithelial malignant cells or by the malignant cells. In contrast, IGF-I is expressed in fibroblasts surrounding normal breast tissue and not in the tumoral tissue [98].

An atypical IGF-IR is coexpressed together with typical IGF-IR in human breast cancer cells MCF-7 cells [60]. As previously mentioned, this receptor is characterized by high affinity binding for both IGF-I and insulin and is responsible for the majority of insulin binding to MCF-7 cells [60]. Further studies are required to clarify the expression of these atypical IGF-IRs in human cancer.

In thyroid cancer, the IGF-IR was overexpressed, when compared to normal tissue. Both in well-differentiated and poorly differentiated thyroid tumors, the IGF-II/IGF-IR signaling loop is present along with an IGF-II/IR-A signaling loop [99]. The IGF-I/IGF-IR has been found to be a major autocrine loop for Ewing's sarcoma, the second most common malignant bone tumor, occurring in children and adolescents [100].

IR Overexpression

Because the IR is expressed at low levels in tissues other than classical insulin targets, its involvement in human cancer was, therefore, unexpected. Early studies, however, had shown that insulin may be associated with increased tumor growth. For example, chemically induced breast tumors in rats were shown to undergo regression when the animals were made diabetic and insulinopenic, while tumor growth could be restored by the administration of exogenous insulin [101]. Human breast cancer cell lines were also shown to bind insulin and to form tumors in nude mice only in the presence of insulin [102]. Similarly, the growth of a murine T-cell lymphoma cell line LB was insulin dependent both in vitro [103] and when xenografted into mice [104]. However, these studies did not provide direct evidence of IR involvement in cancer, and one possible interpretation was that insulin favors tumor growth by cross-talk with the homologous IGF-IR.

Direct evidence that the IR may be overexpressed in malignant cells was obtained in breast cancer [105]. By measuring the IR in a large number of breast cancer tissue specimens, these investigators found that IR content was approximately sevenfold higher in breast cancers than in normal breast tissue. Employing specific monoclonal antibodies to the IR (with either stimulating or blocking activities) provided direct evidence that the mitogenic effect of insulin in breast cancer cells was mediated by the IR, and not by cross-talk with the IGF-IR [106].

More recently, it was observed that IR splicing is also altered in cancer cells, causing an abnormally high IR-A:IR-B ratio [34] (Table 11.1). Indeed, aberrant IR-A expression was found not only in breast cancers [107] but also in other malignancies, including carcinomas of the colon, lung, and thyroid [34,99]. Further studies have shown that an autocrine IGF-II/IR-A loop is often activated in these cancers. In a large proportion of breast carcinomas, this loop is more important than the previously recognized IGF/IGF-IR loop [48,107]. In thyroid cancer, the IR-A:IGF-IR ratio and the importance of the IGF-II/IR-A loop progressively increases going from well-differentiated to poorly differentiated and undifferentiated carcinomas [99]. Similar data were independently reported in ovarian cancer cells [108], choriocarcinomas [109], mesenchymal malignancies such as myosarcomas [44], and solitary fibrous tumors (Y. [110]). In the latter tumors, the IR-A was constitutively activated while IGF-IR and IGF-I were not expressed [110]. Both in choriocarcinomas [109] and in leiomyosarcoma cells [44], autocrine IGF-II stimulated cell invasion through the IR-A because IGF-IR expression was very low. Autocrine secretion of insulin itself was recently reported in atypical teratoid/rhabdoid tumors [111], a group of highly malignant tumors of the central nervous system.

HRs Overexpression

Most human cancers overexpress both the IGF-IRs and the IR [48,95,112] and, therefore, are expected to overexpress HRs. However, few studies have specifically addressed the possible role of HRs in cancer. Studies using a specific ELISA for HRs have investigated the HR content in human carcinomas of the breast and the thyroid gland, as well as in sarcomas (Table 11.1). Both in human breast and thyroid cancer specimens, HRs content exceeded IGF-IR content [48,113]. A high HR-A content was also found in human osteosarcomas [114], a malignancy previously found to overexpress the IGF-IR. In human osteosarcoma cells, IGF-II rather than IGF-I was the predominant autocrine growth factor. IGF-I mediated its biological effects via HRs, IR-A, and IGF-IR.

Mechanisms of IGF-IR and IR Overexpression

Gene amplification [115] is rarely the cause of either IGF-IR or IR overexpression in cancer. Gene amplification was only sporadically reported in breast cancers [116,117], melanoma [118], and pancreatic adenocarcinomas [119]. In contrast, oncogene and/or antioncogene mutations seem to play a major role in determining both IGF-IR and IR overexpression by increasing gene transcription (Fig. 11.3). Major regulators of both the genes include Sp1 transcription factor and p53 [120]. In normal cells, antioncogenes, such as wild type p53 and BRCA1, reduce IGF-IR expression by interacting with and sequestering Sp1, a potent transactivator of

IGF-IR [120,121]. Therefore, tumors with inactivating mutations of p53 or BRCA1 are often characterized by increased IGF-IR promoter activity and IGF-IR upregulation [122]. Similar mechanisms may account for IR overexpression. Inactivating mutations of p53, and hyperexpression of the architectural HMGA proteins (which favors the transacting effect of Sp1, C/EBP, and AP-2 transcription factors in promoting full transactivation of the IR gene) [123], may contribute to IR overexpression in cancer cells. Hormones may also influence receptor content in cancer cells. Recently, we found that both androgens and estrogens markedly upregulate the IGF-IR, but not the IR, in prostate cancer cells by a nongenotropic mechanism [75,76] (Fig. 11.3). However, the entire spectrum of molecular mechanisms leading to IGF-IR and/or IR overexpression in cancer is incompletely understood.

Biological Effects of the IGF-I Receptor Family in Cancer

Overexpression of IGF-IR, IR, and HRs may favor cancer progression by a variety of mechanisms. However, although most of these biological effects are expected to be shared by all three receptor subtypes, most studies have only addressed the involvement of IGF-IR. IGF-IR clearly promotes proliferation and survival in cancer cells [78]. It also protects cancer cells from endoplasmic reticulum stress [124]. Cancer cell migration driven by the IGF-IR has also been extensively characterized in breast cancer [125]. Mechanisms involved may include the modulation of alpha-5beta1 integrin, and the transactivation of the chemokine receptor CXCR4 [125].

Clinical Implications of Receptor Deregulation in Cancer

Although the IGF-IR clearly has a role in both the early stages of tumorigenesis and promoting cancer progression, analysis of its possible prognostic value has yielded conflicting results. One study found no clear prognostic values for IGF-IR expression in breast cancer patients [126]. However, in a large series of breast cancer patients categorized as either high risk or low risk, the latter group had a significantly higher IGF-IR content in tumor specimens than the high-risk group [95]. These findings are in agreement with data showing that high IGF-IR expression in ER-positive cancer is associated with a longer relapse-free survival [127] and overall survival (OS) [128]. In contrast, a high IGF-IR content predicts a shorter RFS in ER-negative breast carcinomas [129]. Moreover, very high IGF-IR content, due to IGF-IR gene amplification, is also associated with a short OS. Recently, one study found that a transcription profile activated by IGF-IR (IGF-IR signature) was associated with poor breast cancer prognosis [130].

Conflicting data are also seen in human prostate cancer. Studies have found no correlation between IGF-IR and cancer invasiveness [131], an inverse correlation [132], or a direct correlation between IGF-IR expression and metastasis [133]. In cell xenografts, progression to androgen independence is associated with increased expression of both the IGF-IR and IGF-I [134]. Similarly, in colon tumors, while some studies suggest that IGF-IR expression increases as the tumor progresses from adenomas to aggressive and metastatic carcinomas [135], other studies have found no relationship between the level of IGF-IR expression and colon cancer prognosis [115].

In thyroid carcinomas, IGF-IR content was increased as compared to normal thyroid tissue, but was similar in well-differentiated and in poorly differentiated carcinomas. Therefore, the prognosis value for measurement of IGF-IR content in these tumors does not appear useful [99]. In agreement with these data, it has been recently reported that phosphorylated IGF-IR is significantly higher in well-differentiated thyroid carcinomas compared to either poorly differentiated or undifferentiated thyroid carcinomas [136].

Taken together, these data suggest that either IGF-IR expression or overexpression is very common in cancers and may play a crucial role in transformation and in the early stages of growth. Some advanced carcinomas may be driven by very high IGF-IR levels, especially when the IGF-IR gene is amplified. However, in late cancer stages, the IGF-IR may be lost or downregulated when cancer cells acquire additional molecular abnormalities. The prognostic value of IR-A overexpression in cancer is also controversial. In patients with lymph node-negative breast carcinomas, tumors with a detectable IR had a better prognosis as compared with those with undetectable IR. However, a very high IR content was associated with a reduced RFS [137]. The relationship between IR expression and favorable prognosis was independently confirmed by a recent study [138].

A possible prognostic role of HRs in cancer has not been specifically evaluated. A recent retrospective study, however, may be relevant to this issue [139]. This study, carried out in a large series of breast cancer patients by immunohistochemistry, found that total IGF-IR content had no prognostic value, while total IR content correlated with a shorter survival. Interestingly, the presence of phosphorylated IGF-IR and/or IR was present in approximately 50% of cases and correlated with a poor outcome. It was not possible to distinguish whether the IGF-IR or IR or HRs were predominantly phosphorylated because the antibody employed did not distinguish between the phosphorylated forms of these receptor subtypes.

Targeting Receptors of the IGF System in Cancer

Because of its permissive role in cell transformation and its deregulated expression in a variety of malignancies, the IGF-IR is considered a promising target for anticancer therapy [140]. In principle, inhibition of the IGF-IR should mostly affect actively dividing cancer cells, which overexpresses the IGF-IR and are highly responsive to IGFs, while sparing noncycling, terminally differentiated cells where the IGF-IR is expressed at low level and has a minor trophic role [140]. Indeed, in line with this assumption, several pharmaceutical companies have developed targeted therapies to the IGF-IR [141,142] that are currently at various stages of development. Numerous preclinical studies carried out in various cancer models have partially supported the efficacy of this approach, especially when combined with conventional anticancer therapies [141,142], but have also revealed mechanisms of resistance to these targeted therapies. One possible mechanism, especially operating in advanced cancers, is the activation of molecular pathways downstream from the IGF-IR, regardless of whatever the IGF-IR is expressed or not. This concept is exemplified by the observation that although R fibroblasts are resistant to transformation by a variety of oncogenes, they can be transformed by v-Src [78].

A major mechanism of resistance to therapies specifically targeting the IGF-IR in cancer cells is the frequent aberrant expression of IR (especially IR-A), and consequently of HRs. It is worth noting that a substantial proportion of human malignancies have a high IR-A:IGF-IR ratio [34,99,105]. In this regard, we previously found that in breast cancer cells with a high IR-A:IGF-IR ratio, IGF-II–induced cell growth could be blocked by inhibiting either IGF-II or the IR-A [107]. Similarly, an IR antibody was able to inhibit growth of thyroid cancer cells with high IR-A:IGF-IR ratio, and the combination of anti-IR and anti-IGF-IR antibodies was most effective [99]. When the IGF-IR was targeted with specific small interfering mRNAs (siRNA) in breast cancer cells, cells showed a reduced sequestration of IR moieties in HRs with a consequent increase in IR homodimers and insulin sensitivity [143].

Also overexpression of IR-A in cancer cells may promote tumor growth not only in response to IGF-II but also in response to circulating insulin, especially in hyperinsulinemic patients. Indeed, hyperinsulinemia has been found as a significant risk factor for a variety of malignancies, including cancer of the breast, pancreas, and colon–rectum [144], and is also associated with a worse prognosis in breast cancer patients [145]. Unfortunately, hyperinsulinemia is a common side effect of therapies with anti-IGF-IR antibodies, which reduce IGF-I feedback effect at the level of the pituitary and cause GH elevation and insulin resistance. This mechanism is also activated by other similar therapies, such as small molecules with tyrosine kinase activity against the IGF-IR [146] or blocking antibodies to IGFs [147]. Monoclonal antibodies specifically reacting with IGF-II do not affect the IGF-I feedback on GH and should avoid hyperinsulinemia [148]. These antibodies, however, do not block the effects of IGF-I and insulin.

Another mechanism of resistance to therapies specifically targeting the homodimeric IGF-IR is represented by HRs. HRs may not be recognized with high affinity by monoclonal antibodies used to target the homodimeric IGF-IR [48]. We previously showed that growth of breast or thyroid cancer cells with a high HR:IGF-IR ratio could be better blocked by an antibody against HRs than homodimeric IGF-IR [113]. Similar results were obtained in mice xenografted with breast cancer cells with either high HR:IGF-IR ratio [149].

In summary, therapies targeting the IGF-IR appear promising anticancer tools; however, there is the need to identify biochemical markers of response. Given the complexity of the IGF system and heterogeneity of receptor subtype expression in tumors, basic information for predicting tumor response to those therapies includes a profiling of IGF system components expressed by the malignant cells.

Conclusion

The IGF-IR is a valuable target for cancer therapy and several IGF-IR inhibitors are currently under evaluation in clinical trials. This novel therapeutical approach to cancer has been stimulated by the seminal observation of Baserga et al. that the IGF-IR plays a crucial role in cell transformation, in the maintenance of the malignant phenotype, and is frequently deregulated in cancer. However, in the past few years, there is increasing awareness of the complexity of the IGF system and that other receptors of the IGF family, namely the IR-A and HRs, may have a relevant role in cancer progression and metastases. The appreciation that there is cross-talk between the classical metabolic branch (the IR) and the mitogenic branch (the IGF-IR) of the IR/IGF-IR family has important implications for both cancer prevention and treatment. In fact, insulin resistance and hyperinsulinemia have been recognized as important risk factors for a variety of malignancies [144]. On the other hand, it should now be considered that IR-A and HR-A are predominantly expressed (as compared to the IGF-IR) in a substantial proportion of cancers and may be an important factor for tumor resistance to anticancer therapies including therapies targeting the IGF-IR. While more studies are needed to find strategies to overcome this resistance, a complete profiling of receptors of the IGF-IR and IR systems in cancer, their activated forms, is likely to be a valuable biomarker for predicting the response to IGF-IR targeted therapies.

Acknowledgments This work was partially supported by grants from the AIRC (Associazione Italiana per la Ricerca sul Cancro) and PRIN-MIUR 2005 (Ministero Italiano Università e Ricerca) to A.B.

References

1. Calle EE, Kaaks R (2004) Overweight, obesity and cancer: epidemiological evidence and proposed mechanisms. Nat Rev Cancer 4:579–591
2. Brogiolo W, Stocker H, Ikeya T et al (2001) An evolutionarily conserved function of the Drosophila insulin receptor and insulin-like peptides in growth control. Curr Biol 11:213–221
3. Ullrich A, Gray A, Tam AW et al (1986) Insulin-like growth factor I receptor primary structure: comparison with insulin receptor suggests structural determinants that define functional specificity. Embo J 5:2503–2512
4. Mynarcik DC, Williams PF, Schaffer L et al (1997) Identification of common ligand binding determinants of the insulin and insulin-like growth factor 1 receptors. Insights into mechanisms of ligand binding. J Biol Chem 272:18650–18655
5. Seino S, Seino M, Nishi S et al (1989) Structure of the human insulin receptor gene and characterization of its promoter. Proc Natl Acad Sci U S A 86:114–118
6. Mosthaf L, Vogt B, Haring HU et al (1991) Altered expression of insulin receptor types A and B in the skeletal muscle of non-insulin-dependent diabetes mellitus patients. Proc Natl Acad Sci U S A 88:4728–4730
7. Hubbard SR, Wei L, Ellis L et al (1994) Crystal structure of the tyrosine kinase domain of the human insulin receptor. Nature 372:746–754

8. Pawson T (1994) Signal transduction. Look at a tyrosine kinase. Nature 372:726–727
9. Cheng I, Stram DO, Penney KL et al (2006) Common genetic variation in IGF1 and prostate cancer risk in the Multiethnic Cohort. J Natl Cancer Inst 98:123–134
10. White MF (1998) The IRS-signalling system: a network of docking proteins that mediate insulin action. Mol Cell Biochem 182:3–11
11. Chiang SH, Baumann CA, Kanzaki M et al (2001) Insulin-stimulated GLUT4 translocation requires the CAP-dependent activation of TC10. Nature 410:944–948
12. Backer JM, Myers MG Jr, Shoelson SE et al (1992) Phosphatidylinositol 3'-kinase is activated by association with IRS-1 during insulin stimulation. Embo J 11:3469–3479
13. Skolnik EY, Lee CH, Batzer A et al (1993) The SH2/SH3 domain-containing protein GRB2 interacts with tyrosine-phosphorylated IRS1 and Shc: implications for insulin control of ras signalling. Embo J 12:1929–1936
14. Kornfeld S (1992) Structure and function of the mannose 6-phosphate/insulinlike growth factor II receptors. Annu Rev Biochem 61:307–330
15. Dhillon AS, Hagan S, Rath O et al (2007) MAP kinase signalling pathways in cancer. Oncogene 26:3279–3290
16. Wellbrock C, Karasarides M, Marais R (2004) The RAF proteins take centre stage. Nat Rev Mol Cell Biol 5:875–885
17. Harrington LS, Findlay GM, Lamb RF (2005) Restraining PI3K: mTOR signalling goes back to the membrane. Trends Biochem Sci 30:35–42
18. Bjornsti MA, Houghton PJ (2004) The TOR pathway: a target for cancer therapy. Nat Rev Cancer 4:335–348
19. Holland EC, Sonenberg N, Pandolfi PP et al (2004) Signaling control of mRNA translation in cancer pathogenesis. Oncogene 23:3138–3144
20. O'Reilly KE, Rojo F, She QB et al (2006) mTOR inhibition induces upstream receptor tyrosine kinase signaling and activates Akt. Cancer Res 66:1500–1508
21. Foster FM, Traer CJ, Abraham SM et al (2003) The phosphoinositide (PI) 3-kinase family. J Cell Sci 116:3037–3040
22. Yin Y, Shen WH (2008) PTEN: a new guardian of the genome. Oncogene 27:5443–5453
23. Zapf A, Hsu D, Olefsky JM (1994) Comparison of the intracellular itineraries of insulin-like growth factor-I and insulin and their receptors in Rat-1 fibroblasts. Endocrinology 134:2445–2452
24. Dupont J, Khan J, Qu BH et al (2001) Insulin and IGF-1 induce different patterns of gene expression in mouse fibroblast NIH-3T3 cells: identification by cDNA microarray analysis. Endocrinology 142:4969–4975
25. Siddle K, Urso B, Niesler CA et al (2001) Specificity in ligand binding and intracellular signalling by insulin and insulin-like growth factor receptors. Biochem Soc Trans 29:513–525
26. Frasca F, Pandini G, Malaguarnera R et al (2007) Role of c-Abl in directing metabolic versus mitogenic effects in insulin receptor signaling. J Biol Chem 282:26077–26088
27. Najjar SM, Blakesley VA, Li Calzi S et al (1997) Differential phosphorylation of pp 120 by insulin and insulin-like growth factor-1 receptors: role for the C-terminal domain of the beta-subunit. Biochemistry 36:6827–6834
28. O'Neill TJ, Zhu Y, Gustafson TA (1997) Interaction of MAD2 with the carboxyl terminus of the insulin receptor but not with the IGFIR. Evidence for release from the insulin receptor after activation. J Biol Chem 272:10035–10040
29. Koval AP, Blakesley VA, Roberts CT Jr et al (1998) Interaction in vitro of the product of the c-Crk-II proto-oncogene with the insulin-like growth factor I receptor. Biochem J 330(Pt 2):923–932
30. Dupont J, Fernandez AM, Glackin CA et al (2001) Insulin-like growth factor 1 (IGF-1)-induced twist expression is involved in the anti-apoptotic effects of the IGF-1 receptor. J Biol Chem 276:26699–26707
31. Mosthaf L, Grako K, Dull TJ et al (1990) Functionally distinct insulin receptors generated by tissue-specific alternative splicing. Embo J 9:2409–2413
32. Yamaguchi Y, Flier JS, Yokota A et al (1991) Functional properties of two naturally occurring isoforms of the human insulin receptor in Chinese hamster ovary cells. Endocrinology 129:2058–2066

33. Kosaki A, Pillay TS, Xu L et al (1995) The B isoform of the insulin receptor signals more efficiently than the A isoform in HepG2 cells. J Biol Chem 270:20816–20823
34. Frasca F, Pandini G, Scalia P et al (1999) Insulin receptor isoform A, a newly recognized, high-affinity insulin-like growth factor II receptor in fetal and cancer cells. Mol Cell Biol 19:3278–3288
35. Benyoucef S, Surinya KH, Hadaschik D et al (2007) Characterization of insulin/IGF hybrid receptors: contributions of the insulin receptor L2 and Fn1 domains and the alternatively spliced exon 11 sequence to ligand binding and receptor activation. Biochem J 403:603–613
36. Yamaguchi Y, Flier JS, Benecke H et al (1993) Ligand-binding properties of the two isoforms of the human insulin receptor. Endocrinology 132:1132–1138
37. Blanquart C, Achi J, Issad T (2008) Characterization of IRA/IRB hybrid insulin receptors using bioluminescence resonance energy transfer. Biochem Pharmacol 76:873–883
38. Nevado C, Benito M, Valverde AM (2008) Role of insulin receptor and balance in insulin receptor isoforms A and B in regulation of apoptosis in simian virus 40-immortalized neonatal hepatocytes. Mol Biol Cell 19:1185–1198
39. Kosaki A, Webster NJ (1993) Effect of dexamethasone on the alternative splicing of the insulin receptor mRNA and insulin action in HepG2 hepatoma cells. J Biol Chem 268:21990–21996
40. Entingh AJ, Taniguchi CM, Kahn CR (2003) Bi-directional regulation of brown fat adipogenesis by the insulin receptor. J Biol Chem 278:33377–33383
41. Sciacca L, Prisco M, Wu A et al (2003) Signaling differences from the A and B isoforms of the insulin receptor (IR) in 32D cells in the presence or absence of IR substrate-1. Endocrinology 144:2650–2658
42. Leibiger B, Leibiger IB, Moede T et al (2001) Selective insulin signaling through A and B insulin receptors regulates transcription of insulin and glucokinase genes in pancreatic beta cells. Mol Cell 7:559–570
43. Morrione A, Valentinis B, Xu SQ et al (1997) Insulin-like growth factor II stimulates cell proliferation through the insulin receptor. Proc Natl Acad Sci U S A 94:3777–3782
44. Sciacca L, Mineo R, Pandini G et al (2002) In IGF-I receptor-deficient leiomyosarcoma cells autocrine IGF-II induces cell invasion and protection from apoptosis via the insulin receptor isoform A. Oncogene 21:8240–8250
45. Pandini G, Medico E, Conte E et al (2003) Differential gene expression induced by insulin and insulin-like growth factor-II through the insulin receptor isoform A. J Biol Chem 278:42178–42189
46. Ullrich A, Bell JR, Chen EY et al (1985) Human insulin receptor and its relationship to the tyrosine kinase family of oncogenes. Nature 313:756–761
47. Soos MA, Siddle K (1989) Immunological relationships between receptors for insulin and insulin-like growth factor I. Evidence for structural heterogeneity of insulin-like growth factor I receptors involving hybrids with insulin receptors. Biochem J 263:553–563
48. Pandini G, Vigneri R, Costantino A et al (1999) Insulin and insulin-like growth factor-I (IGF-I) receptor overexpression in breast cancers leads to insulin/IGF-I hybrid receptor overexpression: evidence for a second mechanism of IGF-I signaling. Clin Cancer Res 5:1935–1944
49. Soos MA, Whittaker J, Lammers R et al (1990) Receptors for insulin and insulin-like growth factor-I can form hybrid dimers. Characterisation of hybrid receptors in transfected cells. Biochem J 270:383–390
50. Soos MA, Nave BT, Siddle K (1993) Immunological studies of type I IGF receptors and insulin receptors: characterisation of hybrid and atypical receptor subtypes. Adv Exp Med Biol 343:145–157
51. Soos MA, Field CE, Siddle K (1993) Purified hybrid insulin/insulin-like growth factor-I receptors bind insulin-like growth factor-I, but not insulin, with high affinity. Biochem J 290(Pt 2):419–426
52. Moxham CP, Duronio V, Jacobs S (1989) Insulin-like growth factor I receptor beta-subunit heterogeneity. Evidence for hybrid tetramers composed of insulin-like growth factor I and insulin receptor heterodimers. J Biol Chem 264:13238–13244
53. Frattali AL, Treadway JL, Pessin JE (1992) Insulin/IGF-1 hybrid receptors: implications for the dominant-negative phenotype in syndromes of insulin resistance. J Cell Biochem 48:43–50

54. Kasuya J, Paz IB, Maddux BA et al (1993) Characterization of human placental insulin-like growth factor-I/insulin hybrid receptors by protein microsequencing and purification. Biochemistry 32:13531–13536
55. Pandini G, Frasca F, Mineo R et al (2002) Insulin/insulin-like growth factor I hybrid receptors have different biological characteristics depending on the insulin receptor isoform involved. J Biol Chem 277:39684–39695
56. Slaaby R, Schaffer L, Lautrup-Larsen I et al (2006) Hybrid receptors formed by insulin receptor (IR) and insulin-like growth factor I receptor (IGF-IR) have low insulin and high IGF-1 affinity irrespective of the IR splice variant. J Biol Chem 281:25869–25874
57. Garcia-de Lacoba M, Alarcon C, de la Rosa EJ et al (1999) Insulin/insulin-like growth factor-I hybrid receptors with high affinity for insulin are developmentally regulated during neurogenesis. Endocrinology 140:233–243
58. Alexandrides TK, Smith RJ (1989) A novel fetal insulin-like growth factor (IGF) I receptor. Mechanism for increased IGF I- and insulin-stimulated tyrosine kinase activity in fetal muscle. J Biol Chem 264:12922–12930
59. Navarro M, Joulia D, Fedon Y et al (2008) The atypical alpha2beta2 IGF receptor expressed in inducible c2.7 myoblasts is derived from post-translational modifications of the mouse IGF-I receptor. Growth Horm IGF Res 18:412–423
60. Milazzo G, Yip CC, Maddux BA et al (1992) High-affinity insulin binding to an atypical insulin-like growth factor-I receptor in human breast cancer cells. J Clin Invest 89:899–908
61. Jonas HA, Cox AJ, Harrison LC (1989) Delineation of atypical insulin receptors from classical insulin and type I insulin-like growth factor receptors in human placenta. Biochem J 257:101–107
62. Jonas HA, Cox AJ (1991) Insulin receptor sub-types in a human lymphoid-derived cell line (IM-9): differential regulation by insulin, dexamethasone and monensin. J Recept Res 11:813–829
63. Werner H, Le Roith D (2000) New concepts in regulation and function of the insulin-like growth factors: implications for understanding normal growth and neoplasia. Cell Mol Life Sci 57:932–942
64. Zhao H, Dupont J, Yakar S et al (2004) PTEN inhibits cell proliferation and induces apoptosis by downregulating cell surface IGF-IR expression in prostate cancer cells. Oncogene 23:786–794
65. Hwang PH, Kim SY, Lee JC et al (2005) PTEN/MMAC1 enhances the growth inhibition by anticancer drugs with downregulation of IGF-II expression in gastric cancer cells. Exp Mol Med 37:391–398
66. Yi HK, Kim SY, Hwang PH et al (2005) Impact of PTEN on the expression of insulin-like growth factors (IGFs) and IGF-binding proteins in human gastric adenocarcinoma cells. Biochem Biophys Res Commun 330:760–767
67. Buckbinder L, Talbott R, Velasco-Miguel S et al (1995) Induction of the growth inhibitor IGF-binding protein 3 by p53. Nature 377:646–649
68. Ahmad T, Farnie G, Bundred NJ et al (2004) The mitogenic action of insulin-like growth factor I in normal human mammary epithelial cells requires the epidermal growth factor receptor tyrosine kinase. J Biol Chem 279:1713–1719
69. Balana ME, Labriola L, Salatino M et al (2001) Activation of ErbB-2 via a hierarchical interaction between ErbB-2 and type I insulin-like growth factor receptor in mammary tumor cells. Oncogene 20:34–47
70. Nahta R, Yuan LX, Zhang B et al (2005) Insulin-like growth factor-I receptor/human epidermal growth factor receptor 2 heterodimerization contributes to trastuzumab resistance of breast cancer cells. Cancer Res 65:11118–11128
71. Roudabush FL, Pierce KL, Maudsley S et al (2000) Transactivation of the EGF receptor mediates IGF-1-stimulated shc phosphorylation and ERK1/2 activation in COS-7 cells. J Biol Chem 275:22583–22589
72. Sisci D, Surmacz E (2007) Crosstalk between IGF signaling and steroid hormone receptors in breast cancer. Curr Pharm Des 13:705–717
73. Umayahara Y, Kawamori R, Watada H et al (1994) Estrogen regulation of the insulin-like growth factor I gene transcription involves an AP-1 enhancer. J Biol Chem 269:16433–16442

74. Dupont J, Karas M, LeRoith D (2000) The potentiation of estrogen on insulin-like growth factor I action in MCF-7 human breast cancer cells includes cell cycle components. J Biol Chem 275:35893–35901
75. Pandini G, Mineo R, Frasca F et al (2005) Androgens up-regulate the insulin-like growth factor-I receptor in prostate cancer cells. Cancer Res 65:1849–1857
76. Pandini G, Genua M, Frasca F et al (2007) 17beta-estradiol up-regulates the insulin-like growth factor receptor through a nongenotropic pathway in prostate cancer cells. Cancer Res 67:8932–8941
77. Sell C, Dumenil G, Deveaud C et al (1994) Effect of a null mutation of the insulin-like growth factor I receptor gene on growth and transformation of mouse embryo fibroblasts. Mol Cell Biol 14:3604–3612
78. Baserga R, Hongo A, Rubini M et al (1997) The IGF-I receptor in cell growth, transformation and apoptosis. Biochim Biophys Acta 1332:F105–F126
79. Kaleko M, Rutter WJ, Miller AD (1990) Overexpression of the human insulinlike growth factor I receptor promotes ligand-dependent neoplastic transformation. Mol Cell Biol 10:464–473
80. Rubini M, Hongo A, D'Ambrosio C et al (1997) The IGF-I receptor in mitogenesis and transformation of mouse embryo cells: role of receptor number. Exp Cell Res 230:284–292
81. Giorgino F, Belfiore A, Milazzo G et al (1991) Overexpression of insulin receptors in fibroblast and ovary cells induces a ligand-mediated transformed phenotype. Mol Endocrinol 5:452–459
82. Ish-Shalom D, Christoffersen CT, Vorwerk P et al (1997) Mitogenic properties of insulin and insulin analogues mediated by the insulin receptor. Diabetologia 40(Suppl 2):S25–S31
83. Drejer K (1992) The bioactivity of insulin analogues from in vitro receptor binding to in vivo glucose uptake. Diabetes Metab Rev 8:259–285
84. Milazzo G, Sciacca L, Papa V et al (1997) ASPB10 insulin induction of increased mitogenic responses and phenotypic changes in human breast epithelial cells: evidence for enhanced interactions with the insulin-like growth factor-I receptor. Mol Carcinog 18:19–25
85. Carboni JM, Lee AV, Hadsell DL et al (2005) Tumor development by transgenic expression of a constitutively active insulin-like growth factor I receptor. Cancer Res 65:3781–3787
86. Jones RA, Campbell CI, Gunther EJ et al (2007) Transgenic overexpression of IGF-IR disrupts mammary ductal morphogenesis and induces tumor formation. Oncogene 26:1636–1644
87. Mathews LS, Hammer RE, Behringer RR et al (1988) Growth enhancement of transgenic mice expressing human insulin-like growth factor I. Endocrinology 123:2827–2833
88. DiGiovanni J, Kiguchi K, Frijhoff A et al (2000) Deregulated expression of insulin-like growth factor 1 in prostate epithelium leads to neoplasia in transgenic mice. Proc Natl Acad Sci U S A 97:3455–3460
89. Hadsell DL, Greenberg NM, Fligger JM et al (1996) Targeted expression of des(1-3) human insulin-like growth factor I in transgenic mice influences mammary gland development and IGF-binding protein expression. Endocrinology 137:321–330
90. Hadsell DL, Murphy KL, Bonnette SG et al (2000) Cooperative interaction between mutant p53 and des(1-3)IGF-I accelerates mammary tumorigenesis. Oncogene 19:889–898
91. Bates P, Fisher R, Ward A et al (1995) Mammary cancer in transgenic mice expressing insulin-like growth factor II (IGF-II). Br J Cancer 72:1189–1193
92. Moorehead RA, Fata JE, Johnson MB et al (2001) Inhibition of mammary epithelial apoptosis and sustained phosphorylation of Akt/PKB in MMTV-IGF-II transgenic mice. Cell Death Differ 8:16–29
93. Peyrat JP, Bonneterre J, Beuscart R et al (1988) Insulin-like growth factor 1 receptors in human breast cancer and their relation to estradiol and progesterone receptors. Cancer Res 48:6429–6433
94. Cullen KJ, Yee D, Sly WS et al (1990) Insulin-like growth factor receptor expression and function in human breast cancer. Cancer Res 50:48–53
95. Papa V, Gliozzo B, Clark GM et al (1993) Insulin-like growth factor-I receptors are overexpressed and predict a low risk in human breast cancer. Cancer Res 53:3736–3740
96. Koda M, Sulkowski S, Garofalo C et al (2003) Expression of the insulin-like growth factor-I receptor in primary breast cancer and lymph node metastases: correlations with estrogen receptors alpha and beta. Horm Metab Res 35:794–801

97. Resnik JL, Reichart DB, Huey K et al (1998) Elevated insulin-like growth factor I receptor autophosphorylation and kinase activity in human breast cancer. Cancer Res 58:1159–1164
98. Rasmussen AA, Cullen KJ (1998) Paracrine/autocrine regulation of breast cancer by the insulin-like growth factors. Breast Cancer Res Treat 47:219–233
99. Vella V, Pandini G, Sciacca L et al (2002) A novel autocrine loop involving IGF-II and the insulin receptor isoform-A stimulates growth of thyroid cancer. J Clin Endocrinol Metab 87:245–254
100. Strammiello R, Benini S, Manara MC et al (2003) Impact of IGF-I/IGF-IR circuit on the angiogenetic properties of Ewing's sarcoma cells. Horm Metab Res 35:675–684
101. Heuson JC, Legros N, Heimann R (1972) Influence of insulin administration on growth of the 7,12-dimethylbenz(a)anthracene-induced mammary carcinoma in intact, oophorectomized, and hypophysectomized rats. Cancer Res 32:233–238
102. Nandi S, Guzman RC, Yang J (1995) Hormones and mammary carcinogenesis in mice, rats, and humans: a unifying hypothesis. Proc Natl Acad Sci U S A 92:3650–3657
103. Pillemer G, Lugasi-Evgi H, Scharovsky G et al (1992) Insulin dependence of murine lymphoid T-cell leukemia. Int J Cancer 50:80–85
104. Sharon R, Pillemer G, Ish-Shalom D et al (1993) Insulin dependence of murine T-cell lymphoma. II. Insulin-deficient diabetic mice and mice fed low-energy diet develop resistance to lymphoma growth. Int J Cancer 53:843–849
105. Papa V, Pezzino V, Costantino A et al (1990) Elevated insulin receptor content in human breast cancer. J Clin Invest 86:1503–1510
106. Milazzo G, Giorgino F, Damante G et al (1992) Insulin receptor expression and function in human breast cancer cell lines. Cancer Res 52:3924–3930
107. Sciacca L, Costantino A, Pandini G et al (1999) Insulin receptor activation by IGF-II in breast cancers: evidence for a new autocrine/paracrine mechanism. Oncogene 18:2471–2479
108. Kalli KR, Falowo OI, Bale LK et al (2002) Functional insulin receptors on human epithelial ovarian carcinoma cells: implications for IGF-II mitogenic signaling. Endocrinology 143:3259–3267
109. Diaz LE, Chuan YC, Lewitt M et al (2007) IGF-II regulates metastatic properties of choriocarcinoma cells through the activation of the insulin receptor. Mol Hum Reprod 13:567–576
110. Li Y, Chang Q, Rubin BP et al (2007) Insulin receptor activation in solitary fibrous tumours. J Pathol 211:550–554
111. Arcaro A, Doepfner KT, Boller D et al (2007) Novel role for insulin as an autocrine growth factor for malignant brain tumour cells. Biochem J 406:57–66
112. Vella V, Sciacca L, Pandini G et al (2001) The IGF system in thyroid cancer: new concepts. Mol Pathol 54:121–124
113. Belfiore A, Pandini G, Vella V et al (1999) Insulin/IGF-I hybrid receptors play a major role in IGF-I signaling in thyroid cancer. Biochimie 81:403–407
114. Avnet S, Sciacca L, Salerno M et al (2009) Insulin receptor isoform A and insulin-like growth factor II as additional treatment targets in human osteosarcoma. Cancer Res 69:2443–2452
115. Shiono S, Ishii G, Nagai K et al (2006) Immunohistochemical prognostic factors in resected colorectal lung metastases using tissue microarray analysis. Eur J Surg Oncol 32:308–309
116. Almeida A, Muleris M, Dutrillaux B et al (1994) The insulin-like growth factor I receptor gene is the target for the 15q26 amplicon in breast cancer. Genes Chromosomes Cancer 11:63–65
117. Papa V, Milazzo G, Goldfine ID et al (1997) Sporadic amplification of the insulin receptor gene in human breast cancer. J Endocrinol Invest 20:531–536
118. Zhang J, Trent JM, Meltzer PS (1993) Rapid isolation and characterization of amplified DNA by chromosome microdissection: identification of IGF1R amplification in malignant melanoma. Oncogene 8:2827–2831
119. Armengol G, Knuutila S, Lluis F et al (2000) DNA copy number changes and evaluation of MYC, IGF1R, and FES amplification in xenografts of pancreatic adenocarcinoma. Cancer Genet Cytogenet 116:133–141

120. Werner H, Shalita-Chesner M, Abramovitch S et al (2000) Regulation of the insulin-like growth factor-I receptor gene by oncogenes and antioncogenes: implications in human cancer. Mol Genet Metab 71:315–320
121. Maor S, Yosepovich A, Papa MZ et al (2007) Elevated insulin-like growth factor-I receptor (IGF-IR) levels in primary breast tumors associated with BRCA1 mutations. Cancer Lett 257:236–243
122. Hudelist G, Wagner T, Rosner M et al (2007) Intratumoral IGF-I protein expression is selectively upregulated in breast cancer patients with BRCA1/2 mutations. Endocr Relat Cancer 14:1053–1062
123. Paonessa F, Foti D, Costa V et al (2006) Activator protein-2 overexpression accounts for increased insulin receptor expression in human breast cancer. Cancer Res 66:5085–5093
124. Novosyadlyy R, Kurshan N, Lann D et al (2008) Insulin-like growth factor-I protects cells from ER stress-induced apoptosis via enhancement of the adaptive capacity of endoplasmic reticulum. Cell Death Differ 15:1304–1317
125. Samani AA, Yakar S, LeRoith D et al (2007) The role of the IGF system in cancer growth and metastasis: overview and recent insights. Endocr Rev 28:20–47
126. Foekens JA, Portengen H, van Putten WL et al (1989) Prognostic value of receptors for insulin-like growth factor 1, somatostatin, and epidermal growth factor in human breast cancer. Cancer Res 49:7002–7009
127. Maor S, Mayer D, Yarden RI et al (2006) Estrogen receptor regulates insulin-like growth factor-I receptor gene expression in breast tumor cells: involvement of transcription factor Sp1. J Endocrinol 191:605–612
128. Bonneterre J, Peyrat JP, Beuscart R et al (1990) Prognostic significance of insulin-like growth factor 1 receptors in human breast cancer. Cancer Res 50:6931–6935
129. Railo MJ, von Smitten K, Pekonen F (1994) The prognostic value of insulin-like growth factor-I in breast cancer patients. Results of a follow-up study on 126 patients. Eur J Cancer 30A:307–311
130. Creighton CJ, Casa A, Lazard Z et al (2008) Insulin-like growth factor-I activates gene transcription programs strongly associated with poor breast cancer prognosis. J Clin Oncol 26:4078–4085
131. Figueroa JA, De Raad S, Speights VO et al (2001) Gene expression of insulin-like growth factors and receptors in neoplastic prostate tissues: correlation with clinico-pathological parameters. Cancer Invest 19:28–34
132. Tennant MK, Thrasher JB, Twomey PA et al (1996) Protein and messenger ribonucleic acid (mRNA) for the type 1 insulin-like growth factor (IGF) receptor is decreased and IGF-II mRNA is increased in human prostate carcinoma compared to benign prostate epithelium. J Clin Endocrinol Metab 81:3774–3782
133. Hellawell GO, Turner GD, Davies DR et al (2002) Expression of the type 1 insulin-like growth factor receptor is up-regulated in primary prostate cancer and commonly persists in metastatic disease. Cancer Res 62:2942–2950
134. Hellawell GO, Brewster SF (2002) Growth factors and their receptors in prostate cancer. BJU Int 89:230–240
135. Hakam A, Yeatman TJ, Lu L et al (1999) Expression of insulin-like growth factor-1 receptor in human colorectal cancer. Hum Pathol 30:1128–1133
136. Chakravarty G, Santillan AA, Galer C et al (2009) Phosphorylated insulin like growth factor-I receptor expression and its clinico-pathological significance in histologic subtypes of human thyroid cancer. Exp Biol Med (Maywood) 234:372–386
137. Mathieu MC, Clark GM, Allred DC et al (1997) Insulin receptor expression and clinical outcome in node-negative breast cancer. Proc Assoc Am Physicians 109:565–571
138. Mulligan AM, O'Malley FP, Ennis M et al (2007) Insulin receptor is an independent predictor of a favorable outcome in early stage breast cancer. Breast Cancer Res Treat 106:39–47
139. Law JH, Habibi G, Hu K et al (2008) Phosphorylated insulin-like growth factor-i/insulin receptor is present in all breast cancer subtypes and is related to poor survival. Cancer Res 68:10238–10246

140. Baserga R, Peruzzi F, Reiss K (2003) The IGF-1 receptor in cancer biology. Int J Cancer 107:873–877
141. Hofmann F, Garcia-Echeverria C (2005) Blocking the insulin-like growth factor-I receptor as a strategy for targeting cancer. Drug Discov Today 10:1041–1047
142. Pollak M (2008) Targeting insulin and insulin-like growth factor signalling in oncology. Curr Opin Pharmacol 8:384–392
143. Zhang H, Pelzer AM, Kiang DT et al (2007) Down-regulation of type I insulin-like growth factor receptor increases sensitivity of breast cancer cells to insulin. Cancer Res 67:391–397
144. Pisani P (2008) Hyper-insulinaemia and cancer, meta-analyses of epidemiological studies. Arch Physiol Biochem 114:63–70
145. Goodwin PJ, Ennis M, Pritchard KI et al (2002) Fasting insulin and outcome in early-stage breast cancer: results of a prospective cohort study. J Clin Oncol 20:42–51
146. Haluska P, Carboni JM, Loegering DA et al (2006) In vitro and in vivo antitumor effects of the dual insulin-like growth factor-I/insulin receptor inhibitor, BMS-554417. Cancer Res 66:362–371
147. Miyamoto S, Nakamura M, Shitara K et al (2005) Blockade of paracrine supply of insulin-like growth factors using neutralizing antibodies suppresses the liver metastasis of human colorectal cancers. Clin Cancer Res 11:3494–3502
148. Feng Y, Zhu Z, Xiao X et al (2006) Novel human monoclonal antibodies to insulin-like growth factor (IGF)-II that potently inhibit the IGF receptor type I signal transduction function. Mol Cancer Ther 5:114–120
149. Pandini G, Wurch T, Akla B et al (2007) Functional responses and in vivo anti-tumour activity of h7C10: a humanised monoclonal antibody with neutralising activity against the insulin-like growth factor-1 (IGF-1) receptor and insulin/IGF-1 hybrid receptors. Eur J Cancer 43:1318–1327
150. Ouban A, Muraca P, Yeatman T et al (2003) Expression and distribution of insulin-like growth factor-1 receptor in human carcinomas. Hum Pathol 34:803–808
151. Guo YS, Narayan S, Yallampalli C et al (1992) Characterization of insulinlike growth factor I receptors in human colon cancer. Gastroenterology 102:1101–1108
152. Iwamura M, Sluss PM, Casamento JB et al (1993) Insulin-like growth factor I: action and receptor characterization in human prostate cancer cell lines. Prostate 22:243–252
153. Nickerson T, Chang F, Lorimer D et al (2001) In vivo progression of LAPC-9 and LNCaP prostate cancer models to androgen independence is associated with increased expression of insulin-like growth factor I (IGF-I) and IGF-I receptor (IGF-IR). Cancer Res 61:6276–6280
154. Huff KK, Kaufman D, Gabbay KH et al (1986) Secretion of an insulin-like growth factor-I-related protein by human breast cancer cells. Cancer Res 46:4613–4619
155. Yee D, Paik S, Lebovic GS et al (1989) Analysis of insulin-like growth factor I gene expression in malignancy: evidence for a paracrine role in human breast cancer. Mol Endocrinol 3:509–517
156. Maiorano E, Ciampolillo A, Viale G et al (2000) Insulin-like growth factor 1 expression in thyroid tumors. Appl Immunohistochem Mol Morphol 8:110–119
157. Michell NP, Langman MJ, Eggo MC (1997) Insulin-like growth factors and their binding proteins in human colonocytes: preferential degradation of insulin-like growth factor binding protein 2 in colonic cancers. Br J Cancer 76:60–66
158. Pietrzkowski Z, Mulholland G, Gomella L et al (1993) Inhibition of growth of prostatic cancer cell lines by peptide analogues of insulin-like growth factor 1. Cancer Res 53:1102–1106
159. Paik S (1992) Expression of IGF-I and IGF-II mRNA in breast tissue. Breast Cancer Res Treat 22:31–38
160. Singh P, Dai B, Yallampalli C et al (1994) Expression of IGF-II and IGF-binding proteins by colon cancer cells in relation to growth response to IGFs. Am J Physiol 267:G608–G617
161. Jehle PM, Fussgaenger RD, Blum WF et al (1999) Differential autocrine regulation of intestine epithelial cell proliferation and differentiation by insulin-like growth factor (IGF) system components. Horm Metab Res 31:97–102
162. Li SL, Goko H, Xu ZD et al (1998) Expression of insulin-like growth factor (IGF)-II in human prostate, breast, bladder, and paraganglioma tumors. Cell Tissue Res 291:469–479

Chapter 12
Insulin Resistance: Clinical Implications for Cancer Treatment and Prevention

Saroj Niraula and Pamela J. Goodwin

Introduction

Obesity is a major threat to health worldwide and if the current trend continues, more than 50% of the world's population is projected to be obese by the year 2030 [1]. As reviewed by Irwin et al. in another chapter [2], obesity has been linked to both cancer risk and cancer outcome. Although obesity, insulin resistance and hyperinsulinemia are interrelated [3], until recently the primary focus of epidemiologic and clinical cancer research has been on obesity. Eugenia Calle et al. [4] provided an elegant demonstration of the association between body size and mortality from cancer in the prospective Cancer Prevention Study II, conducted by the American Cancer Society. Studying over 900,000 American adults, they found that individuals with a body mass index (BMI=weight(kg)/height(m)^2) of at least 40 had death rates from cancer that were 52% higher (for men) and 62% higher (for women) than the rates seen in normal weight individuals. Higher BMI was significantly associated with increased death rates from a number of common cancers, including colon and rectum, breast, uterus and prostate as well as from less common cancers such as liver, gallbladder, pancreas, kidney, stomach, cervix, non-Hodgkin's lymphoma and multiple myeloma. The only cancer demonstrating an inverse association between BMI and future cancer mortality was lung cancer. The results of this study (which combine the effect of obesity on cancer risk and cancer progression) suggest that obesity may contribute to 14% of all deaths from cancer in men and 20% of all deaths from cancer in women, evidence of an important contribution of obesity to cancer death. Similar results were obtained in a recent study by Whitlock et al. [5] in an analysis involving approximately 90,000 subjects that obesity was associated with significantly increased mortality from several causes,

P.J. Goodwin (✉)
Samuel Lunenfeld Research Institute, Mount Sinai Hospital and Princess Margaret Hospital, University of Toronto, Toronto, ON, Canada
e-mail: pgoodwin@mtsinai.on.ca

I.G. Fantus (ed.), *Insulin Resistance and Cancer: Epidemiology, Cellular and Molecular Mechanisms and Clinical Implications*, Energy Balance and Cancer 1, DOI 10.1007/978-1-4419-9911-5_12,

including cancer; with every 5 kg/m^2 increase in BMI, risk of cancer-specific mortality increased by 10%. Furthermore, a recent meta-analysis by Renehan et al. [6] that focused on cancer incidence rather than mortality, reported that increased BMI was associated with increased risk of several different cancers including esophageal, thyroid, colon, rectal, renal, endometrial, gallbladder, breast (post-menopausal) and pancreatic, as well as melanoma, leukaemia, multiple myeloma, and non-Hodgkin lymphoma.

In some cancers, notably colorectal, and to some extent breast, low levels of physical activity (a factor that also contributes to obesity and insulin resistance) have also been associated with increased risk of incidence [7, 8]. In colorectal cancer, physical inactivity appears to influence cancer risk independent of obesity, possibly through a favorable effect on insulin resistance. High levels of physical activity have been linked to a 40–50% reduced risk of colorectal cancer [9], 35–40% reduced risk of prostate cancer [10] and a 25–30% reduced risk of breast cancer [11].

Taken together, these observations linking lifestyle factors such as obesity and physical activity to cancer risk and mortality have stimulated interest in potential roles of insulin and insulin resistance in cancer risk and prognosis. The remainder of this chapter will focus on these factors.

Insulin Resistance and Cancer Risk

Although several mechanisms have been proposed for the association of obesity and physical inactivity with cancer risk and prognosis, including alterations in profiles of sex hormones (e.g., estrogens, androgens, sex hormone binding globulin), inflammation and reduced immune surveillance, the insulin resistance syndrome (IRS) and its associated metabolic changes have been increasingly recognized as potential contributors to this link [9, 11]. Aspects of the IRS that have been postulated as potential mediators of the obesity-cancer link include hyperinsulinemia, increased free IGF-I, increased adipocytokines (including leptin), as well as increased markers of inflammation such as C-reactive protein. Research, reviewed in several other chapters of this volume [12–18], is ongoing to elucidate the biologic basis for the obesity/insulin resistance/cancer risk association and this research is likely to yield important insight in upcoming years.

The evidence linking hyperinsulinemia to the risk of developing cancer is growing, but is not as robust as that relating to obesity. Pisani et al. [19] has recently reviewed this evidence, using a meta-analytic approach. Higher insulin levels were significantly associated with increased risk of colorectal and pancreatic cancer, but less convincingly with breast and endometrial cancers. A meta-analysis has suggested that, compared to nondiabetics, those with diabetes and prediabetes have an increased risk of cancer-related mortality (HR and 95% Confidence Interval (CI) 1.71 (1.35, 2.17) and 1.13 (1.00, 1.28) respectively [20]). Studies published subsequently (e.g., [21] have demonstrated links between hyperinsulinemia and breast cancer risk). Recent reports have raised concerns that use of exogenous insulin may increase risk of colorectal cancer (injected insulin) [22] or lung cancer (inhaled insulin) [23]. In 2009 a number of studies suggested the use of glargine insulin (with known mitogenic properties) may be associated with increased cancer risk [24–26]; however, the potential for bias in the observational designs used and publication of subsequent studies that failed to replicate these findings have raised doubts about the validity of the initial reports [27–29]. Diabetes in adults (usually associated with insulin resistance) has been also linked to a modest increased risk of breast [30–32] but not prostate cancer [33]. A large 14 year prospective cohort study in a Korean population [34], involving 1,298,385 subjects reported a 30% increased likelihood of cancer related death in subjects with high fasting serum glucose concentration (an indirect measure of insulin resistance), compared to those with lower fasting serum glucose after controlling for potential confounders; the association was present in all BMI categories, indicating an effect of insulin resistance beyond that of body weight. Similarly, a pooled analysis of prospective studies involving over 62,000 subjects has suggested an approximate threefold elevation in colorectal cancer mortality among those with insulin resistance or associated biochemical abnormality after adjusting for age, alcohol consumption and smoking [35].

Taken together, these observations suggest that insulin resistance may be an important mediator of the associations of obesity and possibly physical inactivity, with cancer risk and it may be a potential target in cancer prevention.

Insulin Resistance and Cancer Outcomes

Obesity has also been linked to cancer prognosis. The strongest evidence exists for breast cancer. A recent meta-analysis by Protani et al. [36] suggests that compared to nonobese women, obese women have an increased risk of overall and breast cancer-specific mortality (HR 1.33, 95% CI 1.21–1.47 and HR 1.33, 95% CI 1.19–1.50 respectively). Although obesity has been associated with several adverse prognostic characteristics including estrogen receptor negativity, higher grade, larger tumor size and greater axillary nodal involvement, it exerts prognostic effects that are independent of these factors [37]. Obesity has also been associated with hyperinsulinemia in early stage breast cancer. Hyperinsulinemia has, in turn, been associated with insulin resistance (HOMA) and components of the IRS are more common in obese vs. nonobese breast cancer patients [38]. At least seven studies [39–46] have identified high levels of insulin or related factors, such as c-peptide, HOMA or HbA1c, as being associated with adverse prognosis in early stage breast cancer with a two to threefold increased risk of distant recurrence or death in those with the highest insulin levels.

Several studies have shown higher levels of physical activity (associated with improved insulin resistance) around the time of breast cancer diagnosis to be associated with improved cancer outcomes [47–51] (see Table 12.1). These studies collectively report a relative reduction of about 50% in breast cancer-related death with increased physical activity, however, no association between physical activity and breast cancer

Table 12.1 Associations of physical activity with breast cancer survival

Citation	n	Intervention setting	Outcome parameters	Results (HR)
Holmes et al. [152]	2,987	2 years postdiagnosis	Death	0.59 ($p=0.03$)
			BC death	0.50 ($p=0.004$)
			Recurrence	0.57 ($p=0.05$)
Abrahamson et al. [48]	1,264	1 year prediagnosis	Mortality	
			All subjects	0.78 (0.56–1.08)
			BMI ≥ 25	0.70 (0.49–0.99)
			<25	1.08 (0.077–1.52)
Pierce et al. [153]	1,490	2 years postdiagnosis	Mortality, exercise + diet	0.56 (0.31–0.98)
Holick et al. [49]	4,482	5–6 years postdiagnosis	BC mortality	0.53 ($p=0.01$)
			Non-BC mortality	0.52 ($p<0.001$)
Irwin et al. [154]	933	Pre and postdiagnosis	Mortality	
			Pre diagnosis	0.69 ($p=0.045$)
			Post diagnosis	0.33 ($p=0.046$)
Friedenreich et al. [155]	1,231	Prediagnosis	Mortality	
			Moderate	0.56 (0.38–0.82)
			Vigorous	0.74 (0.56–0.98)
West-wright et al. [156]	3,539	Prediagnosis	Mortality	RR
			High-level	0.53 (0.35–0.80)
			Low-level	0.65 (0.45–0.93)
Sternfeld et al. [51]	1,970	Up to 3 years postdiagnosis	Mortality	0.76 ($p=0.20$)
			BC mortality	0.87 ($p=0.41$)
			Recurrence	0.91 ($p=0.78$)
Keegan et al. [157]	4,153	3-year prediagnosis	Mortality (ER positive only)	0.66 (0.51–0.85)
Emaus et al. [43]	1,364	Prediagnosis	Mortality; BMI < 25 and age of diagnosis ≥55 years	0.34 (0.16–0.71)
Bertram et al. [158]	2,361	Postdiagnosis	Mortality, baseline	0.47 ($p=0.01$)
			Adherence at 1 year	0.65 ($p<0.01$)

mortality was found in other smaller studies [51–53]. In some but not all studies, the effect of physical activity was more evident in women with hormone receptor positive disease thereby providing additional support for studies of physical activity in hormone receptor positive breast cancer.

A link between insulin and breast cancer outcomes is biologically plausible given high levels of expression of the insulin receptor on human breast cancer cells [54, 55]. This expression is not downregulated by circulating insulin [54] and strong preclinical evidence suggests that insulin signals, at least in part, through a fetal form of its own receptor (IR-α) and through hybrid insulin/IGF-I receptors to stimulate tumor growth [56]. The presence of phosphorylated insulin or hybrid insulin/IGF-1 receptors (indicating activation) on breast cancer specimens has been associated with worse outcomes in early stage breast cancer, providing empiric evidence of the importance of this pathway [46].

Evidence for an adverse prognostic effect of obesity in other cancers is less convincing. In prostate cancer [57, 58], for example, several studies have suggested that obesity is associated with adverse prognostic factors (e.g., high Gleason score, high grade, more advanced pathologic stage) and with increased risk of biochemical or clinical recurrence, or with mortality [59–64]. However, other studies have not confirmed these associations [65–67]. It is possible obesity exerts prognostic effects only in certain subgroups of patients or when BMI is very high; additional research is needed. Hyperinsulinemia has been linked to adverse prostate cancer prognostic factors in two studies [68, 69] and high C-peptide levels prior to prostate cancer diagnosis have been associated with increased cancer specific mortality in one study [70]. Similar to breast cancer, insulin receptors are expressed in human prostate cancer, providing a biologic link for an adverse prognostic effect of hyperinsulinemia [71].

It has been difficult to consistently demonstrate an association between obesity and outcomes in colorectal cancer. Although some studies [72] demonstrated greater risk of a colon cancer event (recurrence or second primary tumor) in obese patients, mortality effects have been less clear, in part because increased mortality is dominated by noncolon cancer deaths in all but the most obese individuals. Meyerhardt et al. [73] reported adverse prognostic effects of obesity on overall mortality in female but not male colon cancer patients in an early study , however, they failed to replicate their observations in a subsequent study [74]. In separate work, visceral adiposity (more strongly associated with insulin resistance than overall obesity) has been associated with poor disease-free survival in colorectal cancer (HR=1.98; 95% CI, 1.02–3.87) [75].

High levels of C-peptide (a marker of insulin resistance) were associated with increased risk of death in early stage colorectal cancer in a recent report. Furthermore, elevated hemoglobin A1C (a marker of poor glycemic control) has been associated with presentation of colorectal cancer at a more advanced stage and with worse 5 year survival [76, 77]. Two studies [78, 79] have provided evidence that increased levels of physical activity before diagnosis (associated with reduced insulin resistance) may be associated with improved short-term [78] and long-term [79] survival, but another study has revealed no such association with increased physical activity at the time of diagnosis [80]. Physical activity levels at various times postdiagnosis have been consistently associated with decreased mortality from colorectal cancer [81–83].

Cancer treatment may increase insulin resistance in patients receiving glucocorticoids [84] and it may increase risk of the IRS in childhood cancer survivors [85]. Furthermore, in a recent meta-analysis, existing diabetes in cancer patients has been associated with increased overall mortality from cancer (HR 1.41, 95% CI 1.28–1.55) and increased mortality from specific types of cancer, including endometrium (HR, 1.76; 95% CI, 1.34–2.31), breast (HR, 1.61; 95% CI, 1.46–1.78), and colorectum (HR, 1.32; 95% CI, 1.24–1.41) [86]. More recent meta-analysis looking at breast cancer outcome on preexisting diabetes patients has found a significant increase in all cause mortality in diabetics with breast cancer than non-diabetics with breast cancer (HR, 1.49; 95% CI, 1.35–1.65) [87].

With this background, it is apparent that obesity is associated with risk of many types of cancers and that obesity and/or the associated insulin resistance may be associated with outcomes in some groups of cancer patients (notably those with breast, prostate and colon cancer). These observations suggest that interventions to reduce obesity (and insulin resistance) may reduce risk of cancer at a population level, although this has not been proven. Interventions to reduce obesity and/or improve insulin levels may be beneficial in individuals diagnosed with breast and, to a lesser extent, colon and prostate cancer. The contribution of obesity and/or insulin resistance to the outcome of other cancers is less well established.

Potential Interventions to Reduce Insulin Resistance in Cancer Prevention and Treatment

With the exception of a single randomized trial, the Women's Intervention Nutrition Study (WINS) in the adjuvant breast cancer setting (discussed below) [88], there is no level one (randomized) evidence that an intervention that influences obesity or insulin resistance will reduce cancer risk or improve cancer prognosis. As a result, it is not currently possible to recommend any intervention that targets obesity or insulin resistance as a means of reducing cancer risk or improving cancer outcomes. Rigorous evaluation of the approaches discussed here, in the settings of both cancer prevention and cancer treatment, is required before they should be used to prevent or treat cancer. Over time, it is likely information will be available from randomized trials, particularly in the setting of cancer treatment, to develop treatment recommendations in those diagnosed with cancer. In the setting of cancer prevention high costs and the large sample sizes that would be required increase the challenges of conducting randomized trials, although population-based intervention studies evaluating a range of health outcomes may eventually be conducted.

Potential interventions targetting insulin resistance as a means of reducing the burden of cancer can be grouped into two broad categories: (1) lifestyle interventions targeting diet, exercise and/or weight and (2) pharmacologic interventions targeting weight, metabolic parameters of insulin resistance such as insulin levels, or specific tumor attributes such as insulin (and related IGF-I) receptors that may mediate effects of insulin within cancer cells. Selection of the most appropriate interventions for further investigation will depend on the level of evidence linking the intervention target (e.g., insulin, obesity, physical inactivity) to cancer risk and/or prognosis and on the setting in which the intervention will be used (e.g., population-based interventions to lower cancer risk vs. individual interventions in cancer patients to improve outcomes). When the focus is on population based cancer prevention, the absolute benefits of any intervention are likely to be small (even in the presence of a two to threefold elevation in relative risk) because cancer is an infrequent event and risks associated with the intervention must also be small. In practical terms, this means that interventions in this setting will usually be lifestyle based and will less often involve pharmaceutical approaches. However, in the setting of individual subjects, when there is strong evidence that obesity or insulin resistance are associated with cancer risk, greater risk for a preventive strategy may be accepted because the absolute benefits of an effective intervention may be greater – as a result, either lifestyle or pharmacologic interventions (or both) may be appropriate. This situation may exist in patients diagnosed with cancers for which strong evidence exists for a role of obesity and/or insulin resistance (e.g., breast cancer); it may also exist in individuals with obesity or insulin resistance who do not have cancer but are at markedly increased risk for a variety of adverse health outcomes, including cancer.

Lifestyle Interventions

The American Cancer Society has suggested that more than 50% of cancer related deaths could be prevented by modifiable lifestyle factors including diet and exercise [89]. Lifestyle interventions targeting body weight are typically multimodality, including dietary, physical activity and behavioral change. Weight loss and/or increased physical activity have been shown to improve insulin sensitivity in the general population [90–92]. When cancer prevention is the goal, interventions developed for other purposes for use in the general population are potentially relevant; when improvement in cancer outcomes is the goal, more targeted, cancer specific, interventions will likely be necessary.

Lifestyle Interventions in the General Population

Targeting weight loss in the general population is complex – healthy individuals may be difficult to motivate to change (because they do not have an identifiable condition) and the cost of delivering intensive individualized interventions is often prohibitive. Furthermore, social factors linked to obesity, such as poverty or the built environment, may be difficult to modify. As a result, population-based rather than individual interventions may be the optimal approach. Although the impact of such interventions on general health may be considerable, the absolute reduction in risk of specific diseases (e.g., cancer) is likely to be small. Discussion of specific approaches to weight loss in the general population is beyond the scope of this chapter – they are reviewed elsewhere [93–99]. In general, research has shown that multidisciplinary lifestyle approaches that target diet, physical activity and behavior in individuals will lead to weight loss, at least in the short-term (6–12 months), but that weight regain is common over the longer term. Additionally, intensive lifestyle programs involving reduction in body weight and body fat has shown to significantly improve insulin sensitivity and glucose metabolism in obese youths [100]. Bariatric surgery in patients with type II diabetes has been associated with amelioration or resolution of the diabetes [101] and with reduction in cancer mortality [102]. Despite these successes, optimal approaches to the prevention and treatment of obesity have yet to be identified.

There are no randomized trials in the general population that target weight, diet alone or exercise alone as a means of reducing cancer risk. Based on the observational evidence summarized above, it appears possible that weight loss might be effective in reducing risk of some cancers. Furthermore, based on observational data strongly linking reduced physical activity to colon cancer risk and more weakly to breast cancer risk, it is possible increased physical activity in the absence of weight loss might reduce risk of these two common cancers.

Interventions in Glucose Intolerant/Insulin Resistant Populations Without Cancer

The Diabetes Prevention Program Randomized Trial [103, 104] was conducted in 3,234 glucose intolerant but nondiabetic individuals who were randomized to (1) a lifestyle modification program (goals: ≥7% weight loss and at least 150 min of physical activity per week), (2) metformin 850 mg po twice daily or (3) placebo. After a mean follow-up of 2.8 years, weight loss was 5.6, 2.1, and 0.1 kg respectively (maximum weight loss occurred at 6 months), and the incidence of diabetes was reduced by 58% in those randomized to the lifestyle intervention and by 31% in those randomized to metformin, as compared to the control population. The lifestyle intervention also significantly reduced the prevalence of IRS from 51 to 43% ($p<0.001$ compared to placebo). In a second study [105, 106], Finnish investigators randomized 522 overweight subjects with glucose intolerance to an individualized lifestyle intervention (goals: weight loss 5%, reduced fat and increased fiber diet, 30 min of moderate exercise per day) or to a control group. Mean weight loss in the intervention group was 4.2 kg (vs. 0.8 kg in controls), and the risk of diabetes was reduced by 58% in the intervention group (11 vs. 23% in controls, $p<0.001$). During the first year of the study, the prevalence of the metabolic syndrome decreased from 74 to 58% in the intervention group vs. 74–66.7% in the control group ($p=0.018$). At the end of the 3.9 year study, there was a 38% reduction in the age and sex adjusted persistence of the metabolic syndrome in the intervention group (compared to the control group). Insulin levels 2 h after a glucose challenge were reduced by 29 μg/mL (95% CI 21–37) in the intervention group and by 11 μg/mL (95% CI 4–18) in controls ($p=0.001$). Additional reports have documented beneficial effects of lifestyle interventions on insulin resistance, inflammation and markers of cardiovascular complications in patients with metabolic syndrome [107] or severe obesity [108]. Unfortunately, none of these studies have reported the impact of the interventions on cancer.

Taken together, these studies demonstrate that intensive lifestyle interventions targeting caloric intake, physical activity and behavioral change are feasible in defined high risk segments of the population (i.e., glucose intolerant, insulin resistant, obese), and that they result in weight loss, reduce the presence of insulin resistance and reduce the future risk of diabetes. These interventions are of considerable interest as potential means of reducing cancer risk or improving outcomes of certain cancers, however, they involved intensive interactions with participants that would be extremely costly on a large scale. Furthermore, partial weight regain may occur after the first year or two, suggesting metabolic improvements may not be maintained over longer periods of time.

Interventions in Cancer Populations

In cancer populations, considerable research has targeted various aspects of lifestyle, focusing primarily on breast cancer patients, and to a lesser extent on other cancer patients. This work has demonstrated the feasibility of dietary change, physical activity and weight loss, at least in the short-term [109–111]. Many studies and systematic reviews have demonstrated association of physical activity with reduced fatigue, improved quality of life, better physical function and improved physiologic parameters of fitness [112–114]. In individuals with cancer, physical activity has been suggested to increase survival, reduce risk of recurrence and reduce the risk of secondary fatal diseases [115].

Randomized Trials with Cancer Outcomes

Only two randomized trials evaluating the effect of lifestyle interventions on cancer outcomes. Both trials targeted dietary change in women with early breast cancer. The WINS Study [87, 116] enrolled 2,437 postmenopausal women with early stage breast cancer, during the first year after diagnosis. Chemotherapy, if administered, was completed prior to randomization; women with hormone receptor positive tumors received tamoxifen. At 12 months, women on the intervention arm reduced fat intake to 33.3 g/day and those in the control group to 51.3 g/day ($p<0.001$); the intervention group lost 2.1 kg vs. a gain of 0.2 kg in the control group ($p<0.05$). These changes were maintained over the 5 year intervention. With a median follow up of 60 months, relapse-free survival was significantly improved in the intervention group: HR 0.76, 95% CI 0.60–0.98, $p=0.034$. In unplanned post hoc analyses, the effect of the intervention was shown to be greatest in hormone receptor negative (HR 0.58, 95% CI 0.37–0.91) vs. hormone receptor positive breast cancer (HR 0.85, 95% CI 0.63–1.14) and in obese (HR 0.66, 95% CI 0.42–1.04) vs. normal weight women (HR 0.83, 95% CI 0.54–1.27). The fact that women in the intervention arm lost weight makes it difficult to determine whether dietary fat reduction or weight loss (or both) contributed to the improved outcomes. Potential physiologic mediators of the prognostic effect of the intervention (e.g., insulin, estrogen, adipocytokines) have not been reported.

The Women's Healthy Eating and Living Study (WHEL) [117] randomized 3,088 pre and postmenopausal women with breast cancer diagnosed in the previous 4 years to a complex, telephone-based dietary intervention that sought to increase fruit, vegetable and fiber intake while reducing fat intake. Important changes in diet in the expected directions were seen in the intervention arm at 12 months, however, there was attenuation of these changes at 72 months. The intervention did not impact weight nor did it influence disease-free or overall survival at 5 years (HR 0.96, 95% CI 0.80–1.14, $p = 0.63$ and HR 0.91, 95% CI 0.72–1.15, $p = 0.43$ respectively). The absence of prognostic benefit in this study suggests that weight loss may have contributed to the benefit seen in the WINS Study. As in the WINS Study, there has been no report of effects of the intervention on key insulin related physiologic mediators such as insulin and insulin resistance although changes in carotenoids in the expected direction were identified [118]. In subsequent exploratory analyses, the WHEL investigators have reported that dietary intervention was associated with improved breast cancer outcomes in women who did not have hot flashes at baseline (HR 0.69; 95% CI, 0.51–0.93; $p = 0.02$) (but not in those who had hot flashes) [119].

Randomized Trials of the Impact of Physical Activity on Insulin Levels in Cancer Populations

Several studies have evaluated the impact of physical activity on weight in breast cancer survivors. Body weight is usually maintained (unless caloric intake is also restricted), although body composition may be altered (increased muscle mass, reduced fat mass). Recent studies have reported the impact of physical activity on insulin related factors including insulin, IGF-I and IGFBP-3 (see Table 12.2) [120–123]. Mixed aerobic and strengthening physical activity [120] or moderate intensity physical activity [121] were associated with modest reductions in insulin levels (−2.9 vs. −0.3 μU/mL, $p = 0.07$ and −1.75 vs. +3.49 μU/mL, $p = 0.09$ respectively) in two studies and significant reductions in IGF-I and IGFBP-3 were seen in one of these studies [121]. In contrast, two small studies failed to identify effects of weight training [122] or cycling [123] on insulin in breast cancer survivors. The observation that a moderate amount of physical activity may reduce insulin levels in early stage breast cancer patients is consistent with studies conducted in noncancer subjects [124–126] and it suggests that exercise interventions (even in the absence of weight loss) may be a useful means of targeting insulin and insulin resistance, at least in the breast cancer population.

Table 12.2 Effect of exercise interventions on insulin levels in breast cancer patients

Citation	*n*	Intervention	Effect on insulin
Fairey et al. [159]	53	Cycling × 15 weeks	Insulin increased 12.0% in exercise group (exercise vs. control, $p = 0.94$)
Schmitz et al. [119]	85	Weight training × 6 months	Insulin increased 7.2% in exercise group (exercise vs. control, $p = 0.79$)
Ligibel et al. [160]	101	Mixed strength and endurance × 16 weeks	Insulin reduced 28.2% in exercise group $p = 0.03$ (exercise vs. control, $p = 0.07$)
Irwin et al. [161]	75	Moderate intensity physical activity × 6 months	Insulin reduced 7.1% in exercise group (exercise vs. control, $p = 0.09$)

Summary and Future Directions

Lifestyle interventions in glucose intolerant and/or insulin resistant individuals lower insulin levels, reduce insulin resistance and lower the risk of diabetes. In cancer populations, a single randomized trial that targeted dietary fat reduction and also resulted in significant weight loss reported a significant improvement in 5 year relapse-free survival in breast cancer for women participating in the dietary intervention group; the effect was greatest in women with estrogen receptor negative breast cancer and in obese women. A similar effect was not seen in a second dietary intervention study in breast cancer patients in which weight loss did not occur. There is no information regarding the impact of either intervention on potential physiologic mediators, including insulin. Finally, in the breast cancer population, small randomized trials have reported physical activity (either aerobic or mixed aerobic/strength) to be associated with reduced insulin, IGF-I and IGFBP-3 levels.

Future research involving cancer patients is needed to elucidate the impact of lifestyle interventions – weight loss, physical activity and targeted dietary interventions – on factors that may mediate prognostic effects of these interventions and on cancer outcomes. Potential physiologic factors include insulin, insulin resistance, IGFs and their binding proteins as well as selected adipocytokines such as leptin. The impact of these interventions on sex hormones is also of interest for some cancers. Large scale, randomized trials are currently justifiable in the breast cancer population. One pilot study involving over 300 subjects, the lifestyle intervention study in adjuvant treatment of early breast cancer (LISA), that uses a telephone-based modification of the Diabetes Prevention Program intervention is underway; other studies are planned. Such studies should enroll sufficient subjects to provide definitive evidence regarding the impact of weight loss interventions on cancer outcomes and they should examine potential physiologic mediators in associated correlative studies. Future studies should also target the impact of specific physical activity interventions on physiologic mediators and cancer outcomes in selected cancers (discussed above). Studies in individuals at high cancer risk, targeting intermediate physiologic mediators, are also warranted and will be useful in further elucidating the association between insulin/insulin resistance and cancer risk. Finally, given the impact of obesity on health and mortality in general, effective population-based interventions to reduce the prevalence of obesity in the long-term in the general population should be developed.

Pharmacologic Interventions

Obesity, insulin resistance and/or hyperinsulinemia can also be targeted through a number of pharmacologic interventions. Pharmacologic approaches that lead to significant weight loss are likely to result in improvements to insulin resistance. These pharmacologic interventions are beyond the scope of this chapter – they are reviewed elsewhere [95, 127]. None has been tested as a means of preventing cancer or improving cancer outcomes.

Interventions that target insulin resistance and/or circulating insulin levels, as well as those that target insulin/IGF-I receptors on the surface of tumor cells, are of considerable interest and are entering clinical testing in cancer patients. Agents that target insulin levels and/or insulin resistance will be discussed here. IGF-1 receptor targeting has been reviewed [126]. The use of lifestyle or pharmacologic approaches that reduce insulin levels combined with IGF-I receptor blockers may prove to be more efficacious in the cancer treatment setting than either approach used in isolation. As a result, evaluation of their combined effects is of considerable interest. Clinically available agents that target insulin and/or insulin resistance include metformin (a biguanide) and a class of drugs known as thiazolidinediones. Both of these enhance insulin sensitivity and reduce insulin levels, are well tolerated and commonly used to treat type II diabetes.

Metformin

Metformin is an inexpensive oral agent that is commonly used to treat type II diabetes. Its most serious toxicity is lactic acidosis, occurring in 1 per 100,000 patient years of use – risk is significantly reduced when metformin use is avoided in those with hepatic, cardiac or renal compromise, and in those over 80 years of age. Minor gastrointestinal upset is the commonest toxicity, leading to cessation of therapy in approximately 10% of individuals. Modest weight loss is common.

A beneficial effect of metformin in cancer appears to be biologically plausible, particularly in breast and prostate cancers. Metformin may act through (1) indirect, insulin lowering (metabolic) effects in liver and muscle or through (2) direct AMPK and mammalian target of rapamycin (mTOR), mediated effects in tumor cells (see Fig. 12.1). Indirect metabolic effects occur when metformin inhibits transcription of key gluconeogenesis genes in the liver and increases glucose uptake in skeletal muscle, leading to a reduction in levels of circulating glucose, improvement in insulin sensitivity and reduction in the hyperinsulinemia associated with insulin resistance [128]. Activation of AMPK, a central cellular energy sensor mediates these metabolic effects of metformin in liver [129, 130].

Direct effects of metformin occur as a result of inhibition of complex I of the mitochondrial respiratory chain leading to AMPK activation within cancer cells. AMPK activation leads to inhibition of cellular protein synthesis and growth through inhibition of mTOR [131]. In vivo and in vitro research provides evidence of an anticancer effect of metformin. In animal models, metformin reduces growth of mammary tumors and in cell culture it reduces proliferation of glioma, breast, colon and pancreatic cancer cells [132–138].

Several epidemiological studies, combined in a recent meta-analysis have found that use of metformin is associated with a 30% reduction in all types of cancers [139]. Retrospective evidence for a potential clinically important effect of metformin in human cancer has been reported by Jiralerspong et al. [140], who found pathologic complete response (pCR) rates to neoadjuvant systemic therapy in breast

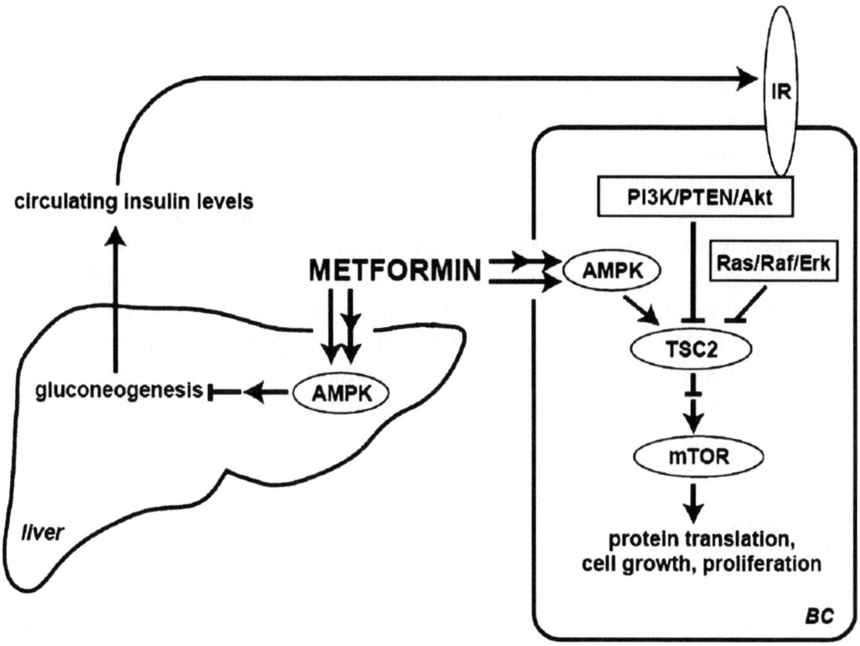

Fig. 12.1 Mechanism of metformin action [90] (figure by Vuk Stambolic PhD, Ontario Cancer Institute, Toronto, Canada) Copyright – *Journal of Clinical Oncology* 2009 (permission will need to be obtained to use this figure)

cancer patients were significantly higher in diabetics receiving metformin ($n=68$, pCR=24%) than in diabetics not receiving metformin ($n=87$, pCR=8%) or in nondiabetics ($n=2{,}374$, pCR=16%). Similar retrospective research has found metforminn use in diabetics to be associated with presentation of lung cancer at an earlier stage, with a greater proportion of cancers being adenocarcinomas, and with improved survival [141]. Hosono et al. [142] have reported a small randomized trial showing that a very low dose of metformin (250 mg daily) reduces proliferation and aberrant crypt foci formation in the rectal epithelium of nondiabetic patients with previous colorectal polyps when compared to placebo. Furthermore, interim data from ongoing "window of opportunity" neoadjuvant studies in breast cancer have provided evidence that metformin administration (in standard clinical dose) to newly diagnosed breast cancer patients is safe and has favorable effects on gene expression, proliferation and apoptosis in the absence of other anticancer treatment [143–145]. Completion of these studies, as well as planned and ongoing studies in the metastatic and adjuvant setting in breast, prostate, pancreatic and endometrial cancers will provide important additional information on the anticancer effects of metformin and help elucidate the clinically important mechanisms of metformin action in diabetic and nondiabetic cancer patients [146, 147].

Thiazolidinediones

Thiazolidinediones are PPAR-gamma activating agents that improve insulin sensitivity and lower insulin levels in subjects with insulin resistance and/or type II diabetes [148]. The mechanisms by which they do this is unclear. One epidemiologic study suggests that lung cancer risk among subjects with diabetes receiving thiazolidinediones is 33% lower than in those not receiving thiazolidinediones, however, a similar association was not seen with risk of colorectal or prostate cancer [149]. A second epidemiological study has shown an association between use of thiazolidinediones and reduced incidence of hepatocellular carcinoma (adjusted OR 0.3 (95% CI, 0.1–0.7) [150]. Although these agents effectively lower insulin and may be associated with lower cancer risk, growing concerns about cardiotoxic effects have reduced enthusiasm for their use in diabetes and as potential anticancer agents [151].

Summary

Obesity has been linked to cancer risk and mortality for a number of common cancers. There is growing evidence that this link between obesity and cancer risk and prognosis is mediated, in many cases, by hyperinsulinemia and insulin resistance. While no studies conducted in cancer patients have demonstrated that reversal of insulin resistance improves cancer risk or cancer outcome, randomized trials in glucose intolerant and/or insulin resistant individuals demonstrate that lifestyle interventions or metformin improve insulin resistance, and reduce risk of subsequent diabetes. It is likely similar interventions would have a similar effect on insulin resistance in individuals at risk for, or diagnosed with, cancer and, as a result, they may also impact cancer. In the cancer setting, only one randomized trial [92] that reduced fat intake and promoted weight loss has identified improvement in cancer outcomes as a result of a lifestyle intervention. No information is available on physiologic mediators of this effect.

Future work should focus on the role of population-based lifestyle interventions designed to reduce obesity, insulin resistance and, potentially, cancer risk (see Table 12.3).Evaluation of effects of weight loss, particularly in breast cancer patients, and to a lesser extent in patients with colon and prostate cancer, is indicated. Furthermore, because of evidence suggesting that exercise interventions, without associated weight loss, may reduce the hyperinsulinemia that has been associated with both cancer risk and poor cancer outcomes, the impact of enhanced physical activity on cancer should be investigated in selected settings as discussed above. Finally, in cancer populations, there is growing evidence that metformin may improve outcomes of some common cancers (notably breast and prostate) through one or both of two mechanisms – an indirect, insulin mediated effect or a direct, AMP kinase/mTOR mediated effect.

At present, there is insufficient evidence from randomized trials to recommend interventions to reduce insulin resistance in individuals at risk for, or diagnosed with,

Table 12.3 Potential areas for research involving intervention to reduce obesity and/or insulin resistance in cancer prevention or treatment

	Cancer prevention	Cancer treatment
Lifestyle intervention		
Weight loss	Cancer risk in general	Breast cancer[a]
	Potential emphasis on breast (postmenopausal), uterine, colorectal, prostate cancers	Potential focus on breast, colorectal, prostate cancer
Enhanced physical activity	Colorectal cancer	Colorectal cancer
	Breast cancer	Breast cancer
Pharmacologic intervention		
Metformin	Potential role in individuals with IRS or diabetes	Breast cancer
		Prostate cancer
		Potential role in colorectal cancer
Other (including thiazolidinediones)	Preclinical	Preclinical

IRS insulin resistance syndrome

[a]One randomized trial [60] demonstrates improved relapse-free survival with an intervention that reduced fat intake and promoted moderate weight loss

cancer as a means of reducing cancer risk or improving cancer outcomes. Given the results of the WINS Study [116], it is reasonable to advise women with early stage breast cancer that reduction in dietary fat intake and loss of a modest amount of weight may reduce risk of relapse. Intensive research is ongoing to explore effects of both lifestyle and pharmacologic interventions in cancer populations.

References

1. Kelly T et al (2008) Global burden of obesity in 2005 and projections to 2030. Int J Obes (Lond) 32(9):1431–1437
2. Pierce JP et al (2007) Re: dietary fat reduction and breast cancer outcome: interim efficacy results from the Women's Intervention Nutrition Study. J Natl Cancer Inst 99(11):900; author reply 900–901
3. Clegg D (2009) Mechanisms of insulin resistance, obesity and metabolic syndrome. In: Fantus IG (ed) Insulin resistance and cancer. Springer, New York
4. Calle EE, Rodriguez C, Walker-Thurmond K et al (2003) Overweight, obesity, and mortality from cancer in a prospectively studied cohort of U.S. adults. N Engl J Med 348:1625–1638
5. Whitlock G et al (2009) Body-mass index and cause-specific mortality in 900 000 adults: collaborative analyses of 57 prospective studies. Lancet 373(9669):1083–1096
6. Renehan AG et al (2008) Body-mass index and incidence of cancer: a systematic review and meta-analysis of prospective observational studies. Lancet 371(9612):569–578
7. Friedenreich CM, Orenstein MR (2002) Physical activity and cancer prevention: etiologic evidence and biological mechanisms. J Nutr 132(11 Suppl):3456S–3464S

8. Friedenreich CM, Cust AE (2008) Physical activity and breast cancer risk: impact of timing, type and dose of activity and population subgroup effects. Br J Sports Med 42:636–647
9. Hursting SD et al (2008) Reducing the weight of cancer: mechanistic targets for breaking the obesity-carcinogenesis link. Best Pract Res Clin Endocrinol Metab 22(4):659–669
10. Moore SC et al (2009) Age-specific physical activity and prostate cancer risk among white men and black men. Cancer 115(21):5060–5070
11. Renehan AG, Roberts DL, Dive C (2008) Obesity and cancer: pathophysiological and biological mechanisms. Arch Physiol Biochem 114(1):71–83
12. Lipscombe L (2009) Insulin, insulin resistance and cancer associations. In: Fantus IG (ed) insulin resistance and cancer. Springer, New York
13. LeRoith D (2009) Animal models of hyperinsulinemia, insulin resistance and cancer. In: Fantus IG (ed) insulin resistance and cancer. Springer, New York
14. Fantus IG (2009) Potential mechanisms linking insulin to cancer. In: Fantus IG (ed) Insulin resistance and cancer. Springer, New York
15. Sonnenberg N (2009) Actions of insulin as a survival and growth factor: Akt/PKB, mTOR and regulation of translation. In: Fantus IG (ed) Insulin resistance and cancer. Springer, New York
16. Cantley LC (2009) Cancer cell metabolism and AMPK: regulation of cell proliferation and apoptosis. In: Fantus IG (ed) Insulin resistance and cancer. Springer, New York
17. Brodt P (2009) Insulin-like growth factors and cancer. In: Fantus IG (ed) Insulin resistance and cancer. Springer, New York
18. Belfiore A (2009) Insulin, IGF receptors and cancer. In: Fantus IG (ed) Insulin resistance and cancer. Springer, New York
19. Pisani P (2008) Hyper-insulinaemia and cancer, meta-analyses of epidemiological studies. Arch Physiol Biochem 114:63–70
20. Zhou XH et al (2010) Diabetes, prediabetes and cancer mortality. Diabetologia 53(9):1867–1876
21. Gunter MJ et al (2009) Insulin, insulin-like growth factor-I, and risk of breast cancer in postmenopausal women. J Natl Cancer Inst 101(1):48–60
22. Vinikoor LC, Long MD, Keku TO et al (2009) The Association between diabetes, insulin use, and colorectal cancer among Whites and African Americans. Cancer Epidemiol Biomark Prev 18:1239–1242
23. von Kriegstein E, von Kriegstein K (2007) Inhaled insulin for diabetes mellitus. N Engl J Med 356(20):2106; author reply 2108
24. Hemkens LG et al (2009) Risk of malignancies in patients with diabetes treated with human insulin or insulin analogues: a cohort study. Diabetologia 52(9):1732–1744
25. Jonasson JM et al (2009) Insulin glargine use and short-term incidence of malignancies-a population-based follow-up study in Sweden. Diabetologia 52(9):1745–1754
26. Mannucci E et al (2010) Doses of insulin and its analogues and cancer occurrence in insulin-treated type 2 diabetic patients. Diabetes Care 33(9):1997–2003
27. Colhoun HM (2009) Use of insulin glargine and cancer incidence in Scotland: a study from the Scottish Diabetes Research Network Epidemiology Group. Diabetologia 52(9):1755–1765
28. Currie CJ, Poole CD, Gale EA (2009) The influence of glucose-lowering therapies on cancer risk in type 2 diabetes. Diabetologia 52(9):1766–1777
29. Home PD, Lagarenne P (2009) Combined randomised controlled trial experience of malignancies in studies using insulin glargine. Diabetologia 52(12):2499–2506
30. Lipscombe LL et al (2006) Diabetes mellitus and breast cancer: a retrospective population-based cohort study. Breast Cancer Res Treat 98(3):349–356

31. Lipscombe LL et al (2006) Increased prevalence of prior breast cancer in women with newly diagnosed diabetes. Breast Cancer Res Treat 98(3):303–309
32. Xue F, Michels KB (2007) Diabetes, metabolic syndrome, and breast cancer: a review of the current evidence. Am J Clin Nutr 86(3):s823–s835
33. Pierce BL et al (2008) Diabetes mellitus and prostate cancer risk. Prostate 68(10):1126–1132
34. Jee SH et al (2008) Body mass index and cancer risk in Korean men and women. Int J Cancer 123(8):1892–1896
35. Trevisan M et al (2001) Markers of insulin resistance and colorectal cancer mortality. Cancer Epidemiol Biomark Prev 10(9):937–941
36. Protani M, Coory M, Martin JH (2010) Effect of obesity on survival of women with breast cancer: systematic review and meta-analysis. Breast Cancer Res Treat 123(3):627–635
37. Goodwin P (2006) Energy balance and prognosis: breast cancer. In: McTiernan A (ed) Cancer prevention and management through exercise and weight control. Taylor and Francis Group, Boca Raton
38. Goodwin PJ et al (2009) High insulin levels in newly diagnosed breast cancer patients reflect underlying insulin resistance and are associated with components of the insulin resistance syndrome. Breast Cancer Res Treat 114(3):517–525
39. Goodwin PJ et al (2002) Fasting insulin and outcome in early-stage breast cancer: results of a prospective cohort study. J Clin Oncol 20(1):42–51
40. Pasanisi P et al (2008) Serum insulin-like growth factor-I and platelet-derived growth factor as biomarkers of breast cancer prognosis. Cancer Epidemiol Biomark Prev 17(7):1719–1722
41. Pollak M et al (2006) Insulin resistance, estimated by serum C-peptide level, is associated with reduced event-free survival for postmenopausal women in NCIC CTG MA.14 adjuvant breast cancer trial. J Clin Oncol ASCO Ann Meet Proc I 24(Suppl 18S):Abstract 524
42. Irwin ML et al (2011) Fasting C-peptide levels and death resulting from all causes and breast cancer: the health, eating, activity, and lifestyle study. J Clin Oncol 29(1):47–53
43. Duggan C et al (2011) Associations of insulin resistance and adiponectin with mortality in women with breast cancer. J Clin Oncol 29(1):32–39
44. Emaus A et al (2010) Metabolic profile, physical activity, and mortality in breast cancer patients. Breast Cancer Res Treat 121(3):651–660
45. Erickson K et al (2011) Clinically defined type 2 diabetes mellitus and prognosis in early-stage breast cancer. J Clin Oncol 29(1):54–60
46. Law JH et al (2008) Phosphorylated insulin-like growth factor-i/insulin receptor is present in all breast cancer subtypes and is related to poor survival. Cancer Res 68(24):10238–10246
47. Holmes MD et al (2005) Physical activity and survival after breast cancer diagnosis. JAMA 293(20):2479–2486
48. Abrahamson PE et al (2006) Recreational physical activity and survival among young women with breast cancer. Cancer 107(8):1777–1785
49. Holick CN et al (2008) Physical activity and survival after diagnosis of invasive breast cancer. Cancer Epidemiol Biomark Prev 17(2):379–386
50. Irwin ML et al (2003) Physical activity levels before and after a diagnosis of breast carcinoma: the health, eating, activity, and lifestyle (HEAL) study. Cancer 97(7): 1746–1757
51. Sternfeld B et al (2009) Physical activity and risk of recurrence and mortality in breast cancer survivors: findings from the LACE study. Cancer Epidemiol Biomark Prev 18(1):87–95

52. Enger SM, Bernstein L (2004) Exercise activity, body size and premenopausal breast cancer survival. Br J Cancer 90(11):2138–2141
53. Borugian MJ et al (2004) Insulin, macronutrient intake, and physical activity: are potential indicators of insulin resistance associated with mortality from breast cancer? Cancer Epidemiol Biomark Prev 13(7):1163–1172
54. Mulligan AM et al (2007) Insulin receptor is an independent predictor of a favorable outcome in early stage breast cancer. Breast Cancer Res Treat 106(1):39–47
55. Mathieu MC et al (1997) Insulin receptor expression and clinical outcome in node-negative breast cancer. Proc Assoc Am Physicians 109(6):565–571
56. Frasca F et al (2008) The role of insulin receptors and IGF-I receptors in cancer and other diseases. Arch Physiol Biochem 114(1):23–37
57. Hsing AW, Sakoda LC, Chua S Jr (2007) Obesity, metabolic syndrome, and prostate cancer. Am J Clin Nutr 86(3):s843–s857
58. Skolarus TA, Wolin KY, Grubb RL 3rd (2007) The effect of body mass index on PSA levels and the development, screening and treatment of prostate cancer. Nat Clin Pract Urol 4(11):605–614
59. Magheli A et al (2008) Impact of body mass index on biochemical recurrence rates after radical prostatectomy: an analysis utilizing propensity score matching. Urology 72(6):1246–1251
60. Motamedinia P et al (2008) Body mass index trends and role of obesity in predicting outcome after radical prostatectomy. Urology 72(5):1106–1110
61. Freedland SJ et al (2008) Obesity and oncological outcome after radical prostatectomy: impact of prostate-specific antigen-based prostate cancer screening: results from the Shared Equal Access Regional Cancer Hospital and Duke Prostate Center databases. BJU Int 102(8):969–974
62. King CR, Spiotto MT, Kapp DS (2009) Obesity and risk of biochemical failure for patients receiving salvage radiotherapy after prostatectomy. Int J Radiat Oncol Biol Phys 73(4):1017–1022
63. Stroup SP et al (2007) Effect of obesity on prostate-specific antigen recurrence after radiation therapy for localized prostate cancer as measured by the 2006 Radiation Therapy Oncology Group-American Society for Therapeutic Radiation and Oncology (RTOG-ASTRO) Phoenix consensus definition. Cancer 110(5):1003–1009
64. Spangler E et al (2007) Association of obesity with tumor characteristics and treatment failure of prostate cancer in African-American and European American men. J Urol 178(5):1939–1944; discussion 1945
65. Paaskesen CE, Borre M (2008) Body mass index and prognostic markers at radical prostatectomy. Scand J Urol Nephrol 42:230–236
66. Merrick GS et al (2007) Obesity is not predictive of overall survival following permanent prostate brachytherapy. Am J Clin Oncol 30(6):588–596
67. Halabi S et al (2007) Inverse correlation between body mass index and clinical outcomes in men with advanced castration-recurrent prostate cancer. Cancer 110(7):1478–1484
68. Lehrer S et al (2002) Serum insulin level, disease stage, prostate specific antigen (PSA) and Gleason score in prostate cancer. Br J Cancer 87(7):726–728
69. Hammarsten J, Hogstedt B (2005) Hyperinsulinaemia: a prospective risk factor for lethal clinical prostate cancer. Eur J Cancer 41(18):2887–2895
70. Ma J et al (2008) Prediagnostic body-mass index, plasma C-peptide concentration, and prostate cancer-specific mortality in men with prostate cancer: a long-term survival analysis. Lancet Oncol 9(11):1039–1047
71. Cox ME et al (2009) Insulin receptor expression by human prostate cancers. Prostate 69(1):33–40

72. Dignam JJ et al (2006) Body mass index and outcomes in patients who receive adjuvant chemotherapy for colon cancer. J Natl Cancer Inst 98(22):1647–1654
73. Meyerhardt JA et al (2003) Influence of body mass index on outcomes and treatment-related toxicity in patients with colon carcinoma. Cancer 98(3):484–495
74. Meyerhardt JA et al (2008) Impact of body mass index and weight change after treatment on cancer recurrence and survival in patients with stage III colon cancer: findings from Cancer and Leukemia Group B 89803. J Clin Oncol 26(25):4109–4115
75. Moon HG et al (2008) Visceral obesity may affect oncologic outcome in patients with colorectal cancer. Ann Surg Oncol 15(7):1918–1922
76. Wolpin BM et al (2009) Insulin, the insulin-like growth factor axis, and mortality in patients with nonmetastatic colorectal cancer. J Clin Oncol 27(2):176–185
77. Siddiqui AA et al (2008) Elevated HbA1c is an independent predictor of aggressive clinical behavior in patients with colorectal cancer: a case-control study. Dig Dis Sci 53(9):2486–2494
78. Nickelsen TN, Jorgensen T, Kronborg O (2005) Lifestyle and 30-day complications to surgery for colorectal cancer. Acta Oncol 44(3):218–223
79. Haydon AM et al (2006) Effect of physical activity and body size on survival after diagnosis with colorectal cancer. Gut 55(1):62–67
80. Dray X et al (2003) Influence of dietary factors on colorectal cancer survival. Gut 52(6):868–873
81. Meyerhardt JA et al (2006) Physical activity and survival after colorectal cancer diagnosis. J Clin Oncol 24(22):3527–3534
82. Meyerhardt JA et al (2009) Interaction of molecular markers and physical activity on mortality in patients with colon cancer. Clin Cancer Res 15(18):5931–5936
83. Meyerhardt JA et al (2009) Physical activity and male colorectal cancer survival. Arch Intern Med 169(22):2102–2108
84. Hickish T et al (2009) Glucose intolerance during adjuvant chemotherapy for breast cancer. J Natl Cancer Inst 101(7):537
85. Siviero-Miachon AA, Spinola-Castro AM, Guerra-Junior G (2008) Detection of metabolic syndrome features among childhood cancer survivors: a target to prevent disease. Vasc Health Risk Manag 4(4):825–836
86. Barone BB et al (2008) Long-term all-cause mortality in cancer patients with preexisting diabetes mellitus: a systematic review and meta-analysis. JAMA 300(23):2754–2764
87. Peairs KS et al (2011) Diabetes mellitus and breast cancer outcomes: a systematic review and meta-analysis. J Clin Oncol 29(1):40–6
88. Chlebowski RT et al (2006) Dietary fat reduction and breast cancer outcome: interim efficacy results from the Women's Intervention Nutrition Study. J Natl Cancer Inst 98(24):1767–1776
89. ACS report: half of cancer deaths could be prevented. CA Cancer J Clin 2005; 55(4):209–210
90. Miller JP et al (1994) Strength training increases insulin action in healthy 50- to 65-yr-old men. J Appl Physiol 77(3):1122–1127
91. Kirwan JP et al (1993) Endurance exercise training reduces glucose-stimulated insulin levels in 60- to 70-year-old men and women. J Gerontol 48(3):M84–M90
92. Craig BW, Everhart J, Brown R (1989) The influence of high-resistance training on glucose tolerance in young and elderly subjects. Mech Ageing Dev 49(2):147–157
93. Gill T, King L, Caterson I (2005) Obesity prevention: necessary and possible. A structured approach for effective planning. Proc Nutr Soc 64(2):255–261
94. Glenny AM et al (1997) The treatment and prevention of obesity: a systematic review of the literature. Int J Obes Relat Metab Disord 21(9):715–737

95. Franz MJ et al (2007) Weight-loss outcomes: a systematic review and meta-analysis of weight-loss clinical trials with a minimum 1-year follow-up. J Am Diet Assoc 107(10):1755–1767
96. Ogden CL et al (2007) The epidemiology of obesity. Gastroenterology 132(6):2087–2102
97. Gill T (2002) Importance of preventing weight gain in adulthood. Asia Pac J Clin Nutr 11(Suppl 3):S632–S636
98. Lemmens VE et al (2008) A systematic review of the evidence regarding efficacy of obesity prevention interventions among adults. Obes Rev 9(5):446–455
99. Van Dorsten B, Lindley EM (2008) Cognitive and behavioral approaches in the treatment of obesity. Endocrinol Metab Clin North Am 37(4):905–922
100. Shaw M et al (2009) Effect of a successful intensive lifestyle program on insulin sensitivity and glucose tolerance in obese youth. Diabetes Care 32(1):45–47
101. Cummings S, Apovian CM, Khaodhiar L (2008) Obesity surgery: evidence for diabetes prevention/management. J Am Diet Assoc 108(4 Suppl 1):S40–S44
102. Sjostrom L et al (2007) Effects of bariatric surgery on mortality in Swedish obese subjects. N Engl J Med 357(8):741–752
103. Knowler WC et al (2002) Reduction in the incidence of type 2 diabetes with lifestyle intervention or metformin. N Engl J Med 346(6):393–403
104. Orchard TJ et al (2005) The effect of metformin and intensive lifestyle intervention on the metabolic syndrome: the Diabetes Prevention Program randomized trial. Ann Intern Med 142(8):611–619
105. Tuomilehto J et al (2001) Prevention of type 2 diabetes mellitus by changes in lifestyle among subjects with impaired glucose tolerance. N Engl J Med 344(18): 1343–1350
106. Ilanne-Parikka P et al (2008) Effect of lifestyle intervention on the occurrence of metabolic syndrome and its components in the Finnish Diabetes Prevention Study. Diabetes Care 31(4):805–807
107. Oh EG et al (2011) Effects of a therapeutic lifestyle modification program on inflammatory chemokines and insulin resistance in subjects with metabolic syndrome. Biol Res Nurs 13(2):182–188
108. Hemmingsson E, Udden J, Rossner S (2011) Diet and physical activity interventions in severely obese adults. JAMA 305(6):563–564; author reply 564
109. Howell A, Chapman M, Harvie M (2009) Energy restriction for breast cancer prevention. Recent Results Cancer Res 181:97–111
110. Rooney M, Wald A (2007) Interventions for the management of weight and body composition changes in women with breast cancer. Clin J Oncol Nurs 11(1):41–52
111. Markes M, Brockow T, Resch KL (2006) Exercise for women receiving adjuvant therapy for breast cancer. Cochrane Database Syst Rev (4):CD005001
112. Schmitz KH et al (2005) Controlled physical activity trials in cancer survivors: a systematic review and meta-analysis. Cancer Epidemiol Biomark Prev 14(7):1588–1595
113. McNeely ML et al (2006) Effects of exercise on breast cancer patients and survivors: a systematic review and meta-analysis. CMAJ 175(1):34–41
114. Knols R et al (2005) Physical exercise in cancer patients during and after medical treatment: a systematic review of randomized and controlled clinical trials. J Clin Oncol 23(16):3830–3842
115. Courneya KS, Friedenreich CM (2007) Physical activity and cancer control. Semin Oncol Nurs 23(4):242–252
116. Blackburn GL, Wang KA (2007) Dietary fat reduction and breast cancer outcome: results from the Women's Intervention Nutrition Study (WINS). Am J Clin Nutr 86(3):s878–s881

117. Pierce JP et al (2007) Influence of a diet very high in vegetables, fruit, and fiber and low in fat on prognosis following treatment for breast cancer: the Women's Healthy Eating and Living (WHEL) randomized trial. JAMA 298(3):289–298
118. Rock CL et al (2009) Longitudinal biological exposure to carotenoids is associated with breast cancer-free survival in the Women's Healthy Eating and Living Study. Cancer Epidemiol Biomark Prev 18(2):486–494
119. Schmitz KH, Ahmed RL, Hannan PJ et al (2005) Safety and efficacy of weight training in recent breast cancer survivors to alter body composition, insulin, and insulin-like growth factor axis proteins. Cancer Epidemiol Biomark Prev 14:1672–1680
120. Ligibel JA et al (2008) Impact of a mixed strength and endurance exercise intervention on insulin levels in breast cancer survivors. J Clin Oncol 26(6):907–912
121. Irwin ML et al (2009) Randomized controlled trial of aerobic exercise on insulin and insulin-like growth factors in breast cancer survivors: the Yale Exercise and Survivorship study. Cancer Epidemiol Biomark Prev 18(1):306–313
122. Schmitz KH et al (2005) Safety and efficacy of weight training in recent breast cancer survivors to alter body composition, insulin, and insulin-like growth factor axis proteins. Cancer Epidemiol Biomark Prev 14(7):1672–1680
123. Fairey AS et al (2003) Effects of exercise training on fasting insulin, insulin resistance, insulin-like growth factors, and insulin-like growth factor binding proteins in post-menopausal breast cancer survivors: a randomized controlled trial. Cancer Epidemiol Biomark Prev 12(8):721–727
124. Goodwin PJ (2008) Insulin in the adjuvant breast cancer setting: a novel therapeutic target for lifestyle and pharmacologic interventions? J Clin Oncol 26(6):833–834
125. Padwal R, Li SK, Lau DC (2004) Long-term pharmacotherapy for obesity and overweight. Cochrane Database Syst Rev (3):CD004094
126. Sachdev D (2010) Targeting the type 1 insulin-like growth factor system for breast cancer therapy. Curr Drug Targets 11:1121–1132
127. Padwal R, Li SK, Lau DC (2004). Cochrane Database Syst Rev CD004094
128. Cusi K, DeFronzo RA (1998) Metformin: a review of its metabolic effects. Diab Rev 6:89–131
129. Zhou G et al (2001) Role of AMP-activated protein kinase in mechanism of metformin action. J Clin Invest 108(8):1167–1174
130. Towler MC, Hardie DG (2007) AMP-activated protein kinase in metabolic control and insulin signaling. Circ Res 100(3):328–341
131. Inoki K, Zhu T, Guan KL (2003) TSC2 mediates cellular energy response to control cell growth and survival. Cell 115(5):577–590
132. Anisimov VN et al (2005) Effect of metformin on life span and on the development of spontaneous mammary tumors in HER-2/neu transgenic mice. Exp Gerontol 40(8–9):685–693
133. Huang X et al (2008) Important role of the LKB1-AMPK pathway in suppressing tumorigenesis in PTEN-deficient mice. Biochem J 412(2):211–221
134. Buzzai M et al (2007) Systemic treatment with the antidiabetic drug metformin selectively impairs p53-deficient tumor cell growth. Cancer Res 67(14):6745–6752
135. Zhuang Y, Miskimins WK (2008) Cell cycle arrest in Metformin treated breast cancer cells involves activation of AMPK, downregulation of cyclin D1, and requires p27Kip1 or p21Cip1. J Mol Signal 3:18
136. Wang LW et al (2008) Metformin induces apoptosis of pancreatic cancer cells. World J Gastroenterol 14(47):7192–7198
137. Beckner ME et al (2005) Glycolytic glioma cells with active glycogen synthase are sensitive to PTEN and inhibitors of PI3K and gluconeogenesis. Lab Invest 85(12):1457–1470

138. Isakovic A et al (2007) Dual antiglioma action of metformin: cell cycle arrest and mitochondria-dependent apoptosis. Cell Mol Life Sci 64(10):1290–1302
139. Decensi A et al (2010) Metformin and cancer risk in diabetic patients: a systematic review and meta-analysis. Cancer Prev Res (Phila) 3(11):1451–1461
140. Jiralerspong S et al (2009) Metformin and pathologic complete responses to neoadjuvant chemotherapy in diabetic patients with breast cancer. J Clin Oncol 27(20):3297–3302
141. Mazzone PJ et al (2010) The effect of metformin and thiazolidinedione use on lung cancer. Chest 138:882A
142. Hosono K et al (2010) Metformin suppresses colorectal aberrant crypt foci in a short-term clinical trial. Cancer Prev Res (Phila) 3(9):1077–1083
143. Niraula S et al (2010) Clinical and biologic effects of metformin in early stage breast cancer [PD03-06]. San Antonio Breast Cancer Symphosium. pp 8–10
144. Bonanni B et al (2010) A randomized pre-surgical trial of metformin in breast cancer. Preliminary feasibility and safety results. San Antonio Breast Cancer Symphosium [PD03-02]
145. Hadad S et al (2009) The effect of neoadjuvant metformin on breast cancer related genes clinical trial – a preliminary result. San Antonio Breast Cancer Symphosium (Abstract# 3145)
146. Goodwin PJ, Ligibel JA, Stambolic V (2009) Metformin in breast cancer: time for action. J Clin Oncol 27(20):3271–3273
147. Cazzaniga M et al (2009) Is it time to test metformin in breast cancer clinical trials? Cancer Epidemiol Biomark Prev 18(3):701–705
148. Blanquicett C, Roman J, Hart CM (2008) Thiazolidinediones as anti-cancer agents. Cancer Ther 6(A):25–34
149. Govindarajan R et al (2007) Thiazolidinediones and the risk of lung, prostate, and colon cancer in patients with diabetes. J Clin Oncol 25(12):1476–1481
150. Hassan MM et al (2010) Association of diabetes duration and diabetes treatment with the risk of hepatocellular carcinoma. Cancer 116(8):1938–1946
151. Tolman KG (2011) The safety of thiazolidinediones. Expert Opin Drug Saf
152. Holmes MD, Chen WY, Feskanich D et al (2005) Physical activity and survival after breast cancer diagnosis. JAMA 293:2479–2486
153. Pierce JP et al (2007) Greater survival after breast cancer in physically active women with high vegetable-fruit intake regardless of obesity. J Clin Oncol 25(17):2345–2351
154. Irwin ML et al (2008) Influence of pre- and postdiagnosis physical activity on mortality in breast cancer survivors: the health, eating, activity, and lifestyle study. J Clin Oncol 26(24):3958–3964
155. Friedenreich CM et al (2009) Prospective cohort study of lifetime physical activity and breast cancer survival. Int J Cancer 124(8):1954–1962
156. West-Wright CN et al (2009) Long-term and recent recreational physical activity and survival after breast cancer: the California Teachers Study. Cancer Epidemiol Biomark Prev 18(11):2851–2859
157. Keegan TH et al (2010) Past recreational physical activity, body size, and all-cause mortality following breast cancer diagnosis: results from the Breast Cancer Family Registry. Breast Cancer Res Treat 123(2):531–542
158. Bertram LA et al (2011) Physical activity, additional breast cancer events, and mortality among early-stage breast cancer survivors: findings from the WHEL Study. Cancer Causes Control 22(3):427–435

159. Fairey AS, Courneya KS, Field CJ et al (2003) Effects of exercise training on fasting insulin, insulin resistance, insulin-like growth factors, and insulin-like growth factor binding proteins in postmenopausal breast cancer survivors: a randomized controlled trial. Cancer Epidemiol Biomark Prev 12:721–727
160. Ligibel JA, Campbell N, Partridge A et al (2008) Impact of a mixed strength and endurance exercise intervention on insulin levels in breast cancer survivors. J Clin Oncol 26:907–912
161. Irwin ML, Varma K, Alvarez-Reeves M et al (2009) Randomized controlled trial of aerobic exercise on insulin and insulin-like growth factors in breast cancer survivors: the Yale Exercise and Survivorship study. Cancer Epidemiol Biomark Prev 18:306–313

Index

A
Adipokines
  adiponectin, 86–87
  angiogenic factors, 87
  collagen VI, 87
  HB-EGF, 86
  HGF, 86
  IL–6, 86
  leptin, 84–85
  murine mammary carcinoma cell line, 84
  polypeptide factors and cytokines, 84
  TNF-α, 85–86
Adiponectin, 86–87
Akt
  apoptosis regulators and pro-death signaling, 184–185
  insulin-induced survival signals
    PI3K signaling pathway, 181, 182
    prosurvival signaling, 182, 183
    Ser473 phosphorylation, 181
  mRNA translation
    canonical apoptosis regulators, 185
    eEF2K, 187
    eIF2, 187
    eIF4A, 185
    eIF4E, 186
    lupus autoantigen RNA binding protein, 186
    mTORC1, 186
    murine lymphoma chemoresistance model, 185
    programmed cell death 4, 186
    Ser92 and Ser203, 186
American Cancer Society, 102
AMP-activated protein kinase (AMPK)
  activators, 194–196
  CAMKK, 197
  cancer therapeutic implications, 205–206
  downstream effects
    cancer cell metabolism, 202–203
    cell growth, proliferation and survival, 198
    epithelial polarity, 201–202
    LKB1 tumor suppressor identification, 198
    metabolism regulation, 198
    mTOR, 199
    p27, 200
    p53, 200
  FDG-PET, 193
  signaling regulation, 203–204
  STK11, 196–197
  structure, 194, 195
  TGF-β–activated kinase–1, 197
  Warburg effect, 193

B
Bladder cancer, 125
Breast cancer, 258
  adipocytes, 77
  adipokines
    adiponectin, 86–87
    angiogenic factors, 87
    collagen VI, 87
    HB-EGF, 86
    HGF, 86
    IL–6, 86
    leptin, 84–85
    murine mammary carcinoma cell line, 84
    polypeptide factors and cytokines, 84
    TNF-α, 85–86

I.G. Fantus (ed.), *Insulin Resistance and Cancer: Epidemiology, Cellular and Molecular Mechanisms and Clinical Implications*, Energy Balance and Cancer 1, DOI 10.1007/978-1-4419-9911-5, © Springer Science+Business Media, LLC 2011

Breast cancer (*cont.*)
anthropometric measures, 112
body fat distribution, 80
chronic diseases, 77
diabetes mellitus, 113–114
diagnosis, 271, 272
dietary restriction, 91
diet-induced obesity, 146–148
dyslipidemia, 113
etiology, 78
hyperglycemia, 116
hyperinsulinemia, 114–116
IGF–1, 112
IGF axis, 216, 225–226
inflammation, 83–84
insulin resistance, 81–83
metabolic syndrome, 113
nutrients/fatty acids
adiposity, 88
dietary factors, 88
exposure timing, 89
obesity, 87
potential mechanism, 89–90
public health policy, 88
types, 89
obesity, 112
physical activity, 90
post-menopausal breast cancer, 79
pre-menopausal breast cancer, 79
prognosis, 81, 116–117
United States, 77
weight loss, 90–91
Western societies, 77

C
Ca^{2+}/CaM-dependent kinase kinase (CAMKK), 197
Cancer cell metabolism, 202–203
Cancer therapeutic implications, 205–206
Carbohydrate metabolism
gluconeogenesis *in vivo* assessment
arteriovenous difference technique, 9
dihydroxyacetone phosphate, 8
glucose 6-phosphate, 8
H3/H2 ratio, 8
^2H_2O method, 8, 9
Krebs cycle, 7
labeled precursor infusion, 9
MIDA, 6, 7
reciprocal pool model, 8
hyperinsulinemia, 28
hyperinsulinemic euglycemic clamp
carbon tracers, 5
dysregulated glucose metabolism, 2
EGP (*See* Endogenous glucose production)
glucose infusion, 2, 3
humans and animal models, 2
hydrogen-labelled tracers, 5
oxidative and non-oxidative metabolism, 6
physiological and isotopic steady states, 4
plasma insulin levels, 2
postabsorptive glucose levels, 5
single pool model, 4
statistical analysis, 6
insulin-mediated glucose metabolism (*see* Insulin-mediated glucose metabolism)
insulin signaling cascade
carbohydrate metabolism, 19
glucose homeostasis, 17
insulin receptor, 16
insulin resistance, 18
IRS–2, 17
IRS–1 Ser 307 phosphorylation, 19
mTOR, 18
phosphotyrosine-binding, 17
PI3K, 17
pleckstrin-homology, 17
protein kinase B, 18
Ras-MAPK pathway, 19–20
SOCS, 18
in vivo insulin sensitivity
clamp variables and indices, 16
fasting insulin, 10
FSIVGTT, 14–15
HOMA and QUICKI, 10–11
hyperglycemic clamp, 16
IPGTT, 14
IST, 15–16
ITT, 12–13
OGTT, 13–14
Carcinogenesis
hormone binding, 53
insulin receptor
allosteric enzyme, 55
cancer, 56–57
α–β dimers, 55, 56
insulin receptor-related receptor, 55, 56
isoforms, 60–61
phosphotyrosine binding domain, 57, 58
pleckstrin homology domain, 57, 58
protein regulation, 59
PTB–1B, 55
PTPases, 59
SH2 proteins, 58
SOCS proteins, 56

PI3K
Akt pathway, 53, 54
heterodimeric components, 63–65
inhibitors, 61–62
PIP_3, 62–63
p85 subunit, 65–67
regulatory and catalytic subunit, 61, 62
Cell transformation and tumorigenesis, 253–254
Colon cancer, 149–150, 258–259
Colorectal cancer
anthropometric measures, 118
clinical features, 118
diabetes mellitus, 118–119
hyperglycemia, 120
hyperinsulinemia, 119–120
metabolic syndrome, 118
obesity, 117–118
prognosis, 120–121
Cowden's syndrome, 164

D
Diabetes mellitus
breast cancer, 113–114
colorectal cancer, 118–119
pancreatic cancer, 121–122
prostate cancer, 124
Diet-induced obesity
breast cancer, 146–148
colon cancer, 149–150
LLC cells, 150
N-nitrosobis–2-oxopropylamine-induced pancreatic cancer, 150
prostate cancer, 148–149
ω–3 PUFA, 150, 151
Sprague–Dawley rats, 150

E
Endogenous glucose production (EGP)
calculation, 5
dose-response curves, 3
gluconeogensis, 3
insulin-mediated suppression, 6
liver and the kidney, 3
postabsorptive Rd, 3
Endometrial cancer, 125–127

F
Fluorine labeled 2-deoxyglucose positron emission tomography (FDG-PET), 193
Forkhead box-protein O1 (FOXO), 21
Frequently sampled intravenous glucose tolerance test (FSIVGTT), 14–15

G
Genetically-induced obesity
db/db mouse, 144
hormone leptin, 142
LA/N-cp rat, 145–146
monogenetic obesity syndromes, 142
ob/ob mouse, 143
pro-opiomelacortin, 142
yellow mice, 142–143
zucker fatty rats, 144–145
Glargine insulin, 271
Glycogen synthase kinase–3 (GSK–3) phosphorylation, 184–185

H
Head and neck squamous cell carcinomas (HNSCCs), 231
Heparin-binding epidermal growth factor-like growth factor (HB-EGF), 86
Hepatocyte growth factor (HGF), 86
Homeostasis model assessment (HOMA), 10–11
Hybrid receptors, 249–250
Hyperglycemia
breast cancer, 116
colorectal cancer, 120
pancreatic cancer, 122–123
Hyperinsulinemia, 271, 273
animal models, 151–152
breast cancer, 114–116, 260
colorectal cancer, 119–120
endogenous insulin, 171
exogenous insulin, 171
glargine, 172
IGF–1R, 163
insulin, 169, 170
adipogenesis, 169
adipokines, 169
Cowden's syndrome, 164
EGFR signaling, 165
estrogen receptors, 166
genetic models, 168
glycogen synthase kinase–3, 167
G-protein activation mechanism, 164
growth hormone, 169
hormone therapy, 167
leptin, 169
mammary epithelial cells, 164
MCF–7 BC cells, 165
PI3K pathway, 163
secretagogues, 172
SHBG, 169
synergism, 166
T-bet transcription factor, 167
Tyr kinase receptors, 163

Hyperinsulinemia (*cont.*)
meta-analytic approach, 270
metabolic regulator, 163
multiple pathophysiological mechanisms, 141
pancreatic cancer, 122
prostate cancer, 124–125
type 2 diabetes, 141

I

IGF-IR overexpression, 256
Insulin, 169, 170
adipogenesis, 169
adipokines, 169
Cowden's syndrome, 164
EGFR signaling, 165
estrogen receptors, 166
genetic models, 168
glycogen synthase kinase–3, 167
G-protein activation mechanism, 164
growth hormone, 169
hormone therapy, 167
IGF–1 signaling nodes (*see* Carcinogenesis)
leptin, 169
mammary epithelial cells, 164
MCF–7 BC cells, 165
obesity concomitants
diet, 161–163
hyperinsulinemia (*see* Hyperinsulinemia)
metabolic syndrome, 161
nutrition and lifestyle, 160
PI3K pathway, 163
secretagogues, 172
sensitization, 173
SHBG, 169
synergism, 166
T-bet transcription factor, 167
Tyr kinase receptors, 163
Insulin-like growth factors (IGF)
cell transformation and tumorigenesis, 253–254
deregulated receptor expressions
adult tissues, 254
biological effects, 258
breast cancer, 258
cell xenografts, 258
colon tumors, 258–259
human malignancies, 254, 255
overexpression, 256–258
thyroid carcinomas, 259
tumorigenesis, 258
downstream signaling
atypical receptors, 250
homodimers and heterodimers, 244, 245
hybrid receptors, 249–250
IGF signaling transduction pathway, 245, 246
insulin metabolic effects, 244
MAPK signaling pathway, 246
metabolism regulation, 244
M6P receptor, 244–245
oncogenes and tumor suppressors, 251–252
PI3K signaling pathway, 247
signal specificity and diversification, 247–249
steroid hormones, 252–253
tyrosine kinase receptors, 252
gene and protein expression
extracellular matrix degrading enzymes, 231
HNSCCs, 231
MMP, 231, 232
PIN, 232
tissue microarray analysis, 233
urokinase plasminogen activator, 232–233
human malignancy epidemiological studies
breast cancer, 216, 225–226
gastrointestinal malignancies, 227–228
genetic and nongenetic factors, 230–231
GH-IGF axis, 215–224
metastatic uveal melanoma, 228–229
NSCLC cancer, 229
prostate cancer, 226–227
SCLC, 229
SILs, 229
ligands, 214–215
targeting receptors, 259–260
Insulin-mediated glucose metabolism
modulators
IKKβ, 25–26
JNK, 26
oxidative stress, 26–27
PKC, 25
p38 MAPK, 27
S6K, 27
tissue-specific mechanisms
adipose tissue, 24
liver, 20–22
skeletal muscle, 22–24
Insulinopenia, 141
Insulin receptor
allosteric enzyme, 55
cancer, 56–57
α–β dimers, 55, 56
insulin receptor-related receptor, 55, 56
isoforms, 60–61

phosphotyrosine binding domain, 57, 58
pleckstrin homology domain, 57, 58
protein regulation, 59
PTB–1B, 55
PTPases, 59
SH2 proteins, 58
SOCS proteins, 56
Insulin resistance
adverse prognostic effect, 273
animal models, 151–152
bladder cancer, 125
breast cancer
anthropometric measures, 112
diabetes mellitus, 113–114
dyslipidemia, 113
hyperglycemia, 116
hyperinsulinemia, 114–116
IGF–1, 112
metabolic syndrome, 113
obesity, 112
prognosis, 116–117
breast cancer diagnosis, 271, 272
cancer prognosis, 274
colorectal cancer
anthropometric measures, 118
clinical features, 118
diabetes mellitus, 118–119
hyperglycemia, 120
hyperinsulinemia, 119–120
metabolic syndrome, 118
obesity, 117–118
prognosis, 120–121
diabetes, 271
endometrial cancer, 125–127
glargine insulin, 271
hyperinsulinemia, 270, 271, 273
IRS, 270
lifestyle interventions
cancer populations, 277–278
complex–healthy individuals, 275
glucose intolerant/insulin resistant populations, 276–277
meta-analytic approach, 270
obesity reduction, 282, 283
pancreatic cancer
diabetes, 121–122
hyperglycemia, 122–123
hyperinsulinemia, 122
obesity, 121
pharmacologic interventions
IGF–1 receptor, 280
metformin, 280–281
thiazolidinediones, 282
phosphorylated insulin, 272
prostate cancer, 273
diabetes, 124
hyperinsulinemia, 124–125
obesity, 123–124
WINS, 274, 283
Insulin resistance syndrome (IRS), 270
Insulin suppression test (IST), 15–16
Interleukin–6 (IL–6), 86
Intraperitoneal glucose tolerance tests (IPGTT), 14

L
Leptin, 84–85
Lewis lung carcinoma (LLC) cells, 150
Lupus autoantigen RNA binding protein, 186

M
Madin-Darby canine kidney (MDCK), 201
Mammalian target of rapamycin (mTOR), 182–184, 199
Mannose 6-phosphate (M6P) receptor, 244–245
Mass isotopomer distribution analysis (MIDA), 6, 7
Matrix metalloproteinases (MMP), 231
MDCK. *See* Madin-Darby canine kidney
Metabolic syndrome, 161
Metastatic uveal melanoma, 228–229
Metformin, 205, 280–281
Mitogen-activated protein kinase (MAPK) signaling pathway, 246
MRLC. *See* Myosin regulatory light chain
mRNA translation
canonical apoptosis regulators, 185
eEF2K, 187
eIF2, 187
eIF4A, 185
eIF4E, 186
lupus autoantigen RNA binding protein, 186
mTORC1, 186
murine lymphoma chemoresistance model, 185
programmed cell death 4, 186
Ser92 and Ser203, 186
Myosin regulatory light chain (MRLC), 201

N
Nicotinamide adenine dinucleotide (NAD+), 196
N-nitrosobis–2-oxopropylamine-induced pancreatic cancer, 150
Non-small cell (NSCLC) cancer, 229

O

Obesity
- breast cancer, 112
- cancer mortality
  - American Cancer Society, 102
  - BMI, 103
  - colon and prostate cancer, 103
  - meta-analysis, 103
  - post-diagnosis weight gain, 103–104
- cancer prognosis, 105–107
- colorectal cancer, 117–118
- large-scale weight loss trial, 107–108
- pancreatic cancer, 121
- prostate cancer, 123–124
- risk, 102

Oral glucose tolerance test (OGTT), 13–14

P

Pancreatic cancer
- diabetes, 121–122
- hyperglycemia, 122–123
- hyperinsulinemia, 122
- obesity, 121

Peutz-Jeghers syndrome (PJS), 196

Phenformin, 205

Phosphatidylinositol (3,4,5) trisphosphate $PI(3,4,5)P_3$, 62

Phosphoinositide 3-kinase (PI3K), 17
- Akt pathway, 53, 54
- heterodimeric components, 63–65
- inhibitors, 61–62
- PIP_3, 62–63
- p85 subunit, 65–67
- regulatory and catalytic subunit, 61, 62
- signaling pathway, 181, 182, 247

Prostate cancer, 226–227, 273
- diabetes, 124
- diet-induced obesity, 148–149
- hyperinsulinemia, 124–125
- obesity, 123–124

Prostatic intraepithelial neoplasia (PIN), 232

Protein tyrosine phosphatases (PTPases), 59

Q

Quantitative insulin sensitivity check index (QUICKI), 10–11

S

Ser/Thr kinase 11 (STK11), 196–197

Sex hormone binding globulin (SHBG), 169

Small cell lung cancer (SCLC), 229

Squamous intraepithelial lesions (SILs), 229

Suppressors of cytokine signaling (SOCS), 18

T

Targeting receptors, 259–260

Thiazolidinediones, 282

Thyroid carcinomas, 259

Tumor necrosis factor-alpha (TNF-α), 85–86

Tyrosine kinase receptors, 252

W

Warburg effect, 193

Women's Intervention Nutrition Study (WINS), 274, 283

MIX
Papier aus verantwortungsvollen Quellen
Paper from responsible sources
FSC® C105338

If you have any concerns about our products,
you can contact us on
ProductSafety@springernature.com

In case Publisher is established outside the EU,
the EU authorized representative is:
Springer Nature Customer Service Center GmbH
Europaplatz 3, 69115 Heidelberg, Germany

Printed by Libri Plureos GmbH
in Hamburg, Germany